Sota Omoigui's
Pain Drugs Handbook
Second Edition

D0927622

Notice

Every effort has been made to ensure that the drug dosage schedules herein are accurate and in accord with the standards accepted at the time of publication. As new research and experience broaden our knowledge, changes in treatment and drug therapy occur. The medications described do not necessarily have specific approval by the Food and Drug Administration for use in the situations and the dosages for which they are recommended. This information is advisory only. Drug package inserts should be consulted for use and dosage as approved by the FDA, for any changes in indications and dosages, and for added warnings and precautions. The ultimate responsibility lies with the prescribing physician.

This publication is now available electronically on the website of State-of-the-Art (S.O.T.A.) Technologies (http://www.medicinehouse.com). All rights reserved. No part of this information may be reproduced or transmitted electronically in any information storage or retrieval system or within any monitoring system without prior permission in writing from S.O.T.A. Technologies (Electronic Publishers).

The Universal Drug Infusion Slide Ruler (patent pending) is now available. It incorporates an infusion data guide and enables infusion calculations for any drug at any dose and at any concentration. It may be obtained by calling S.O.T.A. Technologies (1-800-9-MEDIC-9).

Compounded topical medications may be ordered (by prescription only) from L.A. Pain Clinic. Call 310-675-9121 or 1-800-9-MEDIC-9.

Sota Omoigui's
Pain Drugs Handbook
Second Edition

SOTA OMOIGUI, MD
Medical Director
L.A. Pain Clinic
Hawthorne, California
Assistant Professor of Anesthesiology and
    Pain Medicine
Charles Drew University of Science and
    Medicine
Los Angeles, California

Diplomate of the American Board of
    Anesthesiology (with subspecialty
    certification in Pain Management)
Diplomate of the American Board of Pain
    Medicine

Author:
Sota Omoigui's Anesthesia Drugs Handbook
Pain Relief—The L.A. Pain Clinic Guide
The Universal Drug Infusion Ruler

**Blackwell
Science**

Editorial Offices:
Commerce Place, 350 Main Street, Malden, Massachusetts 02148, USA
Osney Mead, Oxford OX2 0EL, England
25 John Street, London WC1N 2BL, England
23 Ainslie Place, Edinburgh EH3 6AJ, Scotland
54 University Street, Carlton, Victoria 3053, Australia

Other Editorial Offices:
Blackwell Wissenschafts-Verlag GmbH, Kurfürstendamm 57, 10707 Berlin, Germany
Blackwell Science KK, MG Kodenmacho Building, 7-10 Kodenmacho Nihombashi, Chuo-ku, Tokyo 104, Japan

Distributors:

USA
  Blackwell Science, Inc.
  Commerce Place
  350 Main Street
  Malden, Massachusetts 02148
  (Telephone orders: 800-215-1000 or
    781-388-8250;
    fax orders: 781-388-8270)

Canada
  Login Brothers Book Company
  324 Saulteaux Crescent
  Winnipeg, Manitoba, R3J 3T2
  (Telephone orders: 204-224-4068)

Australia
  Blackwell Science Pty, Ltd.
  54 University Street
  Carlton, Victoria 3053
  (Telephone orders: 03-9347-0300;
    fax orders: 03-9349-3016)

Outside North America and Australia
  Blackwell Science, Ltd.
  c/o Marston Book Services, Ltd.
  P.O. Box 269
  Abingdon
  Oxon OX14 4YN
  England
  (Telephone orders: 44-01235-465500;
    fax orders: 44-01235-465555)

Acquisitions: Jim Krosschell
Production: Kevin Sullivan
Manufacturing: Lisa Flanagan
Cover design by Alwyn Velásquez
Typeset by Best-set Typesetter, Ltd., Hong Kong
Printed and bound by Edwards Brothers

Printed in the United States of America
99 00 01 02 5 4 3 2 1

RB127
.046
1999

Library of Congress Cataloging-in-Publication Data

Omoigui, Sota.
  Sota Omoigui's pain drugs handbook / Sota Omoigui.—2nd ed.
    P.   cm.
  Includes bibliographical references and index.
  ISBN 0-632-04419-5
  1. Pain—Treatment. 2. Analgesics. 3. Analgesia. I. Title. II. Title: Pain drugs handbook.
    [DNLM: 1. Analgesics handbooks. 2. Pain—drug therapy handbooks.
  QV 39 056p 1999]
  RB127.046 1999
  615′.783—dc21
DNLM/DLC
for Library of Congress   98-40987
                                                                                CIP

CONSULTING EDITORS

SECOND EDITION

Wally Saika, PharmD
Staff Pharmacist
B & B Pharmacy
Bellflower, California

John O. Dimowo, MD
Staff Anesthesiologist and Pain Management Specialist
St. Joseph Medical Center
Stockton, California

Orobosa Agbonkpolor, MD
Diplomate of the American Board of Internal Medicine
Diplomate of the American Board of Anesthesiology
Medical Co-Director
Methuselah Pain Practice
New Rochelle, New York

FIRST EDITION

Nadrine Balady, PharmD
Associate Director of Pharmacy
Department of Pharmacy
Martin Luther King/Drew Medical Center;
Adjunct Associate Professor of Pharmacy
University of Southern California
Los Angeles, California

Martin S. Mok, MD
Professor of Anesthesiology
Former Director of Research in Pain Management
University of Southern California
Los Angeles, California

To the fond memories of

Frank Whyte

1963–1999

Thomas (Tommy) Asemota

1934–1998

Pa Augustine Omoigui Oviawe

1888–1998

To live in the hearts of those who love you is

to live forever

Requiescat in Pace

PREFACE TO THE SECOND EDITION

The rapid advancement in our knowledge of the patho-physiology and pharmacology of acute and chronic pain necessitates an ongoing update of this drug hand-book. For this edition of *Sota Omoigui's Pain Drugs Handbook*, information on all drugs has been updated, and numerous drugs from diverse classes have been added. These include alendronate, botulinum toxin, celecoxib, cosyntropin, dextromethorphan, dihydro-ergotamine, gabapentin, leflunomide, nabumetone, pamidronate, pentosan polysulfate sodium, ropivacaine, sertraline, and tramadol. There is also a section on com-pounded topical medications, another exciting frontier in our battle to conquer pain. I express my gratitude to Neil Badlani, RPh, and Wally Saika, PharmD, at B & B Pharmacy in Bellflower, California. They were an excel-lent resource in compiling this section.

Special thanks to the consulting editors for their meticulous and professional work. I wish to thank my family, including my parents, Daniel and Grace, and my siblings, Nowa, Ifueko, Eghosa, and Nosa, for their love and support. Finally, I thank my publisher, James Krosschell of Blackwell Science, for his support and assistance. Every day, we are able to help more patients with new knowledge and insight. This book will be a valuable resource to all health care providers, who will inevitably encounter a patient with pain.

Sota Omoigui, MD
February 1999

PREFACE TO THE FIRST EDITION

Pain is interwoven in the fabric of life. In one form or another and at some time or another, we shall all experience pain. Yet one of medicine's great paradoxes is the undertreatment of pain. Recent statistics show that 70% or more of patients do not receive adequate treatment for their pain. Biases, myths, unreasonable fear of drug addiction, and lack of knowledge on the part of health care professionals constitute a barrier to effective pain control.

Nothing tries the human soul so much as pain. Unrelieved pain produces unnecessary suffering that is harmful to physical and psychological well-being. Inadequate treatment of pain slows the healing process, lengthens hospital stays, and increases the size of medical bills.

The Pain Drugs Handbook is a compilation of drugs used singly or in combination with other drugs and techniques in the management of acute, chronic, and cancer pain. Also included are therapeutic guidelines for various pain syndromes and a trade name list for rapid retrieval of generic drug names. Familiarity with the pharmacology of these drugs used singly or in combination will enable better treatment of pain and improvement in the quality of life. This knowledge should complement other efforts at treating the whole person and relieving the stresses in life, which compound the illnesses and malignancies that produce pain.

For many patients, this book comes too late. For millions more, it is my hope that this book shall be a beacon of light in the darkness of their pain and suffering.

Sota Omoigui, MD
October 1994

ACKNOWLEDGMENTS TO THE FIRST EDITION

Professional Support
  Barbara Justice, MD
Electronic Development Team, State-of-the-Art (S.O.T.A.) Technologies, Inc.
  Robert Gramcko, BSc; Anson Chapman, BSc; Eghosa Omoigui, LLM; Kate Gramcko; Kathy Lucarro; Norma Haye, RN
Editorial Review Team
  Ret O.J. Omoigui, MD; Paul Phillips III, MD; Gudarshan Gill, MD; Ricardo Chambi, MD; John Cruikshank, MD; Connie Tran, MD; Ronald Shepperson, MD; Kathy K. Shelley, MA; John Dimowo, MD; Sam Otuwa, MD; Michael Lemon, MD
Drug Tables
  Glenn P.K. Akiona, MD
Secretarial Support
  Mabel Betton, Goldie Garett, Nancy Mattox, Gay Akiona
Mosby–Year Book Publishers
  Susan Gay

Plea of a Patient

When I come to you in pain
'Tis for comfort and not for gain
Should I need a narcotic
Label me not a drug addict
And when the pain is phenomenal
Don't forget the nonsteroidal
With the H_2 blocker
or antiulcer
And if it's time for the adjuvants
Do remember the antidepressants
Seek the cause of my pain
And ponder not if I feign
So when the pain fills me with dread
Please don't say it's in my head
When it's time for eternity
Allow me leave with dignity

**Sota Omoigui, MD and
Eghosa Omoigui, LLM, 1994**

It is better to light a candle than curse the darkness

ABOUT THE AUTHOR

Sota Omoigui, MD, is Medical Director of the L.A. Pain Clinic in Southern California and Assistant Professor of Anesthesiology and Pain Medicine at Charles R. Drew University of Science and Medicine in Los Angeles, California. Dr. Omoigui is the author of *Sota Omoigui's Anesthesia Drugs Handbook*, Third Edition (Blackwell Science, 1999), *The Anesthesia Drugs Handbook*, Second Edition (Mosby–Year Book, 1995), *The Pain Drugs Handbook* (Mosby–Year Book, 1995), *Pain Relief—The L.A. Pain Clinic Guide* (State-of-the-Art Technologies, 1998), and *The Universal Drug Infusion Ruler* (State-of-the-Art Technologies, 1995) and co-author of the Nigerian national anthem (1978). Dr. Omoigui's drug handbooks are used worldwide and have been published in five other languages (Italian, Japanese, Malaysian, Polish, and Portuguese). Dr. Omoigui's research focus is on anesthetic and pain pharmacology, herbal medicine, and development of minimally invasive techniques for neural blockade and relief of chronic pain. He pioneered the technique of audio-capnometry and holds a United States patent for the audio-capnometer monitor and a patent for the process of continuous noninvasive hemometry (measurement of hemoglobin).

ABOUT THE BOOK

Designed for quick access to the most current pain drugs information, *Sota Omoigui's Pain Drugs Handbook*, Second Edition, is a complete clinical guide in a handy portable format. This pocket reference is packed with tables, descriptions, and dosages covering a broad range of drugs and the various routes of administration commonly used in the treatment of acute, chronic, and cancer pain.

Over 120 drugs are listed alphabetically for ease of reference. Each is presented using a standard format: class, use(s), dosing, elimination, preparations, and a brief review of pharmacology. Pharmacokinetics are summarized in a succinct manner: onset of action, peak effect, and duration of action. Interactions, toxicity, guidelines and precautions, and principal adverse reactions are also included for each drug. *Sota Omoigui's Pain Drugs Handbook*, Second Edition, contains therapeutic guidelines, sections on topical compounded medications and on cancer pain management, and a handy appendix with drug tables, CPR algorithms, and pain rating scales.

Electronic Publication

The Pain Drugs Handbook is available electronically on the website of State-of-the-Art (S.O.T.A.) Technologies (http://www.medicinehouse.com).

CONTENTS

Part II   Topical Agents   *625*

Part III   Neurolytic Agent   *641*

Part IV   Cancer Pain   *646*

PART I BY DRUG CLASS

Nonopioid Analgesics

Disease-Modifying Antirheumatic Agent

Local Anesthetic Agents

PAIN SYNDROMES AND THERAPEUTIC GUIDELINES

One or more of the therapies listed under each pain syndrome may be used as indicated. The therapies are not listed in any particular order, and some therapies may have been inadvertently omitted. Safe use of these therapies requires intimate familiarity with the pharmacology and toxicity of the various agents and knowledge of other nonpharmacologic and invasive options used in the management of acute, chronic, and cancer pain.

Readers are invited to send comments to the author (e-mail: sota1@aol.com).

Low Back Pain

Bed rest (<3 days) with a firm, nonsagging mattress
Physical therapy:
  Application of heat (hot packs, hydrotherapy, dry/moist heating pads, diathermy, sauna), ice (brushing with an ice stick), therapeutic exercise, deep massage, spinal manipulation, cold laser therapy, application of pulsed electromagnetic field
Drug therapy:
  Nonsteroidal anti-inflammatory drugs (NSAIDs) with or without sucralfate, H_2 receptor antagonists, or misoprostol

Acetaminophen

Opioid analgesics with or without stool softeners or cathartics

Antidepressant agents (e.g., paroxetine)

Phenothiazines

Skeletal muscle relaxants (e.g., baclofen, tizanidine, clonazepam)

Trigger-point injections with local anesthetics and/or corticosteroids (e.g., methylprednisolone)

Selective nerve root sheath infiltration

Epidural injections with local anesthetics, corticosteroids, and/or opioids

Intrathecal opioids and/or baclofen

Facet joint injections with local anesthetics and/or corticosteroids

Chemodenervation of lumbar paraspinal muscles with botulinum toxin and/or local anesthetic

Psoas compartment block with botulinum toxin and/or local anesthetic

Lumbar sympathetic block with local anesthetics, corticosteroids

Electrical stimulation of the spinal cord or affected nerve

Psychological therapies:

Behavioral modification

Biofeedback

Hypnosis

Surgery:

Diskectomy

Laminectomy

Transcutaneous electrical nerve stimulation (TENS)

Acupuncture

Vertebral adjustments

Psychosocial rehabilitation

Cancer Pain

Drug therapy:

    NSAIDs with or without sucralfate, H_2 receptor antagonists, or misoprostol

    Acetaminophen

    Opioid analgesics (e.g., methadone, morphine) with or without stool softeners or cathartics

    Epidural or intrathecal opioids

    Antidepressant agents (e.g., paroxetine)

    Antihistamines (e.g., hydroxyzine)

    Psychostimulants (e.g., amphetamines)

    Phenothiazines (e.g., methotrimeprazine)

    Butyrophenones (e.g., haloperidol)

    Anxiolytics (e.g., clonazepam)

    Stool softeners (e.g., docusate)

    Corticosteroids for oncolysis, metastatic bone pain, plexus or nerve infiltration, cord compression

    Antiemetics (e.g., metoclopramide, prochlorperazine)

    Oral local anesthetics (e.g., mexiletine)

Somatic and/or sympathetic nerve blocks with local anesthetics, corticosteroids, and/or opioids or with neurolytic agents (e.g., phenol)

Trigger-point injections with local anesthetics and/or corticosteroids (e.g., methylprednisolone)

Electrical stimulation of the spinal cord or affected nerve

Surgery:

    Decompression of tumor

    Cordotomy

Radiotherapy to decrease tumor mass

Chemotherapy to decrease tumor mass

Acupuncture

Psychological therapies:

    Behavioral modification

Biofeedback

Hypnosis

Physical therapy:

Application of heat (hot packs, hydrotherapy, dry/moist heating pads, diathermy, sauna), ice (brushing with an ice stick), therapeutic exercise, cold laser therapy, application of pulsed electromagnetic field

Metastatic Bone Pain

Drug therapy:

Bisphosphonates (e.g., alendronate, pamidronate, clodronate) to inhibit osteoclast activity

Corticosteroid agents (e.g., dexamethasone)

NSAIDs with or without sucralfate, H_2 receptor antagonists, or misoprostol

Opioid analgesics (e.g., methadone, morphine) with or without stool softeners or cathartics

Epidural or intrathecal opioids

Radiopharmaceutical agents (e.g., strontium-89, samarium), which are absorbed into areas of high bone turnover

Calcitonin

Gallium nitrate

Somatic and/or sympathetic nerve blocks with local anesthetics, corticosteroids, and/or opioids or with neurolytic agents (e.g., phenol)

Electrical stimulation of the spinal cord or affected nerve

Radiotherapy to decrease tumor mass

Chemotherapy to decrease tumor mass

Acupuncture

Psychological therapies:

Behavioral modification

Biofeedback

Hypnosis

Physical therapy:

Application of heat (hot packs, hydrotherapy, dry/moist heating pads, diathermy, sauna), ice (brushing with an ice stick), therapeutic exercise, cold laser therapy, application of pulsed electromagnetic field

Neuropathic Pain

Drug therapy:

Antidepressant agents (e.g., paroxetine, topical doxepin)

Anticonvulsants (e.g., gabapentin, carbamazepine)

α_2-Agonists (e.g., tizanidine, clonidine)

Corticosteroids (e.g., prednisone, dexamethasone)

GABA agonists and skeletal muscle relaxants (e.g., baclofen, clonazepam)

Opioid analgesics with or without stool softeners or cathartics

Epidural or intrathecal opioids

NSAIDs with or without sucralfate, H_2 receptor antagonists, or misoprostol

Neuroleptics (e.g., fluphenazine, haloperidol)

Oral local anesthetics (e.g., mexiletine)

Intravenous local anesthetics:

Chloroprocaine

Lidocaine

Procaine

Calcitonin

Topical ketamine, gabapentin, dextromethorphan, dimethyl sulfoxide (DMSO), clonidine, ketoprofen, baclofen

Capsaicin cream
Doxepin cream
Somatic and/or sympathetic nerve blocks with local anesthetics, corticosteroids, and/or opioids or with neurolytic agents (e.g., phenol)
Surgical sympathectomy
Electrical stimulation of the spinal cord
TENS
Acupuncture
Psychological therapies:
Behavioral modification
Biofeedback
Hypnosis

Chronic Regional Pain Syndrome Types I and II (Reflex Sympathetic Dystrophy or Causalgia)

Drug therapy:
Antidepressant agents (e.g., trazodone, paroxetine)
Antispasm α_2-agonist drugs (e.g., tizanidine, clonidine)
Anticonvulsant drugs (e.g., gabapentin, carbamazepine, phenytoin)
Skeletal muscle relaxants (e.g., baclofen, clonazepam)
NSAIDs with or without sucralfate, H_2 receptor antagonists, or misoprostol
Bisphosphonates (e.g., alendronate, pamidronate, clodronate) to inhibit bone resorption
Calcitonin
Topical ketamine, gabapentin, dextromethorphan, DMSO, clonidine, ketoprofen, baclofen
Capsaicin cream
Doxepin cream

Sympathetic nerve blocks with local anesthetics, corticosteroids, or with neurolytic agents (e.g., phenol,
alcohol, hypertonic saline)

Intravenous regional sympathetic blocks with, e.g.:

Guanethidine

Bretylium

Labetalol

Phentolamine

Reserpine

Intravenous local anesthetics:

Chloroprocaine

Lidocaine

Procaine

Ultrasound stimulation of sympathetic ganglion

Psychological therapies:

Behavioral modification

Biofeedback

Hypnosis

Physical therapy:

Application of heat (hot packs, hydrotherapy, dry/
moist heating pads, diathermy, sauna), ice (brushing with an ice stick), therapeutic exercise, deep
massage, spinal manipulation, cold laser therapy,
application of pulsed electromagnetic field

Electrical stimulation of the spinal cord

Hyperbaric oxygen therapy

Surgical sympathectomy

Fibromyalgia or Myofascial Pain

Physical therapy:

Heat and/or cold applications

Spray-and-stretch techniques

Drug therapy:

Transdermal clonidine

NSAIDs with or without sucralfate, H_2 receptor antag-

onists, or misoprostol
Acetaminophen
Opioid analgesics with or without stool softeners or cathartics
Skeletal muscle relaxants (e.g., baclofen, tizanidine, clonazepam)
Trigger-point injections with or without local anesthetics and/or corticosteroids
TENS
Acupuncture
Psychological therapies:
Behavioral modification
Biofeedback
Hypnosis

Neck Pain and Cervical Radiculopathy

Soft cervical collar
Cervical traction
Physical therapy:
Application of heat (hot packs, hydrotherapy, dry/ moist heating pads, diathermy, sauna), ice (brushing with an ice stick), therapeutic exercise, deep massage, spinal manipulation, cold laser therapy, application of pulsed electromagnetic field
Trigger-point injections with local anesthetics and/or corticosteroids (e.g., methylprednisolone)
Chemodenervation of cervical paraspinal muscles with botulinum toxin and/or local anesthetic
Psoas compartment block with botulinum toxin and/or local anesthetic
Cervical epidural injections with local anesthetics and/or corticosteroids
Drug therapy:
Short-term steroid course for radiculopathy (e.g., Medrol Dosepak)

NSAIDs with or without sucralfate, H_2 receptor antagonists, or misoprostol

Acetaminophen

Opioid analgesics with or without stool softeners or cathartics

Antidepressant agents (e.g., paroxetine, trazodone)

Skeletal muscle relaxants (e.g., baclofen, clonazepam, diazepam, tizanidine)

Surgery:

Foraminotomy with posterior decompression of osteophytes

Anterior resection of herniated disk combined with fusion

Acupuncture

Psychological therapies:

Behavioral modification

Biofeedback

Hypnosis

Migraine or Cluster Headache

Avoidance of triggering factors (e.g., monosodium glutamate)

Drug therapy:

Prophylaxis:

Methysergide

NSAIDs with or without sucralfate, H_2 receptor antagonists, or misoprostol

β-Blockers (e.g., propranolol)

Antidepressant agents (e.g., paroxetine, trazodone)

Calcium channel blockers (e.g., verapamil, nifedipine)

Clonidine

Lithium

Corticosteroids (e.g., prednisone)
Antiemetics (e.g., promethazine)
Cyproheptadine
Abortive:
Dihydroergotamine nasal spray or injection
5-HT$_1$-Agonists (e.g., sumatriptan or zolmitriptan)
Isometheptene mucate
Ergotamine
Hydroxyzine
Oxygen (10 L/min)
Intravenous local anesthetics:
Chloroprocaine
Lidocaine
Procaine
Acetaminophen
Anxiolytics (e.g., diazepam)
Opioid analgesics with or without stool softeners or cathartics
Skeletal muscle relaxants (e.g., tizanidine, baclofen)
Cervical facet injections with local anesthetics and/or corticosteroids
TENS
Acupuncture
Physical therapy:
Application of heat (hot packs, hydrotherapy, dry/moist heating pads, diathermy, sauna), ice (brushing with an ice stick), therapeutic exercise, deep massage, spinal manipulation, cold laser therapy, application of pulsed electromagnetic field
Psychological therapies:
Behavioral modification
Biofeedback

Hypnosis
Occipital nerve blocks
Sphenopalatine ganglion blocks

Visceral Pain

Drug therapy:
  NSAIDs with or without sucralfate, H_2 receptor antagonists, or misoprostol
  Opioid analgesics (e.g., methadone, morphine) with or without stool softeners or cathartics
  Epidural or intrathecal opioids
  Calcium channel blocking agents (e.g., diltiazem)
  Benzodiazepines
  Phenothiazines (e.g., chlorpromazine)
  Anticholinergic agents (e.g., IV/SL scopolamine)
  Somatostatin analogue (octreotide)
  Trypsin for pancreatic carcinoma (decreases pancreatic exocrine secretion)
Somatic and/or sympathetic nerve blocks with local anesthetics, corticosteroids, and/or opioids or with neurolytic agents (e.g., phenol)
Electrical stimulation of the spinal cord or affected nerve
Radiotherapy to decrease tumor mass
Chemotherapy to decrease tumor mass
Acupuncture
Psychological therapies:
  Behavioral modification
  Biofeedback
  Hypnosis
Physical therapy:
  Application of heat (hot packs, hydrotherapy, dry/moist heating pads, diathermy, sauna), ice (brushing with an ice stick), therapeutic exercise,

cold laser therapy, application of pulsed electro-magnetic field

Sickle Cell Pain

Drug therapy:
  Strong parenteral opioids for acute pain crisis (starting dose should be guided by what the patient has required in the past)
  Weak opioids (short-term postcrisis)
  NSAIDs with or without sucralfate, H_2 receptor antagonists, or misoprostol
  Acetaminophen
  Antihistamines
  Intravenous local anesthetics:
    Procaine
    Lidocaine
Fluid hydration
Oxygen (nasal cannula) when indicated
Physical therapy:
  Application of heat (hot packs, hydrotherapy, dry/moist heating pads, diathermy, sauna), therapeutic exercise, deep massage, spinal manipulation, application of pulsed electromagnetic field
Psychological therapies:
  Behavioral modification
  Biofeedback
  Hypnosis
TENS
Counseling—to avoid precipitating factors

Primary Dysmenorrhea or Chronic Pelvic Pain

Drug therapy:
  Low-dose contraceptives

NSAIDs with or without sucralfate, H_2 receptor antagonists, or misoprostol

Acetaminophen

Antidepressant agents (e.g., paroxetine, trazodone)

TENS

Psychological therapies:

Behavioral modification

Biofeedback

Hypnosis

Physical therapy:

Application of heat (hot packs, hydrotherapy,
dry/moist heating pads, diathermy, sauna), ice
(brushing with an ice stick), therapeutic exercise,
deep massage

Pelvic plexus nerve blocks with local anesthetics

Pain in HIV Infection and AIDS

Drug therapy:

NSAIDs with or without sucralfate, H_2 receptor antagonists, or misoprostol

Acetaminophen

Opioid analgesics with or without stool softeners or
cathartics

Adjuvant drugs:

Anticonvulsant agents (e.g., gabapentin, carbamazepine, or phenytoin)

Corticosteroids

Skeletal muscle relaxants for leg spasms:

Baclofen

Clonazepam

Dantrolene

Diazepam

Tizanidine

Oral local anesthetics
Antiemetics
Laxatives
Anxiolytics (e.g., clonazepam)
Antidepressant agents (e.g., paroxetine, amitriptyline)
Spinal opioids or baclofen
Topical ketamine, gabapentin, dextromethorphan, DMSO, clonidine, ketoprofen, baclofen
Capsaicin cream
Doxepin cream
Somatic and/or sympathetic nerve blocks with local anesthetics, corticosteroids, and/or opioids or with neurolytic agents (e.g., phenol)
Surgical sympathectomy
Electrical stimulation of the spinal cord
TENS
Acupuncture
Psychological therapies:
Behavioral modification
Biofeedback
Hypnosis

Herpes Simplex or Herpes Zoster

Drug therapy:
Antiviral drugs (e.g., valacyclovir, acyclovir)
Topical or systemic steroids (not for eye infections)
Topical local anesthetics
NSAIDs with or without sucralfate, H_2 receptor antagonists, or misoprostol
Opioid analgesics with or without stool softeners or cathartics
Antidepressant agents (e.g., paroxetine, amitriptyline)
Doxepin cream

> Topical ketamine, gabapentin, dextromethorphan, DMSO, clonidine, ketoprofen, baclofen

Somatic or sympathetic nerve blocks with local anesthetics and/or corticosteroids.

Surgical sympathectomy

Subcutaneous injections of steroid or local anesthetic–steroid mixtures (at areas of eruption)

TENS

Cool wet dressings or drying solutions

Treatment of secondary infection

Postherpetic Neuralgia

Drug therapy:

> Antiviral drugs (e.g., acyclovir)
>
> Topical or systemic steroids (not for eye infections)
>
> Topical local anesthetics
>
> NSAIDs with or without sucralfate, H_2 receptor antagonists, or misoprostol
>
> Opioid analgesics with or without stool softeners or cathartics
>
> Antidepressant agents (e.g., paroxetine, amitriptyline)
>
> Topical ketamine, gabapentin, dextromethorphan, DMSO, clonidine, ketoprofen, baclofen
>
> Capsaicin cream
>
> Doxepin cream
>
> Anticonvulsants (e.g., gabapentin, carbamazepine)
>
> Neuroleptics (e.g., fluphenazine, haloperidol)
>
> Antiarrhythmic agents:
>
> > Mexiletine
> >
> > Lidocaine
>
> Intravenous local anesthetics:
>
> > Chloroprocaine
> >
> > Lidocaine

Procaine
Skeletal muscle relaxants (e.g., baclofen, tizanidine, clonazepam)
Somatic or sympathetic nerve blocks with local anesthetics, corticosteroids, and/or opioids
Surgical sympathectomy
Subcutaneous injections of steroid or local anesthetic–steroid mixtures (in area of intense pain)
TENS
Electrical stimulation of spinal cord or deep brain
Acupuncture
Psychological therapies:
Behavioral modification
Biofeedback
Hypnosis

Trigeminal Neuralgia

Drug therapy:
Anticonvulsant drugs (e.g., gabapentin, carbamazepine)
α_2-Agonists (e.g., tizanidine, clonidine)
GABA agonists and skeletal muscle relaxants (e.g., baclofen, clonazepam)
Anxiolytics (e.g., diazepam)
Antiarrhythmic agents:
Mexiletine
Lidocaine
Antidepressant agents (e.g., paroxetine, amitriptyline)
Phenothiazine agents (e.g., chlorpromazine)
Topical ketamine, gabapentin, dextromethorphan, DMSO, clonidine, ketoprofen, baclofen
Capsaicin cream
Doxepin cream

Trigeminal nerve block with local anesthetic and/or steroid

Percutaneous trigeminal rhizotomy

Retrogasserian radiofrequency thermocoagulation

Retrogasserian injection of glycerol

Microvascular decompression of the trigeminal root

TENS

Acupuncture

Psychological therapies:

Behavioral modification

Biofeedback

Hypnosis

Atypical Facial Pain

Drug therapy:

Anticonvulsant drugs (e.g., gabapentin, carbamazepine)

α_2-Agonists (e.g., tizanidine, clonidine)

GABA agonists and skeletal muscle relaxants (e.g., baclofen, clonazepam)

NSAIDs with or without sucralfate, H_2 receptor antagonists, or misoprostol

Acetaminophen

Opioid analgesics with or without stool softeners or cathartics

Antidepressant agents (e.g., paroxetine)

TENS

Acupuncture

Psychological therapies:

Behavioral modification

Biofeedback

Hypnosis

Postamputation and Phantom Limb Pain

Prevention:
  Regional anesthesia for amputation: incidences of
    phantom pain are significantly less than with
    general anesthesia
Treatment:
  Drug therapy:
    Anticonvulsant drugs (e.g., gabapentin, carba-
      mazepine)
    α_2-Agonists (e.g., tizanidine, clonidine)
    GABA agonists and skeletal muscle relaxants (e.g.,
      baclofen, clonazepam)
    NSAIDs with or without sucralfate, H_2 receptor
      antagonists, or misoprostol
    Acetaminophen
    Opioid analgesics with or without stool softeners
      or cathartics
    Antidepressant agents (e.g., paroxetine)
    Neuroleptic agents (e.g., chlorpromazine)
    β-Blocker agents (e.g., propranolol)
    Vasodilators (e.g., topical nitroglycerin for vascular-
      related pain)
    Topical ketamine, gabapentin, dextromethorphan,
      DMSO, clonidine, ketoprofen, baclofen
    Capsaicin cream
    Doxepin cream
  Sympathetic nerve blocks with local anesthetics
    and/or corticosteroids
  Surgical sympathectomy
  Electrical stimulation of spinal cord or deep brain
  TENS
  Acupuncture
  Psychological therapies:

    Behavioral modification
    Biofeedback
    Hypnosis

Burn Pain

Drug therapy:
    Opioid analgesics
    Ketamine
    Nitrous oxide
Physical therapy:
    Hydrotherapy, therapeutic exercise, deep massage

Pain in Multiple Sclerosis

Drug therapy:
    NSAIDs with or without sucralfate, H_2 receptor antagonists, or misoprostol
    Acetaminophen
    Opioid analgesics with or without stool softeners or cathartics
    Adjuvant drugs:
        Anticonvulsant agents (e.g., carbamazepine and phenytoin)
        Corticosteroids
        Skeletal muscle relaxants for leg spasms:
            Baclofen
            Diazepam
            Dantrolene
            Tizanidine
    Antidepressant agents (e.g., paroxetine, trazodone)
    Spinal opioids or baclofen
Sympathetic nerve blocks with local anesthetics and/or corticosteroids
Surgical sympathectomy

Drugs

/

ACETAMINOPHEN

Class: *para*-Aminophenol Derivative Analgesic Agent

Use(s): Symptomatic treatment of mild to moderate pain or fever.

Dosing: *Pain and fever:* PO/rectal, 325–650 mg (6–12 mg/kg) every 4 hours. Maximum daily dose 4 g; maximum dose for long-term therapy 2.6 g daily.

Administer analgesic regularly (not as needed). Addition of opioid analgesics, antidepressant agents, and nondrug therapies such as transcutaneous electrical nerve stimulation (TENS) may enhance analgesia (see pages xxvi–xliv for drug combinations). In geriatric patients and patients with decreased renal or hepatic function, decrease doses by one-third to one-half.

Elimination: Hepatic, renal.

Preparations

Acetaminophen **(Tylenol, Aceta, Anacin-3, Genapap, Panadol, Uni Ace, Acetaminophen Elixir, Tempra Syrup):** Oral solution: 120 mg/5 mL, 130 mg/5 mL,

160 mg/5 mL, 48 mg/mL, 167 mg/5 mL, 325 mg/5 mL, 100 mg/mL.

Acetaminophen **(Tylenol, Aceta, Dapa, Genapap, Genebs, Uni Ace, Panadol):** Tablets: 325 mg, 500 mg, 650 mg.

Acetaminophen **(Panadol Children's, Tylenol Children's, Genapap Children's, Uni Ace, Tempra):** Tablets, chewable: 80 mg, 160 mg.

Acetaminophen **(Tylenol, Anacin-3, Phenaphen, Halenol, Panadol):** Tablets, film coated: 160 mg, 325 mg, 500 mg.

Acetaminophen **(Tylenol, Aceta, Anacin-3, Genapap, Panadol, Uni Ace, Acetaminophen Elixir):** Oral capsules (with powder for solution): 80 mg, 80 mg/packet, 1 g/packet.

Acetaminophen **(Acephen, Acetaminophen Uniserts, Suppap, Neopap Supprettes):** Rectal suppositories: 120 mg, 125 mg, 325 mg, 650 mg.

Acetaminophen with aspirin **(Gemnisyn):** Tablets: Acetaminophen 325 mg and aspirin 325 mg.

Acetaminophen and codeine phosphate **(Tylenol with Codeine No. 2):** Tablets: Acetaminophen 300 mg and codeine phosphate 15 mg.

Acetaminophen and codeine phosphate **(Tylenol with Codeine No. 3):** Tablets: Acetaminophen 300 mg and codeine phosphate 30 mg.

Acetaminophen and codeine phosphate **(Tylenol with Codeine No. 4):** Tablets: Acetaminophen 300 mg and codeine phosphate 60 mg.

Acetaminophen and codeine phosphate **(Phenaphen with Codeine No. 2):** Capsules: Acetaminophen 325 mg and codeine phosphate 15 mg.

Acetaminophen and codeine phosphate **(Phenaphen**

with Codeine No. 3): Capsules: Acetaminophen 325 mg and codeine phosphate 30 mg.

Acetaminophen and codeine phosphate **(Phenaphen with Codeine No. 4):** Capsules: Acetaminophen 325 mg and codeine phosphate 60 mg.

Acetaminophen and codeine phosphate **(Phenaphen 650 with Codeine):** Capsules: Acetaminophen 650 mg and codeine phosphate 30 mg.

Acetaminophen and codeine phosphate **(Tylenol with Codeine):** Elixir: Acetaminophen 120 mg/5 mL and codeine phosphate 12 mg/5 mL.

Acetaminophen and codeine phosphate **(Capital and Codeine):** Suspension: Acetaminophen 120 mg/5 mL and codeine phosphate 12 mg/5 mL.

Acetaminophen and diphenhydramine citrate **(Excedrin P.M.):** Tablets: Acetaminophen 500 mg and diphenhydramine citrate 38 mg.

Acetaminophen and diphenhydramine citrate **(Excedrin P.M. Caplets):** Tablets, film coated: Acetaminophen 500 mg and diphenhydramine citrate 38 mg.

Acetaminophen and pamabrom **(Midol Teen Menstrual Formula):** Tablets: Acetaminophen 500 mg and pamabrom 25 mg.

Acetaminophen, caffeine, and pyrilamine maleate **(Midol Menstrual Formula):** Tablets: Acetaminophen 500 mg, caffeine 60 mg, and pyrilamine 15 mg.

Acetaminophen and hydrocodone bitartrate **(Anexsia Elixir):** Oral solution: Acetaminophen 167 mg/5 mL and hydrocodone bitartrate 1.67 mg/5 mL.

Acetaminophen and hydrocodone bitartrate **(Lortab Elixir):** Oral solution: Acetaminophen 167 mg/5 mL and hydrocodone bitartrate 2.5 mg/5 mL.

Acetaminophen and hydrocodone bitartrate **(Lortab):** Tablets: Acetaminophen 500 mg and hydrocodone bitartrate 2.5 mg; acetaminophen 500 mg and hydrocodone bitartrate 5 mg; acetaminophen 500 mg and hydrocodone bitartrate 7.5 mg; acetaminophen 500 mg and hydrocodone bitartrate 10 mg.

Acetaminophen and hydrocodone bitartrate **(Lorcet Plus, Anexsia):** Tablets: Acetaminophen 650 mg and hydrocodone bitartrate 7.5 mg.

Acetaminophen and hydrocodone bitartrate **(Lorcet 10/650):** Tablets: Acetaminophen 650 mg and hydrocodone bitartrate 10 mg.

Acetaminophen and hydrocodone bitartrate **(Vicodin):** Tablets: Acetaminophen 500 mg and hydrocodone bitartrate 5 mg.

Acetaminophen and hydrocodone bitartrate **(Vicodin ES):** Tablets: Acetaminophen 750 mg and hydrocodone bitartrate 7.5 mg.

Acetaminophen and hydrocodone bitartrate **(Vicodin HP):** Tablets: Acetaminophen 650 mg and hydrocodone bitartrate 10 mg.

Acetaminophen and hydrocodone bitartrate **(Norco 10/325):** Tablets: Acetaminophen 325 mg and hydrocodone bitartrate 10 mg.

Acetaminophen and oxycodone hydrochloride **(Tylox, Roxilox):** Capsules: Acetaminophen 500 mg and oxycodone 5 mg.

Acetaminophen and oxycodone hydrochloride **(Percocet, Oxycet, Roxicet):** Tablets: Acetaminophen 325 mg and oxycodone 5 mg; acetaminophen 500 mg and oxycodone 5 mg.

Acetaminophen and oxycodone hydrochloride **(Roxi-**

cet): Solution: Acetaminophen 325 mg/5 mL and oxycodone 5 mg/5 mL.

Acetaminophen and propoxyphene hydrochloride **(Genagesic, E-Lor, Wygesic):** Tablets/Capsules: Acetaminophen 650 mg and propoxyphene 65 mg.

Acetaminophen and propoxyphene napsylate **(Darvon-N 50, Darvon-N 100):** Tablets: Acetaminophen 325 mg and propoxyphene 50 mg; acetaminophen 325 mg and propoxyphene 100 mg. Tablets/Capsules: Acetaminophen 650 mg and propoxyphene 65 mg.

Pharmacology

A *para*-aminophenol derivative with analgesic and antipyretic properties similar to those of aspirin, acetaminophen appears to be equipotent with aspirin in inhibiting central prostaglandin synthesis. However, unlike aspirin, acetaminophen does not inhibit peripheral prostaglandin synthesis. The antipyretic activity may be due to inhibition of the action of endogenous pyrogen on the heat-regulating center in the hypothalamus and on peripheral vasodilatation. Acetaminophen is an effective analgesic when used for pain of noninflammatory origin. Acetaminophen may have some weak anti-inflammatory action in some nonrheumatoid conditions, for example, in patients who have had oral surgery. In pain of inflammatory origin (e.g., bone pain), acetaminophen is not the drug of choice.

The analgesic potency is identical to aspirin. Compared with aspirin, acetaminophen produces relatively few side effects within the therapeutic dose range.

Acetaminophen does not produce gastric irritation, does not interfere with platelet function, and has no uricosuric activity. Unlike aspirin, acetaminophen is not well absorbed through the gastric mucosa, but is rapidly absorbed through the small intestine; thus, the rate of absorption is influenced by the gastric emptying time. Acetaminophen allergy is rare and there is no cross-sensitivity between acetaminophen and aspirin. Chronic use or acute overdose of acetaminophen may result in hepatic toxicity due to depletion of glutathione stores and a decrease in glutathione-induced inactivation of a toxic metabolite of acetaminophen. Acetaminophen crosses the placenta but is safe for short-term use during all stages of pregnancy. The drug is excreted in breast milk in low concentrations, with no reported adverse effects in nursing infants.

Pharmacokinetics

Onset of Action: PO, 5–30 minutes.
Peak Effect: PO, 0.5–2.0 hours; rectal, 3–4 hours.
Duration of Action: PO, 3–7 hours.

Interactions

Enhances hypoglycemic effects of sulfonylureas; absorption decreased by concomitant administration of activated charcoal, anticholinergics, or narcotics; increases hypoprothrombinemic effects of oral anticoagulants; increased serum levels of acetaminophen with concomitant administration of diflunisal; increased serum levels of chloramphenicol with administration of acetaminophen; increased analgesic efficacy with concomitant administration of caffeine.

Toxicity

Toxic Range: >200 µg/mL at 4 hours after ingestion or >50 µg/mL at 12 hours after ingestion.

Manifestations: *Chronic:* Anemia; renal damage; GI disturbances, including peptic ulcer, cyanosis, methemoglobinemia. *Acute:* In addition to the previously listed symptoms, hepatic necrosis; acute renal failure; metabolic acidosis; hypoglycemia; nausea; vomiting; abdominal pain; CNS stimulation with excitement and delirium, then CNS depression; stupor; hypothermia; hypotension; coma; circulatory failure.

Antidote: *N*-acetylcysteine. Loading PO 140 mg/kg, then 70 mg/kg every 4 hours for 17 additional doses. Repeat dose if patient vomits within 1 hour of administration, or administer medication through a duodenal tube. *N*-acetylcysteine should be administered within 24 hours of ingestion of acetaminophen. Activated charcoal decreases *N*-acetylcysteine absorption and should be removed by stomach lavage if administered. IV administration of *N*-acetylcysteine may lead to anaphylaxis and is contraindicated.

Management: Discontinue or reduce medication. Correct fluid, electrolyte, and acid-base disturbances. Monitor BUN, blood glucose, SGOT, SGPT, PT, PTT, bilirubin, creatinine, and serum electrolytes. Treat hypoglycemia as indicated. Administer phytonadione for prothrombin times greater than 1.5 times control. Administer fresh frozen plasma for prothrombin times greater than 3 times control. Monitor appropriate parameters if hepatic or renal failure occurs. Support ventilation and circulation (patent airway, oxygen, IV fluids, vasopressors). Airway-protected, ipecac syrup–induced emesis (30 mL or 0.5 mL/kg ipecac syrup followed by 200 mL or 4 mL/kg of water or clear fluid) or gastric lavage (with drug ingestion) followed by administration of activated charcoal (PO 50–100 g or 1–2 g/kg). Hemodialysis or hemoperfusion (generally not recommended). Peritoneal dialysis is ineffective. Symptomatic treatment.

Guidelines/Precautions

1. Acetaminophen may precipitate renal failure in patients with impaired renal function; may precipitate hepatotoxicity and severe hepatic failure in chronic alcoholics due to increase in toxic metabolites.
2. The drug formulation may contain sulfites, which may cause allergic-type reactions, including anaphylaxis, in susceptible individuals.
3. Individuals with phenylketonuria should not use acetaminophen formulations that contain aspartame (Nutra-Sweet), for example, Children's Tylenol and Tempra chewable tablets. Following oral administration, aspartame is metabolized in the GI tract to phenylalanine.
4. Use with caution in patients with anemia because cyanosis may not be apparent despite high concentrations of methemoglobin.
5. Repeat administration of acetaminophen is contraindicated in patients with anemia or cardiac, pulmonary, hepatic, or renal disease.
6. Platelet counts and liver function tests should be performed monthly when administered at high doses for a prolonged period.

Principal Adverse Reactions

Cardiovascular: Hypotension.
Pulmonary: Dyspnea, asthma.
CNS: Stupor, coma, euphoria.
Gastrointestinal: Hepatic dysfunction, jaundice, GI disturbances, nausea, vomiting.
Genitourinary: Dysuria, interstitial nephritis, renal papillary necrosis.
Allergic: Pruritus, urticaria.
Hematologic: Leukopenia, thrombocytopenia, pancytopenia, methemoglobinemia.

ACYCLOVIR HYDROCHLORIDE

Class: Nucleoside Antiviral Agent

Use(s): Treatment of initial and recurrent episodes of herpes zoster (shingles), genital herpes, and chickenpox (varicella).

Dosing: *Initial genital herpes simplex*
PO: 200 mg every 4 hours for 10 days.
Slow IV: 5 mg/kg every 8 hours for 5 days.
Topical: 5% ointment applied every 6 hours (less effective than oral administration; it reduces the duration of viral shedding but has no significant effect on symptoms).
Recurrent herpes simplex
Chronic suppression: PO 400 mg twice daily for up to 12 months.
Intermittent suppression: PO 200 mg every 4 hours for 5 days at the earliest sign of

recurrence. Short-term treatment of recurrent episodes is more appropriate for patients with mild and infrequent disease.

Herpes simplex encephalitis: Slow IV 10 mg/kg every 8 hours for 10–14 days.

Neonatal herpes simplex: Slow IV 10 mg/kg every 8 hours for 10–14 days.

Herpes zoster

Normal host: PO 800 mg every 4 hours for 7–10 days.

Compromised host: Slow IV 10 mg/kg every 8 hours for 7–10 days.

Varicella (chickenpox)

Normal host: PO 20 mg/kg (maximum 800 mg) every 6 hours for 5 days.

Compromised host: Slow IV 10 mg/kg every 8 hours for 7–10 days.

Intravenous administration should be reserved for patients with severe local disease or systemic complication. Dose of acyclovir should be reduced in patients with impaired renal function. Creatinine clearance >50 mL/min: 100% of IV dose at 8-hour intervals. Creatinine clearance 25–50 mL/min or 10–25 mL/min: 100% of IV dose at 12- to 24-hour intervals. Creatinine clearance <10 mL/min: 100% of PO dose at 12-hour intervals.

Elimination: Renal, hepatic.

Preparations

Acyclovir **(Zovirax)**

Tablets: 400 mg, 800 mg.

Capsules: 200 mg.
Oral solution: 40 mg/mL.
Ointment: 5% (in a polyethylene-glycol base).
Injection: 50 mg/mL.

Pharmacology

Acyclovir is a synthetic purine nucleoside analogue with in vitro and in vivo inhibitory activity against human herpes viruses, including herpes simplex types 1 (HSV-1) and 2 (HSV-2), varicella-zoster virus (VZV), Epstein-Barr virus (EBV), and cytomegalovirus (CMV), in decreasing order of potency. The inhibitory activity for these viruses is highly selective. Normal uninfected cells are not affected because they take up less acyclovir and activate it much less efficiently. Thymidine kinase encoded by HSV, VZV, and EBV viruses converts acyclovir into acyclovir monophosphate, a nucleotide analogue. The monophosphate is further converted into diphosphate by cellular guanylate kinase and into triphosphate by a number of cellular enzymes. Acyclovir triphosphate interferes with herpes simplex virus DNA polymerase and inhibits viral DNA replication. Acyclovir triphosphate may inhibit cellular α-DNA polymerase to a lesser degree. The mode of acyclovir phosphorylation in CMV-infected cells may involve virally induced cell kinases or an unidentified viral enzyme. However, acyclovir is not efficiently activated in CMV-infected cells, which may account for the reduced potency of the drug.

In patients with acute genital herpes, herpes zoster, and chickenpox infections, acyclovir significantly reduces the duration of pain and the incidence of new lesion formation. Patients with severe episodes may derive more benefit than those with mild disease. Acyclovir also decreases the frequency and/or severity of recurrences of genital herpes. Acyclovir crosses the placenta and may be excreted in breast milk. It should be used cautiously in pregnant and nursing mothers.

Pharmacokinetics

Onset: Decrease in new lesion formation: PO, 24–48 hours. Relief of pain in herpes zoster: 20 days.
Peak Effect: PO, variable.
Duration of Action: Half-life (PO), 2.6 hours.

Interactions

Serum levels of acyclovir increased by co-administration of probenecid; additive impairment of renal function with concomitant administration of nephrotoxic drugs.

Toxicity

Toxic Range: Not routinely monitored.
Manifestations: Peripheral edema; headache; drowsiness; agitation; hallucinations, disorientation (IV overdose); nausea and vomiting; increased serum creatinine; acute renal failure.
Antidote: No specific antidote.
Management: Discontinue or reduce medication. Support ventilation and circulation (patent airway, oxygen, IV fluids, vasopressors). Fluid diuresis. Hemodialysis until renal function is restored. Symptomatic treatment.

Guidelines/Precautions

1. Exposure of herpes simplex and varicella-zoster isolates to acyclovir may result in the emergence of

less sensitive viruses. Patients should be advised to take particular care to avoid potential transmission of virus if active lesions are present while they are on therapy.

2. Use with caution in patients with impaired renal function and those receiving potentially nephrotoxic drugs.

Principal Adverse Reactions

Cardiovascular: Peripheral edema.
CNS: Headache, drowsiness, fatigue.
Gastrointestinal: Nausea, vomiting, constipation, diarrhea, abdominal pain, medication taste.
Genitourinary: Renal dysfunction.
Allergic: Urticaria, pruritus.
Hematologic: Leukopenia, lymphadenopathy.
Other: Muscle pain.

ALENDRONATE SODIUM

Class: Aminobisphosphonate

Use(s): Treatment and prevention of osteoporosis in postmenopausal women, treatment of Paget's disease of the bone, treatment of hypercalcemia, reduction of the incidence of pathologic fractures, slowing of bone disease progression and reduction of tumor-associated metastatic bone pain, and treatment of reflex sympathetic dystrophy (RSD) and its associated osteoporosis and bone pain.

Dosing: *Treatment of osteoporosis and metastatic bone pain:* PO 10 mg once a day.

Prevention of osteoporosis: PO 5 mg once a day.

Paget's disease: PO 40 mg once a day for 6 months.

Medication must be taken with only water at least half an hour before the first food, beverage, or medication of the day. Other beverages, food, and some medications are likely to reduce the absorption of alendronate. To facilitate delivery to the stomach and reduce the potential for esophageal irritation, alendronate should be swallowed with a full glass of water (6 to 8 oz) upon arising for the day, and patients should not lie down for at least 30 minutes *and* not until after their first food of the day. Failure to follow these instructions may increase the risk of adverse esophageal experiences. Patients should receive supplemental calcium and vitamin D if dietary intake is inadequate.

Elimination: Renal.

Preparations

Alendronate sodium **(Fosamax):** Tablets: 5 mg, 10 mg, 40 mg.

Pharmacology

This aminobisphosphonate binds to bone hydroxyapatite and specifically inhibits the activity of osteoclasts, the bone resorbing cells. Alendronate reduces bone resorption with no direct effect on bone formation, although the latter process is ultimately reduced because bone resorption and formation are coupled during bone turnover. Alendronate thus reduces elevated rates of bone turnover. Alendronate shows preferential localization to sites of bone resorption specifically under osteoclasts. The drug inhibits osteoclast activity but does not interfere with osteoclast recruitment or attachment. The osteoclasts adhere normally to the bone surface but lack the ruffled border that is indicative of active resorption. Dose-dependent inhibition of resorption is manifested by decreases in urinary calcium and urinary markers of bone collagen degradation (such as deoxypyridinoline and cross-linked *N*-telopeptides of type I collagen). Within 6 to 49 days after administration, normal bone is formed on top of the alendronate. When incorporated into bone matrix, alendronate is no longer pharmacologically active. Thus, alendronate must be continuously administered to suppress osteoclasts on newly formed resorption surfaces.

In treatment of metastatic bone disease, alendronate and other bisphosphonates (e.g., pamidronate, clodronate) treat hypercalcemia, reduce tumor-associated pain, reduce the incidence of pathologic fractures, and also slow the progression of bone disease. Administration of bisphosphonates shortly after adjuvant chemotherapy can preserve bone density in female patients with chemotherapy-induced menopause. A related bisphosphonate, clodronate, has been shown to reduce the incidence of bone metastasis in patients with early-stage breast cancer. There was no difference in the incidence of nonskeletal metastatic disease. Alendronate may reduce bone resorption and relieve bone pain in patients with RSD. Osteoporosis and bone resorption in RSD may be partly due to increased deep tissue blood flow secondary to surface or capillary vasoconstriction.

Pharmacokinetics

Onset: 4 weeks.
Peak Effects: 3–6 months.
Duration of Action: 7 months.

Interactions

Absorption decreased with administration of calcium supplements, antacids, and some oral medications; increased incidence of gastrointestinal side effects with concomitant administration of compounds containing aspirin.

Toxicity

Toxic Range: Not routinely monitored.
Manifestations: Hypocalcemia; hypophosphatemia; adverse upper GI events (e.g., upset stomach, heart-burn, esophagitis, gastritis, or ulcer).
Antidote: None.
Management: Discontinue or reduce medication. Administer milk or antacids to bind alendronate. Do not induce vomiting because of the risk of esophageal irritation. The patient should remain fully upright. Administer intravenous or oral calcium to correct hypocalcemia. Support ventilation and circulation (patent airway, oxygen, IV fluids, vasopressors). Symptomatic treatment. Dialysis is not beneficial.

Guidelines/Precautions

1. Gastric and duodenal ulcers, some severe and with complications, have been reported with use of alendronate.

2. Concomitant administration with compounds containing aspirin (but not NSAIDs) may increase the incidence of GI side effects. Use with caution in patients receiving aspirin or NSAIDs.

3. Patients should be instructed that the expected benefits of alendronate may only be obtained when each tablet is swallowed with a full glass of water the first thing upon arising for the day and at least 30 minutes before the first food, beverage, or medication of the day. Patients should not lie down for at least 30 minutes and until after their first food of the day. Tablets should not be chewed or sucked because of the potential for oropharyngeal ulceration. Patients should be specifically instructed that failure to follow these instructions may increase the risk of esophageal problems.

4. Patients should be informed to stop taking alendronate and consult their physician if they develop symptoms of esophageal disease, such as retrosternal pain, difficulty or pain on swallowing, or worsening heartburn.

5. Alendronate is contraindicated in patients with clinically significant hypersensitivity to alendronate or other bisphosphonates.

Principal Adverse Reactions

Gastrointestinal: Nausea, dyspepsia, constipation, esophageal ulcer, gastritis, acid regurgitation, abdominal distension.

Musculoskeletal: Bone, muscle, or joint pain.

CNS: Headache.

ALFENTANIL HYDROCHLORIDE

Class: Narcotic Agonist

Use(s): Treatment of acute pain.

Dosing: *Analgesia*
IV/IM: 250–500 µg (5–10 µg/kg).
Epidural
Bolus: 500–1000 µg (10–20 µg/kg).
Infusion: 100–250 µg/hr (2–5 µg/kg/hr).

Elimination: Hepatic.

Preparations

Alfentanil hydrochloride **(Alfenta):** Injection: 500 µg/
mL.

Dilution for Infusion: IV: 10 mg (20 mL) alfentanil in
250 mL of D5W or normal saline (40 µg/mL). Epidural:
1.5 mg (3 mL) alfentanil in 150 mL local anesthetic or
preservative-free normal saline (10 µg/mL).

Pharmacology

Alfentanil is a phenylpiperidine derivative and potent
opioid analgesic with rapid onset and short duration of
action. It is associated with less sedation when used in
patient-controlled analgesia compared with meperidine
or fentanyl. Repeated doses or continuous infusions do
not result in a significant accumulation. Alfentanil
crosses the placental barrier and may produce depression in the neonate. Significant amounts of the drug may
appear in breast milk, and it should be used with
caution in nursing mothers.

Pharmacokinetics

Onset of Action: IV, 1–2 minutes. IM, <5 minutes. Epidural, 5–15 minutes.
Peak Effect: IV, 1–2 minutes. IM, <15 minutes. Epidural, 30 minutes.
Duration of Action: IV, 10–15 minutes. IM, 10–60 minutes. Epidural, 4–8 hours.

Interactions

Circulatory and ventilatory depressant effects potentiated by narcotics, sedatives, volatile anesthetics, nitrous oxide; ventilatory depressant effects potentiated by amphetamines, MAO inhibitors, phenothiazines, and tricyclic antidepressants; analgesia enhanced and prolonged by α_2-agonists (e.g., clonidine, epinephrine); addition of epinephrine to epidural alfentanil results in increased side effects (e.g., nausea) and prolonged motor block; reduced clearance and prolonged respiratory depression with concomitant use of erythromycin; in higher doses, muscle rigidity sufficient to interfere with ventilation.

Toxicity

Toxic Range: Not routinely monitored.
Manifestations: Somnolence; coma; respiratory arrest; apnea; cardiac arrhythmias; combined respiratory and metabolic acidosis; precipitation of withdrawal symptoms from opioids (abdominal cramps, vomiting, skin crawling, piloerection, nasal stuffiness, lacrimation, yawning, sweating, tremor, myalgia); circulatory collapse; cardiac arrest; death.

Antidote: Naloxone IV/IM/SC 0.4–2.0 mg. Repeat dose every 2 to 3 minutes to a maximum of 10–20 mg.

Management: Discontinue or reduce medication. Support ventilation and circulation (patent airway, oxygen, IV fluids, vasopressors). Administer antidote. Monitor blood gases, pH, and electrolytes. Correct acidosis and electrolyte disturbance (lactic acidosis may require IV sodium bicarbonate 1–2 mEq/kg). Symptomatic treatment. Airway-protected, ipecac syrup–induced emesis (30 mL or 0.5 mL/kg ipecac syrup followed by 200 mL or 4 mL/kg of water or clear fluid) or gastric lavage (with drug ingestion) followed by administration of activated charcoal (PO 50–100 g or 1–2 g/kg).

Guidelines/Precautions

1. Reduce doses in elderly patients and with concomitant use of sedatives and other narcotics.
2. Narcotic effects are reversed by naloxone (IV 0.2–0.4 mg or higher).
3. Excessive bradycardia may be treated with atropine.
4. Neonatal resuscitation may be required with alfentanil usage in labor. Have naloxone available.
5. Epidural alfentanil may cause delayed respiratory depression (up to 8 hours after single dose), pruritus, nausea and vomiting, and urinary retention. Naloxone (IV/IM/SC 0.2–0.4 mg as needed or infusion 5–10 μg/kg/hr) is effective for prophylaxis and/or treatment. Ventilatory support for respiratory depression must be readily available. Antihistamines, such as diphenhydramine (IV/IM 12.5–25 mg every 6 hours as needed), may be used for pruri-

tus. Metoclopramide (IV 10 mg every 6 hours as needed) may be used for nausea and vomiting. Urinary retention that does not respond to naloxone may require straight bladder catheterization. Bethanechol (Urecholine) PO 15–30 mg three times a day or SC 2.5–5 mg three or four times daily as required may be used as an alternative to naloxone. (Bethanechol increases the tone of the detrusor urinae muscle. It should not be given IV or IM, which may result in cholinergic overstimulation. Have atropine available [IV/SC 0.5 mg].)

6. Epidural/intrathecal injections should be avoided when the patient has septicemia, infection at the injection site, or coagulopathy.

7. Patients should be warned that alfentanil may impair their ability to perform hazardous tasks requiring mental alertness or physical coordination (e.g., driving a motor vehicle, operating heavy machinery).

8. Alfentanil is subject to control under the Federal Controlled Substances Act of 1970 as a Schedule II (C-II) drug.

Principal Adverse Reactions

Cardiovascular: Bradycardia, hypotension, arrhythmias.
Pulmonary: Respiratory depression.
CNS: Euphoria, dysphoria, convulsions.
Gastrointestinal: Nausea and vomiting, biliary tract spasm, delayed gastric emptying.
Ocular: Miosis.
Musculoskeletal: Muscle rigidity.
Other: Pruritus.

ALPRAZOLAM

Class: Benzodiazepine

Use(s): Sedative, treatment of panic attacks, antidepressant.

Dosing: *Sedation and panic attacks:* PO 0.25–0.5 mg three times daily. Dosage may be titrated upward in 0.25-mg increments at intervals of 3 days. Maximum dose 4 mg daily.

Depression: PO 2.5–3.0 mg daily in divided doses.

Dose should be decreased in elderly or debilitated patients.

Elimination: Hepatic, renal.

Preparations

Alprazolam **(Xanax):** Tablets: 0.25 mg, 0.5 mg, 1 mg, 2 mg.

Pharmacology

This benzodiazepine produces a dose-related sedation and relief of anxiety. Like other benzodiazepines, the drug is thought to influence the effect of γ-aminobutyric acid (GABA), an inhibitory neurotransmitter, in the brain. Compared with other benzodiazepines, alprazolam has particular efficacy in the treatment of panic disorders and has been demonstrated to have antidepressant effects. In chronic pain syndromes, the pain threshold may be increased by relief of anxiety, agitation, and depression. Alprazolam does not have intrinsic analgesic activity and should be used in combination with analgesics (e.g., opioids, NSAIDs, anti-depressant agents). The drug produces minimal depressant effects on ventilation and circulation in the absence of other CNS depressant drugs. Onset of action is comparable to lorazepam.

Pharmacokinetics

Onset of Action: PO, 20–30 minutes.
Peak Effect: PO, 1–2 hours.
Duration of Action: PO, 6–10 hours.

Interactions

CNS and circulatory depressant effects potentiated by alcohol, narcotics, sedatives, barbiturates, phenothiazines, MAO inhibitors, and volatile anesthetics; decreased requirements for volatile anesthetics; effects antagonized by flumazenil.

Toxicity

Toxic Range: Not routinely monitored.
Manifestations: Respiratory depression, apnea, hypotension, confusion, coma, seizures.
Antidote: Flumazenil.
Management: Discontinue or reduce medication. Support ventilation and circulation (patent airway, oxygen, IV fluids, vasopressors). Administer antidote (flumazenil IV 0.2–2.0 mg). Symptomatic treatment. Airway-protected, ipecac syrup–induced emesis (30 mL or 0.5 mL/kg ipecac syrup followed by 200 mL or 4 mL/kg of water or clear fluid) or gastric lavage (with drug ingestion) followed by administration of activated charcoal (PO 50–100 g or 0.5–1.0 g/kg). Hemodialysis is

not useful. Treat withdrawal hyperactivity with a low-dose barbiturate.

Guidelines/Precautions

1. Intra-arterial injection may produce arteriospasm resulting in gangrene. Treat with local infiltration of phentolamine (5–10 mg in 10 mL normal saline) and, if necessary, sympathetic block.
2. For optimal amnesic effects, administer intravenously 15–20 minutes or orally 2 hours before anticipated operative procedure.
3. Unexpected hypotension and respiratory depression may occur when combined with opioids.
4. Use with caution in elderly patients because excessive sedation and hypoventilation may occur.
5. Not for use in children younger than 12 years.
6. Patients should be warned that alprazolam may impair their ability to perform activities requiring mental alertness or physical coordination (e.g., operating heavy machinery, driving a motor vehicle).
7. Alprazolam is contraindicated in patients with known hypersensitivity to benzodiazepines or any ingredients in the parenteral formulation (i.e., polyethylene glycol, propylene glycol, or benzyl alcohol) and in patients with acute close-angle glaucoma.
8. Alprazolam is subject to control under the Federal Controlled Substances Act of 1970 as a Schedule IV (C-IV) drug.

Principal Adverse Reactions

Cardiovascular: Hypotension, hypertension, bradycardia, tachycardia.

Pulmonary: Respiratory depression.
CNS: Sedation, dizziness, weakness, depression, agitation, amnesia.
Psychological: Hysteria, psychosis.
Gastrointestinal: Change in appetite.
Other: Visual disturbances, urticaria, pruritus.

AMITRIPTYLINE HYDROCHLORIDE

Class: Tricyclic Antidepressant

Use(s): Treatment of neurotic and endogenous depression; migraine prophylaxis; adjunct treatment of neuropathic pain syndromes, including diabetic neuropathy, postherpetic neuralgia, tic douloureux, and cancer pain; anxiety disorders; phobias; panic disorders; enuresis; eating disorders.

Dosing: *Pain syndromes*

Initial: PO 10–25 mg (0.2–0.5 mg/kg) daily at bedtime. Titrate dose upward every 3 to 4 weeks by increments of 10–25 mg as necessary.

Maintenance: PO 10–150 mg (0.2–3.0mg/kg) daily at bedtime. Doses should be decreased if unacceptable side effects occur. Serum levels should be determined if there are signs of toxicity. Doses of 150 mg/day may be required in the management of painful diabetic neuropathy.

Migraine prophylaxis/tension headache: PO 25–75 mg (0.5–1.5 mg/kg) daily.

Depression

Initial: PO 75–100 mg (1.5–2.0 mg/kg) daily in one to four divided doses.

Maintenance: PO, 25–150 mg (0.5–3.0 mg/kg) daily in one to four divided doses. IM, 20–30 mg four times daily. Replace with oral medication as soon as possible. Do not administer intravenously.

Doses for pain are generally smaller than those used for treatment of affective disorders. Medication should be administered on a fixed schedule and not as needed. Administration of the entire daily dose at bedtime may reduce daytime sedation. After symptoms are controlled, dosage should be gradually reduced to the lowest level that will maintain relief of symptoms. When amitriptyline is used in conjunction with a phenothiazine, dosages should first be adjusted by administering each drug separately. Commercial fixed-ratio combinations should be used only when the optimum maintenance dosage ratios have been determined and correspond to the ratios in the commercial preparation.

Analgesia may be enhanced by addition of opioid analgesics (see pages xxvi–xliv for drug combinations), nonsteroidal anti-inflammatory drugs (NSAIDs), and nondrug therapies such as transcutaneous electrical nerve stimulation (TENS). In geriatric patients and patients with decreased renal or hepatic function, decrease doses by one-third to one-half. The possibility for suicide is inherent in depression and may persist until significant remission occurs. The quantity of drug dispensed should reflect this consideration.

Elimination: Hepatic, renal.

Preparations

Amitriptyline hydrochloride **(Elavil, Endep):** Tablets, film coated: 10 mg, 25 mg, 50 mg, 75 mg, 100 mg, 150 mg.

Amitriptyline hydrochloride **(Elavil, Enovil):** Injection: 10 mg/mL.

Amitriptyline hydrochloride and chlordiazepoxide **(Limbitrol):** Tablets, film coated: Amitriptyline hydrochloride 12.5 mg with chlordiazepoxide 10 mg.

Amitriptyline hydrochloride and perphenazine (various; previously **Triavil**): Tablets, film coated: Amitriptyline hydrochloride 10 mg and perphenazine 2 mg; amitriptyline hydrochloride 25 mg and perphenazine 2 mg; amitriptyline hydrochloride 10 mg and perphenazine 4 mg; amitriptyline hydrochloride 25 mg and perphenazine 4 mg; amitriptyline hydrochloride 50 mg and perphenazine 4 mg.

Pharmacology

A dibenzocycloheptene derivative and a tertiary amine tricyclic antidepressant, amitriptyline is structurally related to the phenothiazine antipsychotic agents. Antidepressant activity may be partly due to inhibition of the amine-pump uptake of neurotransmitters (e.g., nor-epinephrine and serotonin) at the presynaptic neuron, down-regulation of β-receptor sensitivity, sedation, and peripheral/central anticholinergic effects. Although blockade of neurotransmitter uptake may occur imme-diately, antidepressant response may take days to weeks. Patients with low serotonin levels may respond better to amitriptyline compared with norepinephrine-deficient patients. Amitriptyline (and other tricyclic anti-depressants) does not inhibit the monoamine oxidase (MAO) system. Amitriptyline is demethylated in the liver to the active metabolite, nortriptyline.

The analgesic effects of amitriptyline (and other anti-depressants) may occur partly through the alleviation of depression, which may be responsible for increased pain suffering, but also by mechanisms that are inde-pendent of mood effects. Serotonin and norepinephrine activity may be increased in descending pain inhibitory pathways. Activation of these pathways decreases the transmission of nociceptive impulses from primary affer-ent neurons to first-order cells in laminae I and V of the spinal cord dorsal horn. Amitriptyline may also poten-tiate the analgesic effect of opioids by increasing their binding efficacy to opioid receptors. Amitriptyline (and other tricyclic antidepressants) may have an antagonis-tic effect on *N*-methyl-D-aspartate (NMDA) receptors and inhibit NMDA receptor activation–induced neuro-plasticity. Spinal NMDA receptor activation is thought to be central to the generation and maintenance of hyperalgesic pain. Amitriptyline has varying degrees of efficacy in different pain syndromes and may be better at relieving the burning, aching, and dyesthetic com-ponent of neuropathic pain. The drug is seldom useful in the management of lancinating, shooting paroxysmal pain. At full antidepressant dosages, amitriptyline (and other tricyclic antidepressants) is especially effective in chronic low back pain with associated major depression. Patients with uncomplicated low back pain (i.e., without major depression) do not respond as well. The antimigraine activity of amitriptyline is relatively independent of its antidepressant effects. Low doses of amitriptyline (and other tricyclic antidepressants) are just as effective for chronic tension headache as the commonly used antianxiety drugs.

Amitriptyline produces varying degrees of sedation and blocks α_1-adrenergic, H_1, and H_2 receptors. Amitriptyline may enhance ulcer healing and is a more potent in vitro antagonist of H_2 receptors than cimetidine. Abnormal EEG patterns may be produced, with decrease in alpha activity and increase in theta activity. The seizure threshold may be lowered. Therapeutic doses do not affect respiration, but toxic doses may lead to respiratory depression. The direct quinidine-like effects may manifest at toxic doses and produce cardiovascular disturbances (e.g., conduction blockade). Amitriptyline does not have addiction liability and its use is not associated with drug-seeking behavior. Withdrawal symptoms, including sleep disruption with vivid dreams, may be precipitated by acute withdrawal. Tolerance develops to the sedative and anticholinergic effects, but there are no reports of tolerance to the analgesic effects. Amitriptyline crosses the placenta, and use in pregnancy may be associated with fetal malformations. The drug is excreted in breast milk and has a potential for serious adverse effects in nursing infants.

Pharmacokinetics

Onset of Action: Analgesic effect: PO, <5 days. Antidepressant effect: PO, 1–2 weeks.
Peak Effect: Antidepressant effect: PO, 2–4 weeks.
Duration of Action: Antidepressant effect: PO, variable.

Interactions

Increased risk of hyperthermia with concomitant administration of anticholinergics (e.g., atropine), phenothiazines, thyroid medications; serum levels and toxic effects of amitriptyline increased by concomitant methylphenidate, fluoxetine, cimetidine, phenothiazines, and haloperidol; ventilatory and circulatory depressant effects of CNS depressant drugs and alcohol potentiated by amitriptyline; increases the pressor and cardiac effects of sympathomimetics (e.g., isoproterenol, phenylephrine, norepinephrine, epinephrine, amphetamine); decreases serum levels and pharmacologic effects of levodopa and phenylbutazone; increases serum levels and toxic effects of dicumarol; onset of therapeutic effects shortened and adverse cardiac effects of amitriptyline increased with concomitant administration of levothyroxine and liothyronine; fatal hyperpyretic crisis or seizures with concomitant use of MAO inhibitors; efficacy of IV regional bretylium (uptake-dependent) and IV regional guanethidine decreased by amitriptyline.

Toxicity

Toxic Range: Not routinely monitored.
Manifestations: *Chronic:* Dream and sleep disturbances, akathisia, anxiety, chills, coryza, malaise,

myalgia, headache, dizziness, nausea and vomiting. *Acute:* In addition to the previously listed symptoms, CNS stimulation with excitement, delirium, hallucinations, hyperreflexia, myoclonus, choreiform movements, parkinsonian symptoms, seizures, hyperpyrexia, then CNS depression with drowsiness, areflexia, hypothermia, respiratory depression, cyanosis, hypotension, coma; peripheral anticholinergic symptoms, including urinary retention, dry mucous membranes, mydriasis, constipation, adynamic ileus; cardiac irregularities, including tachycardia, QRS prolongation; metabolic and/or respiratory acidosis; polyradiculoneuropathy; renal failure; vomiting; ataxia; dysarthria; bullous cutaneous lesions; and pulmonary consolidation.

Antidote: None.

Management: Discontinue or reduce medication. Correct fluid, electrolyte, and acid-base disturbances. Airway-protected, ipecac syrup–induced emesis (30 mL or 0.5 mL/kg ipecac syrup) or gastric lavage (with drug ingestion) followed by administration of activated charcoal (PO 50–100 g or 1–2 g/kg). These purging actions should be performed even if several hours have elapsed after ingestion because the anticholinergic effects may delay gastric emptying, and the drug may also be secreted into the stomach. Control seizures: IV benzodiazepines are the first choice because IV barbiturates may enhance respiratory depression; however, IV barbiturates may be useful in refractory seizures. Control hyperpyrexia with ice packs, cooling, and sponge baths. Support ventilation and circulation (patent airway, oxygen, IV fluids, vasopressors). Continuous EKG monitoring. Treat cardiac arrhythmias with IV lidocaine or propranolol. Digoxin, quinidine, procainamide, and diisopyramide should be avoided because they may further depress myocardial conduction and/or contractility. Temporary pacemakers may be necessary in patients with advanced arteriovenous block, severe bradycardia, and/or life-threatening ventricular arrhythmias unresponsive to drug therapy. Physostigmine (slow IV 1–3 mg) may be used in the treatment of life-threatening anticholinergic toxicity. Routine use of physostigmine is not advisable due to its serious adverse effects (e.g., seizures, bronchospasm, and severe bradyarrhythmias). Hemodialysis or peritoneal dialysis are ineffective because the drug is highly protein bound. Symptomatic treatment. Consider the possibility of multiple drug involvement. Counseling prior to and after discharge for patients who attempted suicide.

Guidelines/Precautions

1. To avoid withdrawal symptoms, the medication should be tapered down over a couple of weeks and not discontinued abruptly.
2. Use with caution in patients with cardiovascular disease, thyroid disease, seizure disorders, and in those in whom excessive anticholinergic activity may be harmful (e.g., patients with benign prostatic hypertrophy, a history of urinary retention, or increased intraocular pressure). The drug should be used in close-angle glaucoma only when the glaucoma is adequately controlled by drugs and closely monitored.
3. Amitriptyline is contraindicated in patients receiving MAO inhibitors (concurrently or within the past

2 weeks), patients in the acute recovery phase following myocardial infarction, and those with demonstrated hypersensitivity to amitriptyline. Cross-sensitivity with other tricyclic antidepressants may occur.

4. Patients should be warned of the possibility of drowsiness that may impair performance of potentially hazardous tasks such as driving an automobile or operating machinery. Persisting daytime drowsiness may be decreased by administering a lower dose, administering the dose earlier in the evening, or substituting a less sedating alternative.

5. For optimum effect, discontinue amitriptyline prior to intravenous regional blockade with guanethidine or bretylium.

Principal Adverse Reactions

Cardiovascular: Postural hypotension, arrhythmias, conduction disturbances, hypertension, sudden death.

Pulmonary: Respiratory depression.

CNS: Confusion, disorientation, extrapyramidal symptoms.

Gastrointestinal: Hepatic dysfunction, jaundice, nausea, vomiting, constipation, decrease in lower esophageal sphincter tone.

Genitourinary: Urinary retention, paradoxical nocturia, urinary frequency.

Ocular: Blurred vision, mydriasis, increased intraocular pressure.

Dermatologic: Pruritus, urticaria, petechiae, photosensitivity.

Hematologic: Leukopenia, thrombocytopenia, eosinophilia, agranulocytosis, purpura.

Endocrinologic: Increased or decreased libido, impotence, gynecomastia, SIADH.
Other: Hyperthermia.

AMOXAPINE HYDROCHLORIDE

Class: Tricyclic Antidepressant

Use(s): Treatment of neurotic and endogenous depression; migraine prophylaxis; adjunct treatment of neuropathic pain syndromes, including diabetic neuropathy, postherpetic neuralgia, tic douloureux, and cancer pain; anxiety disorders; phobias; panic disorders; enuresis; eating disorders.

Dosing: *Pain syndromes*
> Initial: PO 50–150 mg (1–3 mg/kg) daily at bedtime. Titrate dose upward every 3 to 4 weeks by increments of 25–50 mg as necessary.
> Maintenance: PO 50–300 mg (1–6 mg/kg) daily at bedtime. Doses should be decreased if unacceptable side effects occur. Serum levels should be determined if there are signs of toxicity. The higher end of the dose range may be required in the management of painful diabetic neuropathy.

Depression
> Initial: PO 100–150 mg (2–3 mg/kg) daily in one to three divided doses.
> Maintenance: PO 100–400 mg (2–8 mg/kg) daily in one to three divided doses. Doses

that exceed 300 mg should be administered in two to three divided doses.

Doses for pain are generally smaller than those used for treatment of affective disorders. Medication should be administered on a fixed schedule and not as needed. Administration of the entire daily dose at bedtime may reduce daytime sedation. After symptoms are controlled, dosage should be gradually reduced to the lowest level that will maintain relief of symptoms. Analgesia may be enhanced by addition of opioid analgesics (see pages xxvi–xliv for drug combinations), nonsteroidal anti-inflammatory drugs (NSAIDs), and use of nondrug therapies such as transcutaneous electrical nerve stimulation (TENS). In geriatric patients and patients with decreased renal or hepatic function, decrease doses by one-third to one-half and do not exceed 300 mg daily. The possibility for suicide is inherent in depression and may persist until significant remission occurs. The quantity of drug dispensed should reflect this consideration.

Elimination: Hepatic, renal.

Preparations

Amoxapine **(Amoxapine, Asendin):** Tablets: 25 mg, 50 mg, 100 mg, 150 mg.

Pharmacology

A dibenzoazepine derivative and a secondary amine tricyclic antidepressant, amoxapine is a metabolite of loxapine, an antipsychotic agent. Antidepressant activity may be partly due to inhibition of amine-pump uptake of norepinephrine and serotonin at the presynaptic neuron. Like loxapine, amoxapine has substantive neuroleptic activity, blocks the effects of dopamine on dopamine receptors, may cause extrapyramidal side effects, and has been associated with development of neuroleptic malignant syndrome. Amoxapine is moderately sedating and has little anticholinergic activity. Compared with amitriptyline or imipramine, amoxapine may have a more rapid onset of action. Amoxapine does not inhibit the monoamine oxidase (MAO) system.

The analgesic effects of amoxapine (and other antidepressants) may occur partly through the alleviation of depression, which may be responsible for increased pain suffering, but also through mechanisms that are independent of mood effects. Serotonin and norepinephrine activity may be increased in descending pain inhibitory pathways. Activation of these pathways decreases the transmission of nociceptive impulses from primary afferent neurons to first-order cells in laminae I and V of the spinal cord dorsal horn. Amoxapine may also potentiate the analgesic effect of opioids by increasing their binding efficacy to opioid receptors. Amoxapine has varying degrees of efficacy in different pain syndromes and may be better at relieving the burning, aching, and dyesthetic component of neuropathic pain. The drug is seldom useful in the management of lancinating, shooting paroxysmal pain. Patients with low norepinephrine levels may respond better to amoxapine (and the other secondary amines) compared with serotonin-deficient patients.

Amoxapine does not have addiction liability and its

use is not associated with drug-seeking behavior. Withdrawal symptoms, including sleep disruption with vivid dreams, may be precipitated by acute withdrawal. Tolerance develops to the sedative and anticholinergic effects, but there are no reports of tolerance to the analgesic effects. Toxic manifestations of amoxapine differ significantly from those of the other tricyclic antidepressants, with CNS effects, particularly grand mal seizures, occurring more frequently in the absence of serious cardiovascular effects. Amoxapine crosses the placenta and is excreted in breast milk. Usage in pregnant or nursing mothers should occur only if the potential benefit justifies the potential risk.

Pharmacokinetics

Onset of Action: Analgesic effect: PO, <5 days. Antidepressant effect: PO, 4–7 days.
Peak Effect: Antidepressant effect: PO, 2–4 weeks.
Duration of Action: Antidepressant effect: PO, variable.

Interactions

Increased risk of hyperthermia with concomitant administration of anticholinergics (e.g., atropine), phenothiazines, thyroid medications; serum levels and toxic effects of amoxapine increased by concomitant methylphenidate, fluoxetine, cimetidine, phenothiazines and haloperidol; ventilatory and circulatory depressant effects of CNS depressant drugs and alcohol potentiated by amoxapine; increases the pressor and cardiac effects of sympathomimetics (e.g., isoproterenol, phenylephrine, norepinephrine, epinephrine, amphetamine); decreases serum levels and pharmacologic effects of levodopa and phenylbutazone; increases serum levels and toxic effects of dicumarol; onset of therapeutic effects shortened and adverse cardiac effects of amoxapine increased with concomitant administration of levothyroxine and liothyronine; fatal hyperpyretic crisis or seizures with concomitant use of MAO inhibitors; uptake-dependent efficacy of IV regional bretylium decreased by amoxapine.

Toxicity

Toxic Range: Not routinely monitored.

Manifestations: *Chronic:* Dream and sleep disturbances, akathisia, anxiety, chills, coryza, malaise, myalgia, headache, dizziness, nausea and vomiting. *Acute:* In addition to the previously listed symptoms, CNS stimulation with grand mal seizures, excitement, delirium, hallucinations, hyperreflexia, myoclonus, and extrapyramidal symptoms, including tardive dyskinesia and hyperpyrexia, then CNS depression with drowsiness, areflexia, hypothermia, respiratory depression, cyanosis, hypotension, and coma; peripheral anticholinergic symptoms, including urinary retention, dry mucous membranes, mydriasis, constipation, adynamic ileus; sinus tachycardia; metabolic and/or respiratory acidosis; polyradiculoneuropathy; rhabdomyolysis; acute tubular necrosis; acute renal failure; vomiting; ataxia; dysarthria; bullous cutaneous lesions; pulmonary consolidation.

Antidote: None.

Management: Discontinue or reduce medication. Correct fluid, electrolyte, and acid-base disturbances. Airway-protected, ipecac syrup–induced emesis (30 mL or 0.5 mL/kg ipecac syrup) or gastric lavage (with drug ingestion) followed by administration of activated charcoal (PO 50–100 g or 1–2 g/kg). These purging actions should be performed even if several hours have elapsed after ingestion because the anticholinergic effects may delay gastric emptying, and the drug may also be secreted into the stomach. Prophylactic anticonvulsants. Control seizures: IV benzodiazepines are the first choice because IV barbiturates may enhance respiratory depression; however, IV barbiturates may be useful in refractory seizures. Support ventilation and circulation (patent airway, oxygen, IV fluids, vasopressors). Treat renal impairment. Control hyperpyrexia with ice packs and cooling sponge baths. Physostigmine (slow IV 1–3 mg) may be used in the treatment of life-threatening anticholinergic toxicity. Routine use of physostigmine is not advisable due to its serious adverse effects (e.g., seizures, bronchospasm, and severe bradyarrhythmias). Hemodialysis or peritoneal dialysis are ineffective because the drug is highly protein bound. Symptomatic treatment. Consider the possibility of multiple drug involvement. Counseling prior to and after discharge for patients who have attempted suicide.

Guidelines/Precautions

1. To avoid withdrawal symptoms, the medication should be tapered down over a couple of weeks and not discontinued abruptly.
2. Use with caution in patients with cardiovascular disease, thyroid disease, and seizure disorders, and in those in whom excessive anticholinergic activity may be harmful (e.g., patients with benign prostatic hypertrophy, a history of urinary retention, or increased intraocular pressure). The drug should

be used in close-angle glaucoma only when the glaucoma is adequately controlled by drugs and closely monitored.

3. Amoxapime is contraindicated in patients receiving MAO inhibitors (concurrently or within the past 2 weeks) and those with demonstrated hypersensitivity to amoxapine. Cross-sensitivity with other tricyclic antidepressants may occur.

4. Neuroleptic malignant syndrome, a rare but potentially fatal side effect, may manifest with hyperpyrexia, muscle rigidity, altered mental status, and evidence of autonomic instability (irregular pulse or blood pressure, tachycardia, diaphoresis, arrhythmias). Discontinue amoxapine and treat symptomatically and with dantrolene or bromocriptine (PO 2.5–10.0 mg three times a day).

5. Patients should be warned of the possibility of drowsiness that may impair performance of potentially hazardous tasks such as driving an automobile or operating machinery. Persisting daytime drowsiness may be decreased by administering a lower dose, administering the dose earlier in the evening, or substituting a less sedating alternative.

Principal Adverse Reactions

Cardiovascular: Postural hypotension, sinus tachycardia.

Pulmonary: Respiratory depression.

CNS: Confusion, disorientation, extrapyramidal symptoms.

Gastrointestinal: Hepatic dysfunction, jaundice, nausea, vomiting, constipation, decrease in lower esophageal sphincter tone.

Genitourinary: Acute tubular necrosis.
Ocular: Blurred vision, mydriasis, increased intraocular pressure.
Dermatologic: Pruritus, urticaria, petechiae, photosensitivity.
Hematologic: Leukopenia, thrombocytopenia, eosinophilia, agranulocytosis, purpura.
Endocrinologic: Increased or decreased libido, impotence, gynecomastia, SIADH.
Other: Hyperthermia, neuroleptic malignant syndrome.

ASPIRIN

Class: Nonsteroidal Anti-inflammatory Drug

Use(s): Symptomatic treatment of mild to moderate pain, fever, inflammatory conditions (e.g., rheumatic fever, rheumatoid arthritis, osteoarthritis), chronic pain, and cancer pain (especially with bone metastasis).

Dosing: *Pain and fever*
> PO: 325–650 mg (6–12 mg/kg) every 4 hours. Maximum daily dose 6 g.
> PO, extended release: 650 mg (12 mg/kg) every 8 hours. Maximum dose 6 g daily. Do not crush or chew extended release preparations.
> Rectal: 325–650 mg (6–12 mg/kg) every 6 hours. Maximum dose 6 g daily. Use rectal suppositories only. Aspirin tablets may cause irritation and erosion of the rectal mucosa if administered rectally.

> *Inflammatory diseases:* PO 2.4–5.4 g (65 mg/ kg/day or 1.5 g/m²/day) daily in divided doses.
>
> Administer analgesic regularly (not as needed). Addition of opioid analgesics, antidepressant agents, and use of nondrug therapies such as transcutaneous electrical nerve stimulation (TENS) may enhance analgesia (see pages xxvi–xliv for drug combinations). In rheumatoid arthritis or juvenile rheumatoid arthritis, second-line rheumatoid agents may include leflunomide (Arava), etanercept (Enbrel), antimalarials or methotrexate. In geriatric patients and patients with decreased renal or hepatic function, decrease doses by one-third to one-half. The incidence of aspirin-induced gastropathy may be decreased by concomitant administration of antacids or sucralfate (PO 1 g four times daily). Misoprostol (PO 100–200 µg four times daily) may be used to prevent gastric ulcers in high-risk patients.

Elimination: Hepatic, renal.

Preparations

Aspirin **(Children's Aspirin):** Tablets: 65 mg, 75 mg, 81 mg.

Aspirin **(Bayer Children's Aspirin):** Tablets, chewable: 81 mg.

Aspirin **(Aspergum):** Gum tablets: 227.5 mg.

Aspirin **(Aspirin, Norwich):** Tablets: 325 mg, 500 mg, 650 mg.

Aspirin **(Bayer Timed Release, Aspirin SR, Sloprin, ZORprin):** Tablets, extended release: 650 mg, 800 mg.

Aspirin **(Ecotrin, Genacote, Duentric, Easprin, Maxiprin, Megaprin):** Tablets, delayed release (enteric coated): 325 mg, 500 mg, 650 mg, 975 mg.

Aspirin **(Bayer Aspirin, Genprin):** Tablets, film coated: 325 mg, 500 mg.

Aspirin **(Aspirin Uniserts):** Rectal suppositories: 60 mg, 65 mg, 120 mg, 125 mg, 130 mg, 195 mg, 200 mg, 300 mg, 325 mg, 600 mg, 650 mg.

Aspirin with buffers **(Buffaprin, Bufferin, Buffered Aspirin, Buffinol, Buffex):** Tablets: 324 mg with buffers, 325 mg with buffers, 500 mg with buffers, 650 mg with buffers.

Aspirin with buffers **(Ascriptin, Magnaprin, Ascriptin A/D, Tri-buffered Bufferin):** Tablets, film coated: 324 mg with buffers, 325 mg with buffers, 500 mg with buffers.

Aspirin with buffers **(Alka-Seltzer):** Tablets for solution: 325 mg, 500 mg.

Aspirin with acetaminophen **(Gemnisyn):** Tablets: Aspirin 325 mg and acetaminophen 325 mg.

Aspirin with codeine phosphate, caffeine, and butalbital **(Fiorinal with Codeine):** Tablets: Aspirin 325 mg, codeine phosphate 30 mg, caffeine 40 mg, and butalbital 50 mg.

Aspirin with oxycodone **(Percodan-Demi):** Tablets: Aspirin 325 mg and oxycodone hydrochloride 2.25 mg.

Aspirin with oxycodone **(Percodan, Codoxy, Roxiprin):** Tablets: Aspirin 325 mg and oxycodone hydrochloride 4.5 mg.

Aspirin with propoxyphene napsylate **(Darvon Compound):** Tablets: Aspirin 325 mg and propoxyphene napsylate 65 mg.

Aspirin with propoxyphene napsylate **(Darvon-N):** Tablets, film coated: Aspirin 325 mg and propoxyphene napsylate 100 mg.

Aspirin with pentazocine **(Talwin Compound Caplets):** Tablets: Aspirin 325 mg and pentazocine hydrochloride 12.5 mg.

Aspirin with meprobamate **(Equagesic, Equazine-M, Mepro-Analgesic):** Tablets: Aspirin 500 mg and meprobamate 200 mg.

Aspirin with butalbital **(Axotal):** Tablets: Aspirin 650 mg and butalbital 50 mg.

Aspirin with caffeine **(Anacin):** Tablets: Aspirin 400 mg and caffeine 32 mg; aspirin 500 mg and caffeine 32 mg.

Pharmacology

Aspirin, a nonsteroidal anti-inflammatory drug (NSAID), is the salicylate ester of acetic acid. The analgesic and anti-inflammatory activity of aspirin may be mediated by inhibition of the biosynthesis and release of prostaglandins that sensitize C fibers' nociceptors to mechanical stimuli and chemical mediators (e.g., bradykinin, histamine), and which may interfere with the endogenous descending pathways that inhibit pain transmission. Aspirin irreversibly acetylates and inactivates cyclooxygenase (prostaglandin synthetase), an enzyme that catalyzes the formation of prostaglandin precursors (endoperoxides) from arachidonic acid. The antipyretic activity of aspirin may occur secondary to inhibition of pyrogen-induced release of prostaglandins in the central nervous system (including the hypothalamus) and possibly to centrally mediated peripheral vasodilatation. Aspirin acetylates platelet cyclooxygenase and prevents the synthesis of thromboxane A_2, a potent vasoconstrictor and inducer of platelet aggregation. Thus, the drug irreversibly (unlike other salicylates) inhibits platelet aggregation for the life of the platelet (7–10 days) and prolongs bleeding time. Aspirin enhances urinary excretion of uric acid and decreases serum uric acid concentration by inhibiting reabsorption of uric acid in the proximal renal tubule. Low-dose aspirin (PO 300–325 mg one to four times daily) may prevent arterial and possibly venous thrombosis, reduce the risk of death or nonfatal myocardial infarction (MI) in patients with previous infarction or unstable angina pectoris, and reduce the risk of recurring transient ischemic attacks (TIAs) and stroke or death in patients who have had single or multiple TIAs.

Pharmacokinetics

Onset of Action: PO, 5–30 minutes.
Peak Effect: PO, 0.5–2.0 hours; rectal, 3–4 hours.
Duration of Action: PO, 3–7 hours.

Interactions

Incidence of GI side effects and risk of bleeding increased with concomitant NSAIDs, anticoagulant or heparin therapy, and alcohol ingestion; enhances toxicity of lithium, methotrexate, and valproic acid; serum levels of aspirin increased by carbonic anhydrous inhibitors; decreases diuretic effects of spirinolactone; decreased serum concentration of aspirin with concomitant corticosteroids; enhances hypoglycemic effects of sulfonylureas; decreases antihypertensive effects of β-adrenergic blockers and ACE inhibitors; enhances hypotensive effects of nitroglycerin; urinary excretion of aspirin increased by antacids and urinary alkalinizers; absorption delayed by food, milk, and concomitant administration of activated charcoal; prostaglandin-mediated natriuretic effects of spirinolactone and furosemide are antagonized by aspirin.

Toxicity

Toxic Range: >250 μg/mL (mild salicylism); >400–500 μg/mL (severe toxicity).

Manifestations: *Chronic:* Tinnitus, hearing loss, dimness of vision, headache, hyperventilation, GI ulceration, dyspepsia, dizziness, mental confusion, drowsiness, sweating, thirst, nausea and vomiting, diarrhea, tachycardia. *Acute:* In addition to the previously listed symptoms, acid-base and electrolyte disturbance, dehydration, hyperpyrexia, oliguria, acute renal failure, hyperthermia, restlessness, irritability, vertigo, asterixis, tremor, diplopia, delirium, mania, hallucinations, EEG abnormalities, seizures, lethargy, coma.

Antidote: None.

Management: Discontinue or reduce medication. Correct fluid, electrolyte, and acid-base disturbances. Support ventilation and circulation (patent airway, oxygen, IV fluids, vasopressors). Airway-protected, ipecac syrup–induced emesis (30 mL or 0.5 mL/kg ipecac syrup followed by 200 mL or 4 mL/kg of water or clear fluid) or gastric lavage (with drug ingestion)

followed by administration of activated charcoal (PO 50–100 g or 1–2 g/kg). Forced alkaline diuresis with IV sodium bicarbonate (IV furosemide if necessary) after correction of dehydration. Hemodialysis or hemoperfusion. Symptomatic treatment.

Guidelines/Precautions

1. Avoid the use of aspirin in children or teenagers with influenza or chickenpox. There is an increased risk of developing Reye's syndrome, an acute life-threatening condition characterized by vomiting, lethargy, delirium, and coma.
2. Discontinue use of the drug if dizziness, tinnitus, or hearing loss occurs. Tinnitus may herald the approach of salicylate levels to the upper limit of the therapeutic range. The temporary hearing loss remits gradually upon discontinuation of aspirin.
3. Use with caution in patients with hepatic or renal dysfunction, preexisting hypoprothrombinemia, or vitamin K deficiency. Aspirin may precipitate renal failure in patients with impaired renal function, heart failure, or liver dysfunction.
4. Avoid aspirin if possible for 1 week prior to surgery because of the risk of impaired hemostasis.
5. Use with caution in patients with active GI lesions (e.g., erosive gastritis, peptic ulcer) or with a history of recurrent GI lesions, since the drug may cause or aggravate GI bleeding and/or ulcerations.
6. Due to the high sodium content, highly buffered aspirin (e.g., Alka-Seltzer) should be used with

caution, if at all, in patients with cardiac decompensation, hypertension, or other conditions in which a high sodium intake would be harmful.

7. Carefully observe patients with coagulation disorders and those receiving drug therapy that interferes with hemostasis.

8. Patient response to NSAIDs is variable. Patients who do not respond to or cannot tolerate aspirin may be successfully treated with another NSAID.

9. Contraindicated in patients with previously demonstrated hypersensitivity to aspirin or with the complete or partial syndrome of nasal polyps, angioedema, or bronchospastic reactivity to aspirin or other NSAIDs. Patients allergic to tartrazine dye should avoid aspirin.

10. Do not use for obstetric analgesia.

11. Signs and symptoms of infection or other diseases may be masked by the antipyretic and anti-inflammatory effects of aspirin.

12. Monitor stool for blood every 14 days, and monitor BUN, serum creatinine, and urinalysis every 1 to 2 months when administering aspirin at chronic high doses.

13. Aspirin should be used during pregnancy only when the potential benefits justify the possible risks to the fetus. Aspirin and other NSAIDs should generally be avoided during the last trimester (although low doses of aspirin have been useful in the prevention of preeclampsia during this period, and especially during the 1 to 2 weeks before delivery). Should maternal inges-

tion of aspirin occur within 1 to 2 weeks of delivery, the neonate should be closely evaluated for the presence of bleeding.

Principal Adverse Reactions

Cardiovascular: Vasodilatation, pallor, angina.
Pulmonary: Dyspnea, asthma.
CNS: Drowsiness, dizziness, headache, sweating, depression, euphoria.
Gastrointestinal: Ulceration, bleeding, dyspepsia, nausea, vomiting, diarrhea, hepatic dysfunction.
Genitourinary: Dysuria, interstitial nephritis, renal papillary necrosis.
Dermatologic: Pruritus, urticaria.
Hematologic: Prolongation of bleeding time, leukopenia, thrombocytopenia, purpura, decreased plasma iron concentration, shortened erythrocyte survival time.

ATROPINE SULFATE

Class: Anticholinergic

Use(s): Treatment of sinus bradycardia, cardiopulmonary resuscitation, adjunctive therapy in treatment of bronchospasm and peptic ulcer, premedication, reversal of neuromuscular blockade.

Dosing: *Sinus bradycardia and CPR*
Adults: IV/IM/SC, 0.4–1.0 mg. Repeat every 3–5 minutes as indicated. Maximum dose 40 µg/kg.

> Children: IV/IM/SC, 10–20 µg/kg (minimum
> dose 0.1 mg).
>
> *Premedication*
> > Adults: IV/IM, 0.4–1.0 mg. PO, 0.4–0.6 mg
> > every 4–6 hours.
> >
> > Children: IV, 10–20 µg/kg (minimum dose
> > 0.1 mg). PO, 30 µg/kg every 4–6 hours.
> > High-potency injectate solutions (>0.3 mg/
> > mL) may be diluted in 3–5 mL apple juice
> > or carbonated cola beverage.
>
> *Bronchodilatation (inhalation)*
> > Adults: 0.025 mg/kg every 4–6 hours.
> >
> > Children: 0.05 mg/kg every 4–6 hours.
> >
> > Maximum dose 2.5 mg. Dilute to 2–3 mL
> > with normal saline and deliver by com-
> > pressed air nebulizer.
>
> *Reversal of neuromuscular blockade:* IV
> 0.015 mg/kg with anticholinesterase neo-
> stigmine (IV 0.05 mg/kg) or edrophonium
> (IV 0.5–1.0 mg/kg).

Elimination: Hepatic, renal.

Preparations

Atropine sulfate **(Atropine Sulfate)**
> Injection: 0.05 mg/mL, 0.1 mg/mL, 0.3 mg/mL, 0.4 mg/
> mL, 0.5 mg/mL, 0.8 mg/mL, 1 mg/mL.
> Inhalation solution: 0.2%, 0.5%.
> Tablets: 0.4 mg, 0.6 mg.

Atropine sulfate and phenobarbital **(Antrocol)**
> Capsules: Atropine sulfate 0.195 mg and phenobarbi-
> tal 16 mg.
> Tablets: Atropine sulfate 0.195 mg and phenobarbital
> 16 mg.

Oral solution: Atropine sulfate 0.039 mg/mL and phenobarbital 3 mg/mL.

Atropine sulfate and meperidine **(Atropine and
Demerol Carpuject):** Injection: Atropine sulfate
0.4 mg/mL and meperidine 50 mg/mL; atropine sulfate
0.4 mg/mL and meperidine 75 mg/mL.

Atropine sulfate and neostigmine methylsulfate
(Atropine and Neostigmine Min-I-Mix): Parenteral
kit: Atropine sulfate 1.2 mg/mL and neostigmine
1 mg/mL.

Pharmacology

Atropine competitively antagonizes the action of acetylcholine at the muscarinic receptor. It decreases salivary,
bronchial, and gastric secretions and relaxes bronchial smooth muscle. Gastrointestinal tone and motility
are reduced. Lower esophageal sphincter pressure
decreases and intraocular pressure (IOP) increases
(because of pupillary dilation). At doses used for premedication, this increase in IOP is not clinically significant. Large doses may increase body temperature by
preventing sweat secretion. Peripheral vagal blockade
of the sinus and atrioventricular node increases heart
rate. Transient decreases in heart rate by small doses
reflect the central nervous system effect of the drug.
Atropine is a tertiary amine and therefore crosses the
blood-brain barrier. In high doses it stimulates and then
depresses the medullary and higher cerebral centers.

Pharmacokinetics

Onset of Action: IV, 45–60 seconds. Intratracheal,
10–20 seconds. IM, 5–40 minutes. PO, 30 minutes to 2
hours. Inhalation, 3–5 minutes.

Peak Effect: IV, 2 minutes. Inhalation, 1–2 hours.
Duration of Action: IV/IM: Vagal blockade, 1 to 2 hours; antisialogogue effect, 4 hours. Inhalation: Vagal blockade, 3–6 hours.

Interactions

Additive anticholinergic effects with antihistamines, phenothiazines, tricyclic antidepressants, procainamide, quinidine, MAO inhibitors, benzodiazepines, and anti-psychotics; increase in intraocular pressure enhanced by nitrates, nitrites, alkalinizing agents, disopyramide, corticosteroids, and haloperidol; potentiates sympathomimetics; antagonizes anticholinesterases and metoclopramide; may produce central anticholinergic syndrome (hallucinations, delirium, coma).

Toxicity

Toxic Range: Not routinely monitored.
Manifestations: Dry mouth, rapid pulse, rapid respiration, fever, CNS stimulation (central anticholinergic syndrome), seizures, delirium, hallucinations, dilated pupils, blurred vision, circulatory collapse, respiratory failure.
Antidote: No specific antidote.
Management: Discontinue or reduce medication. Support ventilation and circulation (patent airway, oxygen, IV fluids, vasopressors). Symptomatic treatment. Airway-protected, ipecac syrup–induced emesis (30 mL or 0.5 mL/kg ipecac syrup followed by 200 mL or 4 mL/kg of water or clear fluid) or gastric lavage (with drug ingestion) followed by administration of activated charcoal (PO 50–100 g or 1–2 g/kg). Benzodiazepines

(diazepam IV 0.05–0.2 mg/kg, midazolam IV/IM 0.025–0.1 mg/kg) or barbiturates (thiopental sodium IV 0.5–2.0 mg/kg) to control seizures. Physostigmine (slow IV 1–4 mg) to reverse anticholinergic effects. (Use with caution. Physostigmine may cause bradycardia, seizures, or severe bronchospasm. Have atropine available.) Physical cooling to treat hyperpyrexia. Fluids (IV/PO) to maintain urine output.

Guidelines/Precautions

1. Use atropine with caution in patients with tachyarrhythmias, congestive heart failure, acute myocardial ischemia or infarction, fever, esophageal reflux, or GI infections.
2. Contraindicated in patients with obstructive uropathy or obstructive disease of the GI tract.
3. If intravenous access is not available during cardiopulmonary resuscitation, the drug may be diluted 1:1 in sterile normal saline and injected via an endotracheal tube. The absorption rate, duration, and pharmacologic effects of intratracheal drug administration compare favorably with the IV route.
4. May accumulate and produce systemic side effects with multiple dosing by inhalation, especially in the elderly.
5. Treat toxicity with sedation (benzodiazepines) and administration of physostigmine.
6. Infants, small children, and elderly patients are more susceptible to the systemic effects of atropine (e.g., rapid and irregular pulse, fever, excitement, and agitation).

Principal Adverse Reactions

Cardiovascular: Tachycardia, bradycardia (low doses), palpitations.
Pulmonary: Respiratory depression.
CNS: Confusion, hallucinations, drowsiness, excitement, agitation.
Genitourinary: Urinary hesitancy, retention.
Gastrointestinal: Gastroesophageal reflux.
Ocular: Mydriasis, blurred vision, increased intraocular pressure.
Dermatologic: Urticaria.
Other: Decreased sweating, allergic reaction.

BACLOFEN

Class: Skeletal Muscle Relaxant

Use(s): Relief of muscle spasticity and rigidity (e.g., in multiple sclerosis, Parkinson's disease, spinal cord lesions); adjunct treatment of trigeminal neuralgia, pretrigeminal neuralgia, glossopharyngeal neuralgia, vagoglossopharyngeal neuralgia, organic (nontraction) headache, neuropathic pain, and postherpetic neuralgia.

Dosing: *Spasticity, trigeminal neuralgia, organic headache, neuropathic pain*
Initial: PO 5–10 mg three times daily.
Maintenance: PO 5–25 mg three times daily and at night. Doses should be increased by 15-mg increments (smaller in geriatric patients) at 3-day intervals until the

optimum effect is achieved. For muscle relaxation, baclofen doses may be supplemented with tizanidine (Zanaflex).

Severe spasticity of spinal cord origin (spinal cord trauma, multiple sclerosis)

Intrathecal bolus: Screening phase, 50–75 µg. Dilute to a concentration of 50 µg/mL. Administer into the intrathecal space by barbotage over a period of not less than 1 minute. Observe patient for 4–8 hours. If response is inadequate, a repeat dose of 75 µg (in 1.5 mL) may be administered 24 hours later. If inadequate response continues, another repeat dose of 100 µg (in 2 mL) may be administered 24 hours later. Patients who do not respond to the 100-µg dose should not be considered candidates for chronic infusion therapy with an implanted pump.

Epidural bolus: Initial dose, 100–400 µg. Dilute in 3 mL preservative-free normal saline. Titrate dose cautiously and to effect. Use intrathecal preparation of baclofen. Maintenance dose, 100 µg to 30 mg daily twice weekly. Dilute in 3–10 mL preservative-free normal saline. Start with low dose and titrate cautiously to effect. May be administered via an implanted subcutaneous port.

Intrathecal infusion, initial dose: 3–6 µg/hr or administer two times the effective bolus dose over 24 hours. If the bolus dose was effective for longer than 12 hours, then administer one times the bolus dose over 24 hours. No dose increases should be given in the first 24 hours. After the first 24 hours, the daily dose may be increased slowly by 10% to 30% increments once every 24 hours. Patients must be monitored closely in a fully equipped and staffed environment during the screening phase and infusion dose titration period immediately following an implant.

Intrathecal infusion, long-term maintenance: 12–1500 µg/day. Titrate to symptom control. During periodic refills of the infusion pump, the daily dose may be increased by 10% to 40%. The daily dose may be reduced by 10% to 20% if patients experience side effects. A sudden large requirement for dose escalation suggests a catheter complication (i.e., a catheter kink or dislodgment).

Oral baclofen should be used in combination with anticonvulsants or antidepressants in the management of trigeminal neuralgia and organic headaches. Baclofen should be combined with antidepressant agents, opioids, and/or nonsteroidal anti-inflammatory drugs (NSAIDs) in the management of neuropathic pain.

Elimination: Renal.

Preparations

Baclofen **(Lioresal)**
  Tablets: 10 mg, 20 mg.
  Intrathecal injection: 50 μg/mL.
  Intrathecal refill kit: 10 mg/5 mL, 10 mg/20 mL.

Pharmacology

Baclofen is a *p*-chlorophenyl derivative of γ-amino-butyric acid (GABA) and a skeletal muscle relaxant. It inhibits monosynaptic and polysynaptic reflexes at the spinal level, possibly by acting as an inhibitory neuro-transmitter and/or by hyperpolarization of afferent nerve terminals, which inhibits the release of excitatory neurotransmitters such as glutamate and aspartic acid. Baclofen is the drug of choice for muscle spasm in patients with multiple sclerosis and other spinal cord lesions, where it decreases the number and severity of muscle spasms (especially flexor spasms), alleviates associated pain, clonus, and muscle rigidity, and improves mobility. When introduced directly into the intrathecal space, effective cerebral spinal fluid (CSF) concentrations of baclofen are achieved with resultant plasma concentrations 100 times less than those occur-ring with oral administration. Intrathecal baclofen is effective in the treatment of severe chronic spasticity in patients who do not respond adequately and/or do not tolerate high oral doses. Either baclofen or diazepam (the drug of second choice) is preferable to intrathecal injections of sclerosing agents (e.g., phenol), rhizotomy, or cordotomy. Intrathecal baclofen may suppress the allodynic dyesthetic pain from spinal lesions. Baclofen, like carbamazepine and phenytoin, depresses excitatory transmission and facilitates segmental inhibition in the trigeminal nucleus. Oral baclofen has been shown to be effective in the treatment of trigeminal neuralgia and nonvascular headache. Baclofen may relieve the episodic and allodynic pain in postherpetic neuralgia. The levoform of baclofen may be more effective than the readily available racemic D-l form. In large doses, baclofen may produce generalized CNS depression, including sedation, ataxia, and respiratory and cardiovascular depression.

Pharmacokinetics

Onset of Action: Antispastic effects: PO, hours to weeks; intrathecal bolus, 30 minutes to 1 hour; intrathecal infusion, 6–8 hours.

Peak Effect: Antispastic: PO, variable; intrathecal bolus, 4 hours; intrathecal infusion, 24–48 hours.

Duration of Action: Antispastic effects: PO, variable; intrathecal bolus, 4–8 hours; epidural bolus, 24–96 hours.

Interactions

Potentiates CNS depressant effects of alcohol, barbiturates, narcotics, volatile anesthetics; additive muscle relaxant effects when coadministered with tizanidine.

Toxicity

Toxic Range: Not routinely monitored.

Manifestations: Hypotension, bradycardia, respiratory depression, coma, vomiting, muscle hypotonia, salivation, drowsiness, confusion, blurred vision, seizures, elevated serum lactate dehydrogenase and AST (SGOT) concentrations.

Antidote: No specific antidote. Slow IV physostigmine (1–2 mg over 5–10 minutes) may reverse respiratory depression and drowsiness. Repeat dose of IV 1 mg may be given in 30–60 minutes if the patient shows a positive response to the initial dose. Monitor the patient closely. Use with caution, as physostigmine may cause serious side effects (e.g., cardiac conduction disturbances, bradycardia, and/or seizures). Flumazenil may be used but is also not a reliable antagonist. Administer IV 0.2–1.0 mg (4–20 µg/kg) at a rate of 0.2 mg per minute. Titrate to patient response. Dose may be repeated at 20-minute intervals. Maximum single dose is 1 mg. Maximum total dose is 3 mg in any one hour. The patient must be monitored closely because of the possible induction of seizures.

Management: Discontinue or reduce medication. Support ventilation and circulation (patent airway, oxygen, IV fluids, vasopressors). Administer physostigmine or flumazenil. Airway-protected, ipecac syrup–induced emesis (30 mL or 0.5 mL/kg ipecac syrup followed by 200 mL or 4 mL/kg of water or clear fluid) or gastric lavage (with drug ingestion) followed by administration of activated charcoal (PO 50–100 g or 1–2 g/kg). If lumbar puncture is not contraindicated, withdraw 30–40 mL of CSF to reduce CSF baclofen concentration. This may be safer and more effective than physostigmine. Symptomatic treatment.

Guidelines/Precautions

1. Deterioration in seizure control may occur in epileptic patients receiving baclofen. The EEG should be monitored periodically.
2. Use with caution in patients who must use spasticity to maintain an upright posture or balance in locomotion or whenever spasticity is utilized to obtain increased function.

3. Abrupt withdrawal may lead to hallucinations, seizures, and acute exacerbation of spasticity.
4. Dosage should be reduced gradually if the drug is to be discontinued.
5. Patients should be warned that baclofen may impair their ability to perform activities requiring mental alertness or physical coordination (e.g., operating heavy machinery or driving a motor vehicle).

Principal Adverse Reactions

Cardiovascular: Tachycardia, bradycardia, hypotension, palpitations, angina, syncope.
Pulmonary: Dyspnea, respiratory depression.
CNS: Drowsiness, fatigue, vertigo, dizziness, hypotonia, mental depression, excitation, headache, hallucinations, euphoria, anxiety, dysarthria, strabismus.
Gastrointestinal: Nausea and vomiting, constipation, diarrhea, taste disorders, abdominal pain.
Musculoskeletal: Muscle pain.
Other: Rash, pruritus.

BOTULINUM TOXIN TYPE A

Class: Chemical Denervating Agent

Use(s): Treatment of involuntary muscle spasm and tremors associated with dystonias (e.g., spasmodic torticollis, blepharospasm, strabismus, limb dystonia, paraspinal muscle spasm, thoracic outlet syndrome).

Dosing: *Strabismus, blepharospasm:* 1.25–2.5 units per muscle. Volume of 0.05–0.15 mL per muscle.

Spasmodic rotational torticollis with or without retrocollis: Contralateral sternocleidomastoid/ipsilateral and contralateral trapezius, 50–100 units per muscle. Inject 5 U/0.2 mL per muscle site. Dilution: 25 U/mL. With presence of head tilt, inject ipsilateral splenius capitis with 15–30 units per muscle, 5 units per muscle site, at a dilution of 25 U/mL.

Scalene compartment block—interscalene brachial plexus approach: 100 units in 10–20 mL preservative-free normal saline.

Psoas/quadratus lumborum compartment block—lumbar plexus block: 100–200 units in 10–20 mL preservative-free normal saline. For bilateral blocks, inject 50–100 units on each side.

Paravertebral nerve block—lumbar plexus block: 100 units in 10 mL preservative-free normal saline. For bilateral blocks, inject 50 units on each side.

Piriformis compartment block—lumbar plexus block: 100–200 units in 2 mL preservative-free normal saline. For bilateral blocks, inject 50–100 units on each side.

Trigger-point injections (e.g., trapezius muscle): 100–200 units in 4–10 mL preservative-free normal saline. Inject 0.5–2.0 mL (5–25 units) in each trigger point on each side.

Treatment of facial lines—corrugator superciliaris, frontalis, orbicularis oculi muscle: 5–10 units (0.2–0.8 mL) in each target muscle. Use dilution of 25 U/mL.

Botulinum toxin should be infiltrated at various sites in muscle belly. Addition of local anesthetics may make injection more comfortable, but the effect on the efficacy of botulinum toxin is undetermined. Electromyographic guidance is required for injection into the small extraocular muscles.

Elimination: Muscle.

Preparations

Botulinum toxin type A **(Botox):** Vial: 100 units of vacuum-dried *Clostridium botulinum* toxin type A. Store the lyophilized product in a freezer at or below −5°C. Administer Botox within 4 hours after the vial is removed from the freezer and reconstituted. During these 4 hours, reconstituted Botox should be stored in a refrigerator (2° to 8°C). Reconstituted Botox should be clear, colorless, and free of particulate matter.

Dilution for Infusion: 100 units in 1–10 mL preservative-free normal saline (10–100 U/mL). Inject diluent into the vial gently. Botox is denatured by bubbling or similar violent agitation. Discard the vial if a vacuum does not pull the diluent into the vial.

Pharmacology

Botulinum toxin type A (Botox) blocks neuromuscular conduction by binding to receptor sites on motor nerve terminals, entering the nerve terminals, and inhibiting the release of acetylcholine. When injected intramuscularly at therapeutic doses, Botox produces a localized chemical denervation muscular paralysis. When the muscle is chemically denervated, it atrophies and may develop extrajunctional acetylcholine receptors. There is evidence that the nerve can sprout and reinnervate the muscle, with the weakness thus being reversible. Botox may affect muscle pairs (e.g., in strabismus) by inducing an atrophic lengthening of the injected muscle and a corresponding shortening of the muscle's antagonist. The paralytic effect on muscles injected with Botox is useful in reducing excessive abnormal contractions associated with muscle spasm. Paralysis of injected muscles begins 1 to 2 days after injection and increases in intensity for the first week. The paralysis lasts for 2 to 6 weeks and gradually resolves over a similar time period. Overcorrections lasting over 6 months have been rare. About one-half of patients will require subsequent doses because of inadequate paralytic response of the muscle to the initial dose or because of mechanical factors such as large deviations or restrictions.

Pharmacokinetics

Onset of Action: <48 hours.
Peak Effect: 2 weeks.
Duration of Action: 2–6 months.

Interactions

Effects of botulinum toxin may be potentiated by aminoglycoside antibiotics or any other drugs that interfere with neuromuscular transmission.

Toxicity

Toxic Range: LD_{50}: 3000 U/70 kg.
Manifestations: Weakness.
Antidote: No specific antidote. Additional information may be obtained by calling Allergan (800-433-8871).

Management: Discontinue injection. Support ventilation and circulation (patent airway, oxygen, IV fluids, vasopressors). Symptomatic treatment.

Guidelines/Precautions

1. To avoid antibody formation, wait about 3 months between injections and limit total dose to less than 400 units.

2. Reduced blinking from Botox injection of the orbicularis muscle can lead to corneal exposure, persistent epithelial defect, and corneal ulceration, particularly in patients with facial nerve disorders. Careful testing of corneal sensation in eyes previously operated upon, avoidance of injection into the lower lid area to prevent ectropion, and vigorous treatment of any epithelial defect should be employed. These may require protective drops, ointments, therapeutic soft contact lenses, or closure of the eye by patching or other means.

3. Sedentary patients should be cautioned to resume activity slowly and carefully following the administration of Botox.

4. During the administration of Botox for the treatment of strabismus, retrobulbar hemorrhages sufficient to compromise retinal circulation have occurred from needle penetrations into the orbit. Appropriate instruments to decompress the orbit should be accessible. Ocular (globe) penetration by needles has also occurred. An ophthalmoscope to diagnose this condition should be available.

5. As with all biologic products, epinephrine and other precautions as necessary should be available should an anaphylactic reaction occur.

Principal Adverse Reactions

Musculoskeletal: Soreness at injection site.

Cardiovascular: Hypotension, transitory hypertension and arrhythmias, anginal attacks, anaphylactic shock.

Ocular: Swelling of the eyelid skin, spatial disorientation, double vision, ptosis, irritation/tearing, photophobia, keratitis, ecchymosis.

Pulmonary: Shortness of breath.

Gastrointestinal: Dysphagia (injection into sternocleidomastoid muscle with spread to esophagus).

Other: Low-grade temperature, flu-like syndrome, diffuse skin rash.

BRETYLIUM TOSYLATE

Class: Antiarrhythmic

Use(s): Treatment of ventricular fibrillation and arrhythmias, treatment of sympathetic mediated pain (SMP).

Dosing: *Arrhythmias*

> IV loading/IM, ventricular tachycardia: 5–10 mg/kg over 15 minutes; may be repeated in 1 to 2 hours.
>
> IV loading, ventricular fibrillation: 5–10 mg/kg over 1 minute (every 15–30 minutes to maximum of 30 mg/kg).
>
> Infusion: 1–2 mg/min.
>
> Therapeutic level: 0.5–1.0 µg/mL.
>
> *Sympathetic mediated pain*
>
> IV regional sympathetic block: 1–2 mg/kg; dilute in 40–50 mL of 0.5% lidocaine or

normal saline (upper extremity) or 50–
60 mL of 0.5% lidocaine or normal saline
(lower extremity). Initial series of blocks
may be repeated every 4 days and then
every 2 to 3 weeks as indicated. Methylprednisolone (80 mg) may be added to
the solution to decrease the postmanipulation edema. Administer 500 mL of
fluid immediately after tourniquet release
to prevent orthostasis.

Elimination: Renal.

Preparations

Bretylium tosylate **(Bretylol, Bretylium Tosylate):**
Injection: 50 mg/mL.
Bretylium tosylate in 5% dextrose **(Bretylol, Bretylium
Tosylate):** Injection for IV infusion: 1 mg/mL, 2 mg/
mL, 4 mg/mL.

Dilution for Infusion: 2 g in 500 mL D5W or normal
saline (4 mg/mL).

Pharmacology

A class III antiarrhythmic agent, bretylium initially releases norepinephrine from sympathetic ganglia and
postganglionic adrenergic neurons. This initial action
may account for increased heart rate, irritability, and
blood pressure. Subsequently, there is inhibition of
release of norepinephrine in response to sympathetic
nerve stimulation. The adrenergic blockade depends
on uptake of bretylium by adrenergic neurons and may
lead to orthostatic hypotension and bradycardia. Cardiac performance is not significantly changed, but

pulmonary artery pressure may be increased. Bretylium increases the ventricular fibrillation threshold and suppresses ventricular arrhythmias. The electrophysiologic effects include an increase in action potential duration and effective refractory period, an increase in ventricular conduction velocity, and a decrease in the disparity between normal and damaged cells. In high concentrations, bretylium has local anesthetic and neuromuscular blocking properties. Intravenous regional administration alleviates peripheral manifestations of sympathetic mediated pain (chronic regional pain syndrome) by adrenergic blockade and alteration of the sensitivity of peripheral nociceptors. However, bretylium is not as effective as guanethidine, and the duration of pain relief is much shorter.

Pharmacokinetics

Onset of Action: IV antifibrillatory, several minutes. IV/IM suppression of ventricular arrhythmia, 20 minutes to 2 hours.
Peak Effect: IV antifibrillatory, 20 minutes to 2 hours. IV/IM suppression of ventricular arrhythmia, 6–9 hours.
Duration of Action: IV/IM (antiarrhythmic effect), 6–24 hours. IV regional (pain relief in SMP), 1 day to 10 weeks.

Interactions

Initial release of norepinephrine may worsen arrhythmias caused by cardiac glycoside toxicity; resistance to antiadrenergic effects in patients receiving tricyclic antidepressants (which block the uptake of bretylium).

Toxicity

Toxic Range: Not routinely monitored.
Manifestations: Hypotension, nausea, vomiting.
Antidote: No specific antidote.
Management: Discontinue or reduce medication. Support ventilation and circulation (patent airway, oxygen, IV fluids, vasopressors). Symptomatic treatment. Avoid the use of sympathomimetics (e.g., epinephrine), which may aggravate the toxic effects.

Guidelines/Precautions

1. Use with caution in patients with pheochromocytoma, aortic stenosis, and pulmonary hypertension.
2. Severe hypotension should be treated with appropriate fluid therapy and vasopressor agents such as dopamine or norepinephrine.
3. In intravenous regional blocks, when normal saline is used as the diluent, the cuff may be deflated cautiously after 10 minutes. If a local anesthetic is used as the diluent (e.g., lidocaine 0.5%), the cuff should be deflated after 40 minutes and no less than 20 minutes. Between 20 and 40 minutes, the cuff may be deflated, reinflated immediately, and finally deflated after a minute to reduce the sudden absorption of local anesthetic into the systemic circulation.
4. Bretylium is contraindicated in patients with allergy to corn products, who may manifest cross-allergy to bretylium.

Principal Adverse Reactions

Cardiovascular: Hypotension, transitory hypertension and arrhythmias, anginal attacks.

Pulmonary: Shortness of breath.
CNS: Dizziness, syncope.
Gastrointestinal: Nausea, vomiting, diarrhea, abdominal pain.
Other: Rash, hiccups.

BUPIVACAINE HYDROCHLORIDE

Class: Local Anesthetic

Use(s): Local and regional anesthesia, sympathetic blockade.

Dosing: *Infiltration, peripheral nerve block:* 1–20 mL (0.25–0.5% solution).
Caudal: 37.5–150.0 mg (15–30 mL of 0.125–0.5% solution). Children, 0.4–0.7–1.0 mL/kg (L2-T10-T7 level of anesthesia). At higher volumes (>0.6 mL/kg) utilize lower concentrations (0.125–0.25% solutions). Maximum safe dose: 2–3 mg/kg.
Brachial plexus block: 75–250 mg (30–50 mL of 0.375–0.5% solution). Children, 0.5–0.75 mL/kg. With high doses (>2 mg/kg), add epinephrine 1:200,000 to decrease systemic toxicity (in the absence of any contraindications). Regional blockade may be potentiated by the addition of tetracaine (0.5–1.0 mg/kg), fentanyl (1–2 µg/kg), or preservative-free morphine (0.05–0.1 mg/kg).
Scalene compartment block—interscalene brachial plexus approach: 20 mL of 0.25–

0.5% solution with or without steroid (e.g., 40–80 mg triamcinolone).

Stellate ganglion block: 10–20 mL of 0.25% solution (25–50 mg) with or without epinephrine 1:200,000.

Psoas/quadratus lumborum compartment block—multiple paravertebral nerve block—lumbar plexus block: 10–20 mL of 0.25–0.5% solution with or without steroid (e.g., 40–80 mg triamcinolone). For bilateral blocks, inject each side with 10–15 mL of 0.125% solution with steroid (e.g., 20–40 mg of triamcinolone).

Paravertebral nerve block: 2–4 mL per segment of 0.25–0.5% solution with or without epinephrine 1:200,000. Total dose should not exceed maximum safe dose of 2–3 mg/kg.

Piriformis compartment block—lumbar plexus block: 10–20 mL of 0.25–0.5% solution with or without steroid (e.g., 40–80 mg triamcinolone). For bilateral blocks, inject each side with 5–10 mL of 0.125% solution with steroid (e.g., 20–40 mg of triamcinolone).

Trigger-point injections (e.g., trapezius muscle): 10 mL of 0.25–0.75% solution with or without steroid (e.g., 40–80 mg triamcinolone).

Lumbar sympathetic block: 10–15 mL of 0.25% solution (25–50 mg) with or without epinephrine 1:200,000.

Posterior tibial nerve sympathetic block: 2–2.5 mL of 1% solution (20–25 mg) with or without epinephrine 1:200,000 and with or without steroids (e.g., triamcinolone ace-tonide). Note: The posterior tibial sympathetics control 85% of the sympathetics to the foot, including all four muscle layers and the vital structures of the sole of the foot. Such selective sympathectomy may be preferable to a lumbar paravertebral block for reflex sympathetic dystrophy (RSD) of the foot.

Celiac plexus block: 20–25 mL of 0.25% solution (25–50 mg) with or without epinephrine 1:200,000.

Epidural

Bolus: 50–150 mg (0.125–0.75% solution). Children, 0.5–2.5 mg/kg or 0.3–0.5 mL/kg (0.125–0.5% solution).

Infusion: 2–12 mL/hr (0.04–0.125% solution) with or without epidural narcotics (e.g., sufentanil 0.4 μg/mL or fentanyl 2 μg/mL). Children, 0.04–0.35 mL/kg/hr.

Infusion (chronic malignant pain): 3–20 mg daily (0.00625–0.0625% solution). When used in combination with epidural morphine infusions, dilute the daily amount of bupivacaine in the daily volume of the morphine infusion:

$$\text{Total Amount of Bupivacaine for Infusion Solution} = \frac{\text{Total Daily Amount of Bupivacaine}}{\text{Total Daily Volume of Morphine}} \times \text{Total Volume of Infusion Solution}$$

For example, a patient is receiving epidural morphine diluted in a total volume of 250 mL preservative-free normal saline at 1 mg/day and 2 mL/hr. If the patient is to receive bupivacaine at 10 mg/day, then the total amount of bupivacaine to add to the infusion will be $(10/48) \times 250 = 52.08$ mg. This is approximately equivalent to adding 6.9 mL of 0.75% bupivacaine solution or 10.4 mL of 0.5% bupivacaine solution to the infusion solution. Final concentration of bupivacaine in the infusion solution is 0.02%, or 0.2 mg/mL.

The rate of onset and potency of local anesthetic action may be enhanced by carbonation. (Add 0.1 mL of 7.5% or 8.4% sodium bicarbonate with 20 mL of 0.25% bupivacaine. Do not use if there is precipitation.)

Intrathecal

Bolus: 7–15 mg (0.75% solution). Children, 0.5 mg/kg with a minimum of 1 mg.

Infusion (chronic malignant pain): 1–5 mg daily (0.1–0.75% solution). When used in combination with intrathecal morphine infusions, dilute the daily amount of bupivacaine in the daily volume of the morphine infusion (see the equation above).

Interpleural

Bolus: 100 mg (20 mL of 0.25–0.5% solution) [0.4 mL/kg].

Infusion: 5–7 mL/hr [0.125 mL/kg/hr] (0.125–0.25% solution).

Intra-articular: <100 mg (20–40 mL of 0.25% solution). If desired add morphine 0.5–1.0 mg.

Maximum safe dose: 2 mg/kg without epinephrine; 2–3 mg/kg with epinephrine. Solutions containing preservatives should not be used for epidural or caudal block. Except where contraindicated, vasoconstrictor drugs (e.g., epinephrine, phenylephrine) may be added to increase effect and prolong local or regional anesthesia. For dosage/route guidelines, see the "Dosing" section of Epinephrine (p. 204). Do not use vasoconstrictor drugs for IV regional anesthesia or local anesthesia of end organs (digits, penis, ears).

Elimination: Hepatic, pulmonary.

Preparations

Bupivacaine hydrochloride **(Marcaine, Sensorcaine):** Injection: 0.25%, 0.5%, 0.75% with and without epinephrine 1:200,000.

Dilution for Infusion: Epidural use only. 20 mL 0.25% in 20 mL preservative-free normal saline (0.125% solution).

Pharmacology

This amino amide local anesthetic stabilizes neuronal membranes by inhibiting ionic fluxes required for the initiation and conduction of impulses. The progression of anesthesia is related to the diameter, myelination, and conduction velocity of affected nerve fibers, with the order of loss of function being as follows: 1) autonomic, 2) pain, 3) temperature, 4) touch, 5) proprioception, and 6) skeletal muscle tone. The onset of action is reasonably rapid, and duration is significantly longer than with any other commonly used local anesthetic. Addition of epinephrine improves the quality of analgesia, but only marginally increases the duration of effect of bupivacaine concentrations ≥0.5%. Hypotension results from loss of sympathetic tone as in spinal or epidural anesthesia. Compared with other amides, there is more cardiotoxicity with intravascular injection. Epidural bupivacaine provides long-acting neural blockade. Impulse transmission is blocked at the nerve roots and dorsal root ganglia. When administered by infusion, tachyphylaxis may occur, possibly due to an increase in blood flow within the epidural space or an increase in size of the pain field at the spinal cord level. Tachyphylaxis may be circumvented by incremental dosing or addition of epidural/intrathecal narcotics. Systemic absorption of bupivacaine (and other long-acting amides) is less than that of lidocaine (and other short-acting amides) due to greater nonspecific binding in the fat of the epidural space.

Pharmacokinetics

Onset of Action: Infiltration, 2–10 minutes. Epidural, 4–17 minutes. Intrathecal, <1 minute.
Peak Effect: Infiltration/epidural, 30–45 minutes. Intrathecal, 15 minutes.
Duration of Action: Infiltration/epidural/intrathecal, 200–400 minutes (prolonged with epinephrine). Interpleural, 12–48 hours. Celiac plexus, few days to >12 months.

Interactions

Reduced clearance with concomitant use of β-blocking agents or cimetidine; benzodiazepines, barbiturates, and volatile anesthetics increase seizure threshold; reduced dose requirements in pregnant patients; duration of anesthesia prolonged by vasoconstrictor agents (e.g., epinephrine), α_2-agonists (e.g., clonidine), and narcotics (e.g., fentanyl); alkalinization increases rate of onset and potency of local or regional anesthesia; myocardial depressant effects (hypotension and bradycardia) potentiated by calcium channel blockers (e.g., nifedipine); prior use of epidural chloroprocaine antagonizes the effects of epidural bupivacaine.

Toxicity

Toxic Range: Not routinely monitored.
Manifestations: Seizures, arrhythmias, circulatory collapse, respiratory depression, cardiac arrest.
Antidote: No specific antidote.
Management: Discontinue or reduce medication. Support ventilation and circulation (patent airway, oxygen, IV fluids, vasopressors). Benzodiazepines (diazepam IV 0.05–0.2 mg/kg, midazolam IV/IM 0.025–0.1 mg/kg) or barbiturates (thiopental sodium IV 0.5–2.0 mg/kg) to control seizures. Prolonged cardiopulmonary resuscitation with cardiac arrest: Sodium bicarbonate IV 1–2 mEq/kg to treat cardiac toxicity (sodium channel blockade); bretylium IV 5 mg/kg; DC cardioversion/ defibrillation for ventricular arrhythmias. Remove ingested drug by induced emesis followed by activated charcoal. Hypersensitivity reaction: Remove from further exposure and treat dermatitis. Exchange transfusions in newborns with toxicity.

Guidelines/Precautions

1. Bupivacaine is not recommended for obstetrical paracervical block. It induces uterine vasoconstriction and may cause fetal bradycardia and death.

Calcium channel antagonists (e.g., verapamil, nifedipine) may attenuate bupivacaine-induced vasoconstriction.

2. Do not use for IV regional anesthesia. High plasma concentrations may occur following tourniquet release and result in refractory cardiac arrest and death.

3. Concentrations above 0.5% are not recommended for use in obstetrics due to incidence of intractable cardiac arrest. The increased cardiac toxicity of bupivacaine (compared with lidocaine or mepivacaine) results from a greater decrease in myocardial contractility and depression of cardiac conduction.

4. Cauda equina syndrome with permanent neurologic deficit has been reported in patients receiving greater than 15mg of a 0.75% bupivacaine solution with a continuous spinal technique.

5. Intravenous access is essential during major regional block.

6. Use with caution in patients with hypovolemia, severe congestive heart failure, shock, and all forms of heart block.

7. Bupivacaine is contraindicated in patients with hypersensitivity to amide-type local anesthetics.

8. The recommended volumes for brachial plexus block are consistent with available data on plasma levels (subtoxic) after brachial plexus block. The risks of systemic toxicity may be decreased by adding epinephrine to the local anesthetic and avoiding IV injection, which may result in an immediate toxic reaction.

9. The level of sympathetic blockade (bradycardia

with block above T5) determines the degree of hypotension (often heralded by nausea and vomiting) following epidural or intrathecal bupivacaine (or other local anesthetic). Fluid hydration (10–20 mL/kg normal saline or lactated Ringer's solution), vasopressor agents (e.g., ephedrine), and left uterine displacement in pregnant patients may be used for prophylaxis and/or treatment. Administer atropine to treat bradycardia.

10. Epidural motor blockade may be reversed by the epidural injection of 20 mL of 0.9% saline.

11. Epidural, caudal, or intrathecal injections should be avoided when the patient has hypovolemic shock, septicemia, infection at the injection site, or coagulopathy.

Principal Adverse Reactions

Cardiovascular: Hypotension, arrhythmias, cardiac arrest.

Pulmonary: Respiratory impairment, arrest.

CNS: Seizures, tinnitus, blurred vision.

Allergic: Urticaria, angioneurotic edema, anaphylactoid symptoms.

Epidural/Caudal/Spinal: High spinal, hypotension, urinary retention, lower extremity weakness and paralysis, loss of sphincter control, headache, backache, cranial nerve palsies, slowing of labor.

BUPRENORPHINE HYDROCHLORIDE

Class: Narcotic Partial Agonist

Use(s): Treatment of acute, chronic, and cancer pain; opiate detoxification.

Dosing: *Analgesia*

      IM/IV/Sublingual: 0.3–0.6 mg (6–12 µg/kg) every 6–8 hours.

      Infusion: 25–250 µg/hr.

      Epidural

        Bolus: 50–60 µg (1 µg/kg).

        Infusion: 5–50 µg/hr.

      Patient-controlled analgesia IV: Bolus, 0.1 mg (0.002 mg/kg); lockout interval 10–20 minutes.

    Opiate detoxification: Sublingual, 0.6–8.0 mg daily.

The sublingual dosage form of buprenorphine is currently (at the time of press) not commercially available in the United States.

Administer analgesic regularly (not as needed). Due to impaired elimination, accumulation and excess sedation may occur in patients with renal or hepatic dysfunction. Analgesia may be enhanced by addition of adjuvant drugs, for example, nonsteroidal anti-inflammatory drugs (NSAIDs) and antidepressant agents (see pages xxvi–xliv for drug combinations), and use of nondrug therapies such as transcutaneous electrical nerve stimulation (TENS).

Elimination: Hepatic, renal.

Preparations

Buprenorphine hydrochloride **(Buprenex):** Injection: 0.3 mg/mL.

Dilution for Infusion

Epidural

    Bolus: 60 µg in 10 mL local anesthetic or (preservative-free) normal saline.

    Infusion: 500 µg in 100 mL local anesthetic or (preservative-free) normal saline (5 µg/mL).

Pharmacology

A thebaine derivative partial agonist that is structurally related to morphine but pharmacologically similar to the other opioid partial agonists, buprenorphine is 30 times as potent as morphine and has a high affinity for µ- and κ-receptors. Slow dissociation from the µ-receptors may account for the prolonged duration of analgesia, the unpredictability of reversal by opiate antagonists, and possibly the limited physical dependence potential observed with the drug. Unlike pentazocine or butorphanol, buprenorphine is relatively free of psychotomimetic effects. Narcotic antagonist activity is approximately equipotent with naloxone and may be mediated via δ- and µ-receptors. Buprenorphine exhibits ceiling effect at high doses (>1.2 mg) for respiratory depression and analgesia. Antagonism of buprenorphine agonist activity may not occur once the drug binds to opiate receptors in the CNS, and buprenorphine-induced respiratory depression may not respond to naloxone. The respiratory stimulant doxapram may be more suitable in such situations.

    Administration of naloxone in patients receiving prolonged therapy with buprenorphine does not precipitate withdrawal. Conversely, buprenorphine may precipitate withdrawal in patients who are opiate dependent. Cardiovascular effects of parenteral buprenorphine include slight changes in heart rate, blood pressure, stroke volume, and cardiac output. Buprenorphine produces minimal nausea, vomiting, or constipation. Buprenorphine crosses the placental barrier and may produce depression in the neonate. The drug may appear in breast milk and should be used with caution in nursing mothers. Epidural buprenorphine is associated with dose-dependent increases in sedation and centrally mediated respiratory depression that may be difficult to reverse with even very high doses of naloxone. Buprenorphine attenuates opiate (and possibly cocaine) craving and causes only minimal withdrawal upon abrupt discontinuation. The drug may be preferable to methadone, which produces dependence and can produce withdrawal when discontinued. It is also preferable to α_2-agonists such as clonidine, which attenuate (by decreasing central adrenergic hyperarousal) but do not totally eliminate withdrawal and which may produce hypotension.

Pharmacokinetics

Onset of Action: IV, <1 minute; IM, 15 minutes.
Peak Effect: IV, 5–20 minutes; IM, 1 hour.
Duration of Action: IV/IM/SL, 6 hours.

Interactions

Potentiates CNS and circulatory depressant effects of benzodiazepines, other narcotic analgesics, volatile anesthetics, phenothiazines, sedative-hypnotics, alcohol, and tricyclic antidepressants; analgesia is enhanced and prolonged by narcotic and non-narcotic analgesics (e.g., aspirin, acetaminophen) and α_2-agonists (e.g., clonidine); concomitant administration with fentanyl produces satisfactory analgesia of prolonged duration and minimal respiratory depression.

Toxicity

Toxic Range: Not routinely monitored.

Manifestations: Somnolence, coma, respiratory arrest, apnea, cardiac arrhythmias, combined respiratory and metabolic acidosis, precipitation of withdrawal symptoms from opioids (abdominal cramps, vomiting, skin crawling, piloerection, nasal stuffiness, lacrimation, yawning, sweating, tremor, myalgia), circulatory collapse, cardiac arrest, death.

Antidote: Naloxone IV/IM/SC 0.4–2.0 mg; repeat dose every 2 to 3 minutes to a maximum of 10–20 mg. Or doxapram slow IV 0.5–1.5 mg/kg; repeat in 5 minutes. Maximum dose: 2 mg/kg. If withdrawal symptoms are precipitated by buprenorphine, administer opioid agonists and benzodiazepines, and treat withdrawal symptomatically.

Management: Discontinue or reduce medication. Support ventilation and circulation (patent airway, oxygen, IV fluids, vasopressors). Administer antidote. Monitor blood gases, pH, and electrolytes. Correct acidosis and electrolyte disturbance (lactic acidosis may require sodium bicarbonate IV 1–2 mEq/kg). Symptomatic treatment. Airway-protected, ipecac syrup–induced emesis (30 mL or 0.5 mL/kg ipecac syrup followed by 200 mL or 4 mL/kg of water or clear fluid) or gastric lavage (with drug ingestion) followed by administration of activated charcoal (PO 50–100 g or 1–2 g/kg).

Guidelines/Precautions

1. Reduce dosage in elderly patients and with concomitant use of narcotics and sedative hypnotics.

2. Prescribe or supply an antiemetic (e.g., metoclo-pramide) for use in the event of nausea and/or vomiting.

3. Constipation may be more difficult to control than pain. Prevent and/or treat by daily administration of laxatives and stool softeners, for example, Colace (docusate sodium) 100–300 mg/day. Do not administer bulk-forming agents that contain methylcellulose, psyllium, or polycarbophil. Temporary arrest in the passage through the gastro-intestinal tract may lead to fecal impaction or bowel obstruction.

4. Tolerance may develop in all patients taking nar-cotic analgesics for more than a couple of weeks. It may be a function of dose, frequency, and route of administration because IV and spinal infusions of narcotics are associated with rapid development of tolerance. The first sign is a decrease in duration of effective analgesia. To delay the development of tolerance, add adjuvant drugs (e.g., NSAIDs, antidepressant agents, dex-tromethorphan), switch to alternative opioids (starting at one-half the equianalgesic dose), or supplement with nondrug therapies such as TENS.

5. Physical dependence may occur infrequently. Withdrawal symptoms may manifest by anxiety, nervousness, irritability, chills alternating with hot flashes, diaphoresis, insomnia, abdominal cramps, nausea, vomiting, and myoclonus. To avoid with-drawal, doses should be reduced slowly (e.g., dose reduction of 75% every 2 days). Withdrawal should be treated symptomatically.

6. Abuse liability for buprenorphine is less than that

for morphine or codeine. Cross-tolerance may occur between buprenorphine and other opiate agonists, such as morphine.

7. Drug combinations with adjuvant drugs enhance analgesia (see pages xxvi–xliv). Adjuvant drug therapies also include regional blockade, trigger-point injections (with local anesthetics and steroids), and intravenous regional anesthesia.

8. Adjuvant nondrug therapies include TENS and modalities such as ice or heat application, ultrasound, and soft tissue mobilization.

9. Patients should be warned that buprenorphine may impair their ability to perform hazardous tasks requiring mental alertness or physical coordination (e.g., driving a motor vehicle, operating heavy machinery).

10. Epidural injections should be avoided when the patient has septicemia, infection at the injection site, or coagulopathy.

11. Buprenorphine is subject to control under the Federal Controlled Substances Act of 1970 as a Schedule V (C-V) drug.

Principal Adverse Reactions

Cardiovascular: Hypertension, hypotension, tachycardia, bradycardia.

Pulmonary: Respiratory depression.

CNS: Sedation, dizziness, headache, euphoria, confusion, hallucinations.

Gastrointestinal: Nausea, vomiting.

Ocular: Miosis.

Dermatologic: Pruritus, injection site reaction, rash.

Autonomic: Flushing, dry mouth, sensitivity to cold.

BUTORPHANOL TARTRATE

Class: Narcotic Agonist-Antagonist

Use(s): Treatment of acute pain, chronic pain, migraine headaches.

Dosing: *Pain*

Nasal spray: 1 mg (one spray). Children, 20–25 μg/kg. May repeat in 1 hour. Two-dose sequence may be repeated every 3–4 hours as indicated.

IM: 1–4 mg (0.02–0.08 mg/kg) every 3–4 hours.

IV: 0.5–2.0 mg (0.01–0.04 mg/kg) every 3–4 hours.

Patient-controlled analgesia IV: Bolus 0.2–0.3 mg (4–6 μg/kg); lockout interval 5–15 minutes.

Epidural: Bolus 1–2 mg (0.02–0.04 mg/kg).

Migraine: Nasal spray: 1 mg (one spray). May repeat in one hour. Two-dose sequence may be repeated every 3–4 hours as indicated.

Due to impaired elimination, accumulation and excess sedation may occur in patients with renal or hepatic dysfunction. Analgesia may be enhanced by addition of adjuvant drugs such as nonsteroidal anti-inflammatory drugs (NSAIDs) and antidepressant agents (see pages xxvi–xliv for drug combinations) and use of nondrug therapies.

Elimination: Hepatic, renal.

Preparations

Butorphanol **(Stadol)**
  Injection: 1 mg/mL, 2 mg/mL.
  Nasal spray: 10 mg/mL or 1 mg/metered spray.

Dilution for Infusion: Epidural bolus: Dilute 1–2 mg in 10 mL local anesthetic or preservative-free normal saline.

Pharmacology

A synthetic benzomorphan derivative, butorphanol is a potent opioid agonist-antagonist with analgesic potency 3.5 to 7 times that of morphine or 30 to 40 times that of meperidine. Butorphanol is a competitive antagonist at μ-receptors and an agonist at δ- and κ-receptors. Psychotomimetic effects of butorphanol may result from agonist effects at σ-receptors. Butorphanol has a ceiling effect for respiratory depression and analgesia at high doses (>30–60 μg/kg). Butorphanol is not recommended for patients with cancer pain and may precipitate withdrawal in patients who have received opioids on a long-term basis. Respiratory depression and psychotomimetic effects of butorphanol may be reversed by naloxone. Butorphanol crosses the placental barrier and may produce depression in the neonate. The drug may appear in breast milk and should be used with caution in nursing mothers. Usefulness of epidural butorphanol is limited by the dose-dependent increases in sedation that are secondary to vascular uptake and activation of κ-receptors in the central nervous system.

Pharmacokinetics

Onset of Action: IV, 1–5 minutes. IM, 10 minutes. Nasal, <15 minutes.

Peak Effect: IV, 5–10 minutes. IM, 30–60 minutes. Nasal, 1–2 hours.

Duration of Action: IV, 2–4 hours. IM/Epidural, 3–4 hours. Nasal, 4–5 hours.

Interactions

Decreases effectiveness of parenteral and epidural/spinal opioid agonists; may precipitate withdrawal in opioid-dependent patients; additive effects with phenothiazines, droperidol, barbiturates, and other tranquilizers.

Toxicity

Toxic Range: Not routinely monitored.

Manifestations: Somnolence, coma, respiratory arrest, apnea, cardiac arrhythmias, combined respiratory and metabolic acidosis, precipitation of withdrawal symptoms from opioids (abdominal cramps, vomiting, skin crawling, piloerection, nasal stuffiness, lacrimation, yawning, sweating, tremor, myalgia), circulatory collapse, cardiac arrest, death.

Antidote: Naloxone IV/IM/SC 0.4–2.0 mg. Repeat dose every 2 to 3 minutes to a maximum of 10–20 mg. If withdrawal symptoms are precipitated by butorphanol, administer opioid agonists and benzodiazepines and treat withdrawal symptomatically.

Management: Discontinue or reduce medication. Support ventilation and circulation (patent airway, oxygen, IV fluids, vasopressors). Administer antidote. Monitor blood gases, pH, and electrolytes. Correct acidosis and electrolyte disturbance (lactic acidosis may require sodium bicarbonate IV 1–2 mEq/kg). Symptomatic treatment. Airway-protected, ipecac syrup–induced emesis (30 mL or 0.5 mL/kg ipecac syrup followed by 200 mL or 4 mL/kg of water or clear fluid) or gastric lavage (with drug ingestion) followed by administration of activated charcoal (PO 50–100 g or 1–2 g/kg).

Guidelines/Precautions

1. May cause respiratory depression.
2. In patients who have been chronically receiving opiate agonists, butorphanol may precipitate withdrawal symptoms as a result of opiate antagonist effect. Such patients should have an adequate period of withdrawal from opioid drugs prior to beginning butorphanol therapy.
3. Patients should be warned that butorphanol may impair their ability to perform hazardous tasks requiring mental alertness or physical coordination (e.g., driving a motor vehicle, operating heavy machinery).
4. Butorphanol crosses the placental barrier, and usage in labor may rarely produce depression of respiration in the neonate. This has been associated with administration of a dose within 2 hours of delivery, use of multiple doses, use with additional analgesics or sedative drugs, or use in preterm pregnancies. Resuscitation may be required; have naloxone available.
5. Drug increases cardiac work and should be used with caution in patients with ischemic disease.
6. Undesirable side effects of epidural butorphanol include delayed respiratory depression, pruritus, nausea and vomiting, and urinary retention. Naloxone (IV/IM/SC 0.2–0.4 mg as required or infusion

5–10 µg/kg/hr) is effective for prophylaxis and/or treatment. Ventilatory support for respiratory depression must be readily available. Antihistamines, for example, diphenhydramine (IV/IM 12.5–25.0 mg every 6 hours as needed) may be used in treating pruritus. Metoclopramide (IV 10 mg every 6 hours as needed) may be used in treating nausea and vomiting. Urinary retention that does not respond to naloxone may require straight bladder catheterization. Bethanechol (Urecholine) PO 15–30 mg three times daily or SC 2.5–5 mg three or four times daily as required may be used as an alternative to naloxone. (Bethanechol increases the tone of the detrusor urinae muscle. It should not be given IV or IM, which may result in cholinergic overstimulation. Have atropine available [IV/SC, 0.5 mg].)

7. Epidural/intrathecal injections should be avoided when the patient has septicemia, infection at the injection site, or coagulopathy.

8. Nasal butorphanol is subject to control under the Federal Controlled Substances Act of 1970 as a Schedule IV (C-IV) drug.

Principal Adverse Reactions

Cardiovascular: Hypertension, hypotension, palpitations.

Pulmonary: Respiratory depression.

CNS: Euphoria, hallucinations, sedation, headache.

Gastrointestinal: Nausea, vomiting.

Ocular: Miosis.

Autonomic: Flushing, dry mouth, sensitivity to cold.

CAPSAICIN

Class: Topical Analgesic

Use(s): Temporary relief of pain from rheumatoid arthritis and osteoarthritis; postmastectomy pain; relief of neuralgias (e.g., diabetic neuropathy, postherpetic neuralgia, phantom limb pain); treatment of psoriasis vulgaris and hemodialysis-associated pruritus.

Dosing: *Pain:* Topical (0.025–0.075% cream) three to five times daily. Apply thin film of cream. No residue should remain. Less frequent use (less than three times daily) may decrease clinical efficacy and increase local discomfort. Avoid contact with eyes and broken or irritated skin. For postherpetic neuralgia, apply to skin only after zoster lesions have healed. Transient burning may occur on application but generally disappears in several days.

Psoriasis: Topical (0.01–0.025% cream) four to six times daily.

Elimination: Hepatic.

Preparations

Capsaicin **(Zostrix):** Capsaicin 0.025%; tubes: 0.7 oz, 1.5 oz, 3.0 oz.

Capsaicin **(Zostrix HP):** Capsaicin 0.075%; tubes: 1 oz, 2 oz.

Pharmacology

Capsaicin is a naturally occurring substance derived from plants of the Solanaceae family (red peppers), with the chemical name *trans*-8-methyl-*N*-vanillyl-6-noneamide. The precise mechanism of action is not fully understood, but capsaicin renders skin and joints insensitive to pain by initial release and then depletion of substance P (the principal chemical mediator) in peripheral sensory neurons and in joint tissues. Initial exposure to capsaicin induces an intense excitation, after which the neurons become temporarily inactive. Capsaicin decreases substance P–induced activation of inflammatory mediators involved with the pathogenesis of rheumatoid arthritis. Capsaicin may provide effective relief of burning, shooting neuropathic pain and pain associated with inflammatory joint diseases. Capsaicin does not appear to act directly on central cells in the brain and spinal cord.

Pharmacokinetics

Onset: 14–28 days (up to 4 weeks).
Peak Effect: Variable.
Duration of Action: 3–6 hours.

Interactions

May induce cough in patients receiving ACE inhibitors.

Toxicity

Toxic Range: Not routinely monitored.
Manifestations: Erythematous ulcers, burning.
Antidote: None.
Management: Discontinue or reduce concentration of medication. Symptomatic treatment.

Guidelines/Precautions

1. Wash hands immediately following application of cream. Do not bandage areas of application tightly.

2. Avoid mixing capsaicin cream with other topical medications.
3. Capsaicin may cause transient burning on initial application. Local reactions diminish with continued therapy but can be persistent and severe in some patients.

Principal Adverse Reactions

Dermatologic: Burning, stinging, erythema, pruritus.

CARBAMAZEPINE

Class: Anticonvulsant

Use(s): Anticonvulsant; antidepressant; treatment of lancinating neuropathic pain, for example, trigeminal neuralgia (tic douloureux) and other cranial neuralgias, postsympathectomy neuralgia, diabetic neuropathy, postherpetic neuralgia, phantom limb pain, the thalamic syndrome or lightning tabetic pain, and migraine.

Dosing: *Pain or depression*

Initial: Tablets/Tablets XR, PO 100 mg (2 mg/kg) twice daily.

Oral suspension, PO 50 mg (1 mg/kg) four times daily.

Dosage should be increased by up to 200 mg daily at weekly intervals until the optimal response is obtained. (Normal dose range 600–1600 mg daily.)

Blood counts (reticulocyte, leukocyte, and platelet counts) should be monitored at the start of therapy and monthly or bimonthly for the first 6 months of therapy. It is advisable to obtain informed consent before institution of carbamazepine for chronic pain management, given the potential for side effects. Analgesia may be enhanced by combination with other anticonvulsants (e.g., phenytoin, gabapentin), benzodiazepines (e.g., diazepam), antidepressant agents (e.g., paroxetine), skeletal muscle relaxants (e.g., baclofen), and use of nondrug therapies such as transcutaneous electrical nerve stimulation (TENS). Therapeutic range (analgesic effects): 3–14 µg/mL (up to 21.2 µg/mL in one report).

Anticonvulsant (adults and children older than 12 years)

Tablets/Tablets XR: Initial dose: PO 200 mg two times daily.

Oral suspension: Optional loading dose PO 8 mg/kg (rapid control of seizures), *or* Initial dose PO 100 mg four times daily.

Dosage should be increased by up to 200 mg daily at weekly intervals. Use a 2 times daily regimen of Tegretol XR or a 3 or 4 times daily regimen of the other formulations until the optimal response is obtained. Maximum recommended dose: 1000 mg/day in children aged 13–15 years and 1200 mg/day in patients older than 15 years (some patients have required 1600–2400 mg daily).

Maintenance: PO 800–1200 mg daily. Adjust to minimum effective dose. Use a 2 times daily regimen of Tegretol XR or a 3 or 4 times daily regimen of the other formulations until the optimal response is obtained.

Anticonvulsant (children 6–12 years)

Tablets/Tablets XR: Initial dose: PO 100 mg two times daily.

Oral suspension, optional loading dose PO 8 mg/kg (rapid control of seizures), *or* Initial dose PO 50 mg four times daily.

Dosage should be increased by up to 100 mg daily at weekly intervals. Use a 2 times daily regimen of Tegretol XR or a 3 or 4 times daily regimen of the other formulations until the optimal response is obtained. Maximum recommended dose 1000 mg/day.

Maintenance: PO 400–800 mg daily. Adjust to minimum effective dose. Use a 2 times daily regimen of Tegretol XR or a 3 or 4 times daily regimen of the other formulations. Therapeutic range (anticonvulsant effects): 3–14 µg/mL.

When converting patients from Tegretol tablets to Tegretol XR, the same total daily dose should be administered. Tegretol is superior to the generic form of carbamazepine. For predictable therapeutic efficacy, do no prescribe generic formulation of anticonvulsant drugs.

Elimination: Hepatic.

Preparations

Carbamazepine **(Tegretol, Epitol)**
    Oral suspension: 20 mg/mL.
    Tablets: 200 mg.
Carbamazepine **(Tegretol, Carbamazepine chewable):** Tablets, chewable: 100 mg.

Pharmacology

An iminostilbene derivative that is structurally related to the tricyclic antidepressants, carbamazepine has sedative, anticholinergic, antidepressant, muscle relaxant, antiarrhythmic, and antidiuretic effects. The anticonvulsant activity is mainly due to limitation of seizure propagation by reduction of posttetanic potentiation (PTP) of synaptic transmission. Blockade of voltage-operated sodium channels leads to decreased electrical activity and a subsequent reduction in release of the excitatory neurotransmitter glutamate. Carbamazepine is reserved for refractory seizure disorders, including partial seizures with complex symptoms, and for patients who have inadequate response to other anticonvulsants such as phenytoin, phenobarbital, or primidone. Carbamazepine is ineffective in the management of petit mal seizures or myoclonic and akinetic seizures. Carbamazepine may suppress the sharp lancinating and paroxysmal electrical shooting qualities common in neuropathic pain, such as in idiopathic trigeminal neuralgia, by decreasing synaptic transmission. It is more effective than phenytoin. Carbamazepine is not as useful for the more chronic aching pains, such as in posttraumatic trigeminal pain. The antidepressant activity is comparable to the tricyclic antidepressants and may contribute to the analgesic effects. Carbamazepine crosses the placenta and has been associated with birth defects. The drug is distributed in breast milk. It should be avoided in pregnancy and nursing mothers except in situations when discontinuation of therapy may pose a serious threat to the mother.

Pharmacokinetics

Onset of Action: Analgesic effects: 3–4 days.
Peak Effect: Anticonvulsant effects: PO, 2–8 hours.
Duration of Action: Anticonvulsant effects: 25–65 hours (half-life).

Interactions

Serum level and toxic effects increased by verapamil, erythromycin, fluoxetine cimetidine, isoniazid, and propoxyphene; serum levels decreased by chronic alcohol abuse, reserpine, phenytoin, phenobarbital, primidone, ethosuximide, and valproic acid; oral absorption decreased by charcoal; seizures precipitated with use of tricyclic antidepressants; decreases serum level and effects of doxycycline, coumarin anticoagulants, theophylline; may potentiate antidiuretic effects of vasopressin, lyepressin, and desmopressin.

Toxicity

Toxic Range: Initial signs of toxicity (ataxia, dizziness) may be observed at levels >10 μg/mL.
Manifestations: Tachycardia, hypotension, hypertension, conduction disturbances, nystagmus, ataxia, nausea and vomiting, psychomotor disturbances, agitation, irritability, coma, respiratory arrest.
Antidote: No specific antidote.
Management: Discontinue or reduce medication. Support ventilation and circulation (patent airway,

oxygen, IV fluids). Airway-protected, ipecac syrup–induced emesis (30 mL or 0.5 mL/kg ipecac syrup followed by 200 mL or 4 mL/kg of water or clear fluid) or gastric lavage (with drug ingestion) followed by administration of activated charcoal (PO 50–100 g or 1–2 g/kg). Monitor EKG to detect and treat arrhythmias. Symptomatic treatment.

Guidelines/Precautions

1. A trial of withdrawal of carbamazepine therapy in chronic pain may be attempted after 4 to 6 months of therapy. Patients occasionally may maintain pain relief once they are off the medication.
2. Monitor serum blood levels to achieve optimal therapeutic effect. In one report, pain relief was correlated with carbamazepine serum levels of 21.2 μmol per liter.
3. Transient leukopenia is to be expected and is not an indication to discontinue therapy if pain relief is evident (unless leukocyte counts are less than 3000 or if the absolute neutrophil count drops below 1500).
4. Carbamazepine may be associated with exfoliative dermatitis and the Stevens-Johnson syndrome as a non-dose-related hypersensitivity reaction. Discontinue the drug if a rash occurs. Prolonged use may be associated with mental and physical sluggishness.
5. Patients should be warned that carbamazepine may impair their ability to perform activities requiring mental alertness or physical coordination (e.g., operating heavy machinery, driving a motor vehicle).

6. Abrupt withdrawal in epileptic patients may precipitate status epilepticus. Reduce dosage, discontinue, or substitute other anticonvulsant
   medications gradually.
7. Contraindicated in patients with a history of bone
   marrow depression, hypersensitivity to tricyclic
   antidepressants, and concomitant use of
   monoamine oxidase (MAO) inhibitors. Discontinue
   MAO inhibitors for a minimum of 14 days before
   carbamazepine administration.

Principal Adverse Reactions

Cardiovascular: Hypotension, hypertension, congestive heart failure, atrial and ventricular conduction depression, arrhythmias.

CNS: Ataxia, confusion, dizziness, tremors, headaches,
peripheral neuropathy, activation of latent psychosis.

Gastrointestinal: Nausea, vomiting, epigastric pain,
constipation.

Genitourinary: Urinary frequency, acute urinary retention, azotemia, renal failure, impotence.

Dermatologic: Stevens-Johnson syndrome, lupus erythematosus, rash, hypertrichosis.

Hematologic: Thrombocytopenia, leukopenia, agranulocytosis, aplastic anemia.

Other: Hyperglycemia, gingival hyperplasia.

CELECOXIB

Class: Nonsteroidal Anti-inflammatory Drug

Use(s): Symptomatic treatment of osteoarthritis and
rheumatoid arthritis

Dosing: *Osteoarthritis:* PO 200 mg once daily or 100 mg twice daily.

Rheumatoid arthritis: PO 100–200 mg twice daily.

Celecoxib capsules may be administered without regard to meals. Dose adjustment in the elderly is generally not necessary. However, for patients less than 50 kg in body weight, initiate therapy at the lowest recommended dose.

Administer medication regularly, not as necessary. Addition of opioid analgesics and antidepressant agents and the use of nondrug therapies (e.g., TENS) may enhance analgesia (see pages xxvi–xliv for drug combinations).

Elimination: Hepatic

Preparations

Celecoxib **(Celebrex):** Capsules: 100 mg, 200 mg.

Pharmacology

This nonsteroidal anti-inflammatory drug (NSAID) was designed using advance molecular technology. Celecoxib in clinical trials was as effective as naproxen in treating arthritis pain and inflammation. In osteoarthritis patients, celecoxib improved pain, stiffness, and patient functions such as walking and bending. The analgesic and anti-inflammatory activity of celecoxib is partly due to the inhibition of prostaglandin synthesis and/or release secondary to the inhibition of cyclooxygenase-2 isoenzyme (COX-2). Cyclooxygenase enzyme (prostaglandin G/H synthetase) catalyzes the formation of prostaglandin precursors, such as endoperoxide intermediate prostaglandin G_2 (PGG$_2$), from arachidonic acid. PGG$_2$ is reduced by peroxidase activity to another endoperoxide intermediate, prostaglandin H_2 (PGH$_2$). These endoperoxide intermediates are the common precursors for the synthesis of prostaglandins, prostacyclins, and thromboxanes. The inhibition of COX and thus prostanoid synthesis by classic NSAIDs is associated with side effects such as irritation and ulcer formation in the upper gastrointestinal tract and impairment of kidney function. It has been recognized recently that mammalian cells express two forms of COX activity. COX-1 isoenzyme is expressed in many normal tissues and is the major form present in platelets, the kidney, and the gastrointestinal tract. COX-2 isoenzyme is induced in response to pro-inflammatory cytokines, lipopolysaccharide (LPS), and growth factors and is subjected to repression by glucocorticosteroids. This second form is generally not detected in healthy tissues but is found in elevated levels in inflammatory exudates. This has led to the hypotheses that COX-1 is mainly associated with homeostasis (including cytoprotection in the stomach and regulation of kidney function), and COX-2 with the edematous, nociceptive and pyretic effects of inflammation. Most classic NSAIDs including diclofenac, naproxen, and ibuprofen show little specificity of inhibition toward COX isoforms. Uniquely, celecoxib at therapeutic concentration does not inhibit COX-1. Ulcerogenic-sparing COX-2 inhibition does not inhibit cytoprotective stomach PGE$_2$ production in contrast to nonspecific NSAIDs. Celecoxib is better tolerated than the classic NSAIDs and equipotent doses are associated with less gastric mucosal abnormalities. The antipyretic activity of celecoxib may occur secondary to inhibition of pyrogen-induced release of prostaglandins in the central nervous system (including the hypothalamus) and possibly to centrally mediated peripheral vasodilation. Celecoxib (like other NSAIDs) exhibits a ceiling effect for analgesia. Exceeding recommended doses results in increased toxicity without improvement in analgesia. Inhibition of prostaglandin synthesis may result in decreased uterine tone, contractility, and prolonged gestation in the parturient and premature closure of the ductus arteriosus in the fetus. Celecoxib has no effect on platelet aggregation or bleeding time and unlike aspirin cannot be used for cardiovascular prophylaxis.

Pharmacokinetics

Onset of Action: 15–30 minutes.
Peak Effect: 24–48 hours.
Duration of Action: Half-life, 11 hours.

Interactions

Risks of bleeding increased with concomitant NSAIDs, anticoagulant or heparin therapy, alcohol ingestion; decreases antihypertensive effects of β-adrenergic blocking agents, ACE inhibitors; decreases the natriuretic effect of furosemide and thiazides in some patients; rate of GI side effects increased with concomitant aspirin; serum levels of celecoxib increased by concomitant fluconazole; serum level and toxic effects of lithium increased by concomitant celecoxib; GI absorption of celecoxib delayed by food, milk, and aluminum/magnesium-containing antacids.

Toxicity

Toxic Range: Not routinely monitored.

Manifestations: *Acute:* Drowsiness, nausea, vomiting, lethargy, paresthesia, disorientation, epigastric pain, GI bleeding.

Antidote: None.

Management: Discontinue or reduce medication. Correction of fluid, electrolyte, and acid-base disturbances. Support ventilation and circulation (patent airway, oxygen, IV fluids, and vasopressors). Airway-protected, ipecac syrup–induced emesis (30 mL or 0.5 mL/kg ipecac syrup followed by 200 mL or 4 mL/kg of water or clear fluid) or gastric lavage (with drug ingestion) followed by administration of activated charcoal (PO 50–100 g or 1–2 g/kg). Symptomatic treatment. Forced diuresis, alkalinization of urine, hemodialysis, or hemoperfusion may not be useful due to high protein binding of celecoxib.

Guidelines/Precautions

1. Serious clinically significant upper GI bleeding has been observed in patients receiving celecoxib, albeit infrequently.

2. Use with caution in patients with active GI lesions (e.g., erosive gastritis, peptic ulcer), a history of recurrent GI lesions, hepatic/renal dysfunction, preexisting hypoprothrombinemia, and vitamin K deficiency. Co-therapies and co-morbid conditions that may increase the risk for GI bleeding include treatment with oral corticosteroids, treatment with anticoagulants, long duration of NSAID therapy, smoking, alcoholism, old age, and poor general health status.

3. Celecoxib may decrease glomerular filtration rate and cause peripheral edema. The drug should be used cautiously in patients with heart failure,

    hypertension, and conditions associated with fluid retention.

4. Renal prostaglandins may have a supportive role in maintaining renal perfusion in patients with pre-renal conditions. Celecoxib should be avoided in such patients as it may cause a dose-dependent decrease in prostaglandin formation and thus precipitate renal decompensation.

5. Observe carefully patients with coagulation disorders and those receiving drug therapy that interferes with hemostasis.

6. Avoid the use of celecoxib during pregnancy (especially during the third trimester) or during labor and delivery. Celecoxib and other NSAIDs inhibit prostaglandin synthesis, which may cause dystocia, interfere with labor, and delay parturition. Prostaglandin synthesis inhibitors may also have adverse effects on the fetal cardiovascular system (e.g., premature closure of ductus arteriosus), or may produce primary pulmonary hypertension or fetal death.

7. Patient response to NSAIDs is variable. Patients who do not respond to or cannot tolerate celecoxib may be successfully treated with another NSAID.

8. Celecoxib may be used with low-dose aspirin. However, concomitant administration of both drugs may result in an increased rate of GI ulcerations or other complications.

9. Celecoxib is contraindicated in patients with previously demonstrated hypersensitivity to celecoxib or with the complete or partial syndrome of nasal polyps, angioedema, or bronchospastic reactivity to aspirin or other NSAIDs.

10. Celecoxib should not be given to patients who have demonstrated allergic-type reactions to sulfonamides.
11. The antipyretic and anti-inflammatory effects of celecoxib may mask signs and symptoms of infection or other diseases.

Principal Adverse Reactions

Cardiovascular: Congestive heart failure, peripheral edema, fluid retention, hypertension, tachycardia, arrhythmias.

Pulmonary: Dyspnea, bronchospasm.

CNS: Drowsiness, dizziness, headache, anxiety, confusion.

Gastrointestinal: Abdominal pain, diarrhea, dyspepsia, flatulence, nausea, gastritis, hepatic dysfunction, elevated liver enzymes.

Genitourinary: Renal dysfunction, acute renal failure, azotemia, cystitis, hematuria.

Dermatologic: Pruritus, urticaria.

Hematologic: Anemia, ecchymosis, epistaxis, thrombocytopenia.

Other: Tinnitus, blurred vision, taste perversion.

CHLORDIAZEPOXIDE HYDROCHLORIDE

Class: Benzodiazepine

Use(s): Sedative, treatment of acute alcohol withdrawal.

Dosing: *Sedation*

PO: 5–10 mg (0.1–0.2 mg/kg) three or four times daily.

IM: Initial, 50–100 mg (1–2 mg/kg) then

> maintenance 25–50 mg (0.5–1.0 mg/kg)
> three or four times daily.
>
> *Withdrawal symptoms:* IM/IV/PO: 50–100 mg
> (IM or IV: dilute in supplied diluent, 5 mL
> normal saline, or sterile water). Repeat
> every 2–4 hours if necessary. Maximum
> daily dose 300 mg. Do not use intramuscu-
> lar diluent for intravenous administration.

Elimination: Hepatic.

Preparations

Chlordiazepoxide **(Libritabs):** Tablets: 10 mg, 25 mg.

Chlordiazepoxide hydrochloride **(Librium, Sereen):**
Capsules: 5 mg, 10 mg, 25 mg.

Chlordiazepoxide hydrochloride **(Librium):** Injection:
100 mg. (5 mL dry filled ampule containing 100 mg
chlordiazepoxide and a 2 mL ampule of special intramuscular diluent. Solution is unstable. Prepare just
before use. Discard unused portions.)

Chlordiazepoxide hydrochloride and amitriptyline
hydrochloride **(Limbitrol):** Tablets: Chlordiazepoxide hydrochloride 5 mg and amitriptyline hydrochloride 12.5 mg.

Chlordiazepoxide hydrochloride and amitriptyline
hydrochloride **(Limbitrol DS):** Tablets: Chlordiazepoxide hydrochloride 10 mg and amitriptyline
hydrochloride 25 mg.

Chlordiazepoxide hydrochloride and esterified estrogens **(Menrium):** Tablets: Chlordiazepoxide hydrochloride 5 mg and esterified estrogens 0.2 mg;
chlordiazepoxide hydrochloride 5 mg and esterified
estrogens 0.4 mg; chlordiazepoxide hydrochloride
10 mg and esterified estrogens 0.4 mg.

Chlordiazepoxide hydrochloride and clindinium bromide **(CDP Plus, Clindex, Clinibrax, Clinoxide, Clipoxide, Librax, Lidoxide):** Tablets: Chlordiazepoxide hydrochloride 5 mg and clindinium bromide 2.5 mg.

Pharmacology

This benzodiazepine increases γ-aminobutyric acid (GABA) neurotransmission in the CNS. The drug exerts antianxiety, sedative, and appetite-stimulating effects. Chlordiazepoxide may possess some peripheral anticholinergic activity. In chronic pain syndromes, relief of anxiety and agitation may increase the pain threshold. Chlordiazepoxide should be used in combination with potent analgesics (e.g., opioids, NSAIDs, antidepressant agents).

Pharmacokinetics

Onset: IV, 1–5 minutes; IM/PO, 15–30 minutes.
Peak Effect: IV, 5 minutes; IM/PO, 45 minutes.
Duration of Action: IV, 15 minutes to 1 hour; IM/PO, 2–6 hours.

Interactions

Potentiates CNS and circulatory depressant effect of narcotics, alcohol, sedative-hypnotics, phenothiazines, monoamine oxidase (MAO) inhibitors; reduces requirements for volatile anesthetics; elimination decreased by cimetidine, propranolol; effects antagonized by flumazenil.

Toxicity

Toxic Range: Not routinely monitored.
Manifestations: Respiratory depression, apnea, hypotension, confusion, coma, seizures.

Antidote: Flumazenil IV 0.2–2.0 mg.

Management: Discontinue or reduce medication. Support ventilation and circulation (patent airway, oxygen, IV fluids, vasopressors). Administer antidote. Symptomatic treatment. Airway-protected, ipecac syrup–induced emesis (30 mL or 0.5 mL/kg ipecac syrup followed by 200 mL or 4 mL/kg of water or clear fluid) or gastric lavage (with drug ingestion) followed by administration of activated charcoal (PO 50–100 g or 0.5–1.0 g/kg). Hemodialysis is not useful. Treat withdrawal hyperactivity with low-dose barbiturate.

Guidelines/Precautions

1. Reduce dosage in elderly patients and with concomitant use of narcotics and other sedatives.
2. Paradoxical reactions (excitement, stimulation) may occur in hyperactive aggressive children and psychiatric patients.
3. Patients should be warned that chlordiazepoxide may impair their ability to perform activities requiring mental alertness or physical coordination (e.g., operating heavy machinery, driving a motor vehicle).
4. Chlordiazepoxide is subject to control under the Federal Controlled Substances Act of 1970 as a Schedule IV (C-IV) drug.

Principal Adverse Reactions

Cardiovascular: Hypotension, tachycardia.
Pulmonary: Hypoventilation, apnea.
CNS: Drowsiness, ataxia, confusion, extrapyramidal symptoms (rarely).
Hematological: Agranulocytosis.
Other: Hepatic dysfunction.

CHLOROPROCAINE HYDROCHLORIDE

Class: Local Anesthetic

Use(s): Regional anesthesia; systemic analgesia for treatment of painful conditions such as neuropathic pain, reflex sympathetic dystrophy, burn or sickle cell pain, and pruritus.

Dosing: *Infiltration/Peripheral nerve block:* <40 mL (1–2% solution).

Epidural: Bolus, 200–750 mg (10–25 mL of a 2% or 3% solution). Approximately 1.5–2.0 mL/kg for each segment to be anesthetized. Repeat doses at 40- to 60-minute intervals. Infusion, 20–30 mL/hr (0.5–1.0% solution).

Caudal: 10–25 mL of a 2% or 3% solution. Children, 0.4–0.7–1.0 mL/kg (L2-T10-T7 level of anesthesia). Repeat doses at 40- to 60-minute intervals.

Rate of onset and potency of local anesthetic action may be enhanced by carbonation. (Add 1 mL of 8.4% sodium bicarbonate with 30 mL of 2–3% chloroprocaine. Do not use if there is precipitation.) Maximum safe dose: 10 mg/kg (without epinephrine); 15 mg/kg (with epinephrine). Use only preservative-free solution for epidural or caudal anesthesia. Except where contraindicated, vasoconstrictor drugs may be added to increase effect and prolong local or regional anesthesia. For dosage/route guidelines, see "Dosing" under Epinephrine (p. 204). Do not use vasoconstrictor drugs for local anesthesia of end organs (digits, penis, ears).

> *Systemic analgesia and pruritus:* Slow IV
> 10–20 mg/kg (3% 2-chloroprocaine solution
> without preservatives). Administer over 30
> minutes. Observe for symptoms of toxicity
> (e.g., hypotension, slurred speech, drowsi-
> ness) and adjust rate accordingly.

Elimination: Plasma cholinesterase.

Preparations

Chloroprocaine hydrochloride **(Nesacaine, Chloroprocaine HCL):** Injection, with methyl paraben: 1%
and 2% preservative-containing solution.

Chloroprocaine hydrochloride **(Nesacaine-MPF):** Injection, methyl paraben free: 2% and 3% preservative-
free solutions.

Dilution for Infusion: Epidural use only. 12.5 mL
(2%) in 37.5 mL preservative-free normal saline (0.5%
solution).

Pharmacology

A benzoic acid ester and short-acting local anesthetic,
chloroprocaine stabilizes the neuronal membrane and
prevents the initiation and transmission of impulses. It
is rapidly hydrolyzed by plasma pseudocholinesterase,
with one of the metabolites being *para*-aminobenzoic
acid. Epinephrine prolongs the duration of action by
reducing the rate of absorption and plasma concentration. Decreased myocardial contractility and peripheral
vasodilatation with toxic blood concentrations result in
decreased arterial pressure and cardiac output. Chloroprocaine is ineffective for topical anesthesia and is not
recommended for IV regional anesthesia because of the

high incidence of thrombophlebitis. When administered intravenously, chloroprocaine may produce central analgesia. This may be due to local anesthetic effects, inhibition of release of neurotransmitters (e.g., substance P, ATP) from nociceptive afferent C fibers, modulation of information transfer along primary afferents, and central sympathetic blockade with decrease in pain-induced reflex vasoconstriction. Epidural chloroprocaine may decrease the duration of analgesia of epidural narcotics, possibly due to a specific antagonism of μ-(G) receptor-mediated analgesia.

Pharmacokinetics

Onset of Action: Infiltration/Epidural, 6–12 minutes.
Peak Effect: Infiltration/Epidural, 10–20 minutes.
Duration of Action: Infiltration/Epidural, 30–60 minutes (prolonged with epinephrine).

Interactions

Prolongs the effect of succinylcholine; metabolite (PABA) inhibits the action of sulfonamides and aminosalicylic acid; toxicity enhanced by cimetidine, anticholinesterases (which inhibit degradation); benzodiazepines, barbiturates, and volatile anesthetics increase seizure threshold; duration of local or regional anesthesia prolonged by vasoconstrictor agents (e.g., epinephrine); alkalinization increases rate of onset and potency of local or regional anesthesia; epidural chloroprocaine antagonizes the analgesic effect of epidural bupivacaine, narcotics, and α_2-agonists.

Toxicity

Toxic Range: Not routinely monitored.

Manifestations: Seizures, arrhythmias, circulatory collapse, respiratory depression, cardiac arrest.

Antidote: No specific antidote.

Management: Discontinue or reduce medication. Support ventilation and circulation (patent airway, oxygen, IV fluids, vasopressors). Benzodiazepines (diazepam IV 0.05–0.2 mg/kg, midazolam IV/IM 0.025–0.1 mg/kg) or barbiturates (thiopental sodium IV 0.5–2.0 mg/kg) to control seizures. Prolonged cardiopulmonary resuscitation with cardiac arrest: Sodium bicarbonate IV 1–2 mEq/kg to treat cardiac toxicity (sodium channel blockade); bretylium IV 5 mg/kg; DC cardioversion/defibrillation for ventricular arrhythmias. Remove ingested drug by induced emesis followed by activated charcoal. Hypersensitivity reactions: Remove from further exposure and treat dermatitis. Exchange transfusions in newborns with toxicity.

Guidelines/Precautions

1. Do not use for spinal anesthesia.
2. Use with caution in patients with severe disturbances of cardiac rhythm, shock, or heart block.
3. Reduce doses in obstetric and elderly patients.
4. The potential for allergic reaction is increased with repeated use.
5. Contraindicated in patients with hypersensitivity to chloroprocaine or ester-type local anesthetics and in patients with allergy to suntan lotion (contains PABA derivatives).
6. Occasional cases of severe back pain have occurred after epidural anesthesia with chloroprocaine. Contributing factors include use of a formulation of chloroprocaine containing disodium

edetate (EDTA), large volume (>20 mL), and low pH of the commercial solution (pH may be increased with carbonation).

7. The level of sympathetic blockade (bradycardia with block above T5) determines the degree of hypotension (often heralded by nausea and vomiting) following epidural administration of chloroprocaine. Fluid hydration (10–20 mL/kg normal saline or lactated Ringer's solution), vasopressor agents (e.g., ephedrine), and left uterine displacement in pregnant patients may be used for prophylaxis and/or treatment. Administer atropine to treat bradycardia.

8. Epidural motor blockade may be reversed by the epidural injection of 20 mL of 0.9% saline.

9. Epidural, caudal, or intrathecal injections should be avoided when the patient has hypovolemic shock, septicemia, infection at the injection site, or coagulopathy.

10. Persistent neurologic damage or prolonged sensory or motor deficits have been reported following accidental spinal anesthesia with large doses of chloroprocaine solutions containing sodium bisulfite or methyl paraben.

Principal Adverse Reactions

Cardiovascular: Hypotension, arrhythmias, bradycardia.
Pulmonary: Respiratory depression, arrest.
CNS: Seizures, tinnitus, tremors.
Allergic: Urticaria, pruritus, angioneurotic edema.
Epidural/Caudal/Spinal: High spinal; arachnoiditis; backache; loss of perineal sensation and sexual function; permanent motor, sensory, and/or autonomic (sphincter control) deficit of lower segments; slowing of labor.

CHLORPROMAZINE HYDROCHLORIDE

Class: Phenothiazine

Use(s): Antipsychotic, antiemetic, relief of hiccups, treatment of phantom limb pain, adjunct treatment of neuropathic pain (e.g., diabetic neuropathy, postherpetic neuralgia).

Dosing: *Emesis and hiccups*

> PO/IM: 10–50 mg (0.25–0.55 mg/kg) three or four times daily. Maximum IM dosage for children: 40 mg/day (<5 years old), 75 mg/day (5–12 years old).
>
> Rectal: 50–100 mg (1.1 mg/kg).
>
> IV: 25–50 mg (0.25–0.55 mg/kg). Dilute to 1 mg/mL with normal saline. Give at rate of 1 mg/min.
>
> *Neuropathic and phantom limb pain:* PO 25–100 mg one to five times daily. Observe for hypotension with parenteral administration.
>
> Dosage recommendations for other oral forms of the drug may be applied to Spansule sustained release capsules on the basis of total daily dosage in milligrams.

Elimination: Hepatic.

Preparations

Chlorpromazine hydrochloride **(Thorazine)**
  Tablets: 10 mg, 25 mg, 50 mg, 100 mg, 200 mg.
  Spansule capsules, sustained release: 30 mg, 75 mg, 150 mg.
  Oral solution: 2 mg/mL.

Oral concentrate: 30 mg/mL, 100 mg/mL.
Suppositories: 25 and 100 mg.
Injection: 25 mg/mL.

Pharmacology

Chlorpromazine is a phenothiazine tranquilizer with strong antiemetic, antiadrenergic, anticholinergic, and sedative effects. The drug has weak antiserotonergic, antihistaminic, and ganglion-blocking activity. The neuroleptic actions are most likely due to antagonism of dopamine as a synaptic neurotransmitter in the basal ganglia and limbic portions of the forebrain. Moderate extrapyramidal side effects are evidence of interference with the normal actions of dopamine. The strong antiemetic effects are mediated by dopamine receptor blockade in the medullary chemoreceptor trigger zone. Chlorpromazine may lower the seizure threshold and cause EEG changes. Therapeutic doses have little effect on respiration, but the drug may enhance respiratory depression produced by other CNS depressants.

Chlorpromazine may be useful in chronic pain syndromes by altering the perception of pain and, where applicable, relieving psychosis and/or anxiety. Chlorpromazine is occasionally useful in postherpetic neuralgia and other neuropathies in which burning dyesthetic pain and lancinating sensations are prominent features. Unlike the anticonvulsant drugs, chlorpromazine may be helpful in the management of both qualities of pain. Due to the risk of serious adverse effects, such as permanent tardive dyskinesia, chlorpromazine is not a drug of first choice for neuropathic pain. It should be used after initial therapy with antidepressants, narcotics, and/or nonsteroidal anti-inflammatory drugs (NSAIDs). It is advisable to obtain informed consent before instituting chlorpromazine therapy for chronic pain management.

Pharmacokinetics

Onset: Antipsychotic/Antiemetic effects: IV/IM, within 30 minutes; PO, 30–60 minutes.
Peak Effect: Antipsychotic/Antiemetic effects: PO, 2–3 hours.
Duration of Action: Antipsychotic/Antiemetic effects: PO, 4–6 hours; PO sustained release, 10–12 hours; IM, 3–4 hours.

Interactions

Potentiates depressant effects of barbiturates, narcotics, anesthetics; additive anticholinergic effects with atropine, glycopyrrolate, and other anticholinergics; decreases hepatic metabolism and increases serum levels and pharmacologic/toxic effects of tricyclic antidepressants; neuronal uptake and antihypertensive effects of guanethidine inhibited; paradoxical hypotension with epinephrine; may potentiate neuromuscular blockade in conjunction with polypeptide antibiotics; interferes with metabolism of phenytoin and may precipitate toxicity; lithium reduces bioavailability; mephentermine, epinephrine, and thiazide diuretics potentiate chlorpromazine-induced hypotension; concomitant administration of propranolol increases plasma levels of both drugs.

Toxicity

Toxic Range: Not routinely monitored.

Manifestations: Hypotension, tardive dyskinesia (rhythmic involuntary movements of the tongue, face, mouth, or jaw), extrapyramidal symptoms (akathisia, cogwheel rigidity, oculogyric crisis), neuroleptic malignant syndrome (hyperpyrexia, muscle rigidity, altered mental status, autonomic instability).

Antidote: No specific antidote.

Management: Discontinue or reduce medication. Support ventilation and circulation (patent airway, oxygen, IV fluids, vasopressors). Phenylephrine or norepinephrine should be used to treat hypotension. Epinephrine should not be used because it may paradoxically further lower the blood pressure. Treat extrapyramidal symptoms with anticholinergic antiparkinsonian agents (e.g., benztropine IV/PO 1–2 mg two or three times daily, or trihexyphenidyl PO 5–15 mg daily) or with H_1 receptor antagonists such as diphenhydramine (IV/PO 25 mg). Treat neuroleptic malignant syndrome symptomatically and with dantrolene (IV 1.0–2.5 mg/kg every 6 hours for up to 2 days). Symptomatic treatment.

Guidelines/Precautions

1. Chlorpromazine may suppress laryngeal reflex, with possible aspiration of vomitus.
2. The drug may lower seizure threshold.
3. Use cautiously in geriatric patients; patients with glaucoma, prostatic hypertrophy, or seizure disorders; and children with acute illnesses (e.g., chickenpox, measles).
4. Neuroleptic malignant syndrome, a rare but potentially fatal side effect, may manifest with hyperpyrexia, muscle rigidity, altered mental status, and

evidence of autonomic instability (irregular pulse or blood pressure, tachycardia, diaphoresis, arrhythmias). Discontinue chlorpromazine and treat symptomatically and with dantrolene or bromocriptine (PO 2.5–10.0 mg three times daily).

5. Extrapyramidal reactions may consist of dystonic reactions, feelings of motor restlessness (akathisia), and parkinsonian signs and symptoms. Dystonic reactions occur more frequently in children, especially those with acute infections, whereas parkinsonian symptoms predominate in geriatric patients. Therapy should include discontinuation of chlorpromazine or reduction in dosage, and treatment with an anticholinergic antiparkinsonian agent (e.g., benztropine, trihexyphenidyl) or with diphenhydramine (IV/PO 25 mg). Maintenance of an adequate airway should be instituted if necessary.

6. Do not use epinephrine to treat chlorpromazine-associated hypotension. Phenothiazines cause a reversal of epinephrine's vasopressor effects (α-adrenergic effects of epinephrine are blocked, leaving unopposed β activity) and a further lowering of blood pressure. Treat the drug-induced hypotension with norepinephrine or phenylephrine.

Principal Adverse Reactions

Cardiovascular: Hypotension, tachycardia.
CNS: Extrapyramidal reactions, seizures, syncope, drowsiness.
Allergic: Urticaria, photosensitivity.
Hematologic: Agranulocytosis, hemolytic anemia.
Other: Neuroleptic malignant syndrome.

CHOLINE SALICYLATE

Class: Nonsteroidal Anti-inflammatory Drug

Use(s): Symptomatic treatment of mild to moderate pain, fever, inflammatory conditions (e.g., rheumatic fever, rheumatoid arthritis, osteoarthritis), chronic pain, and cancer pain (especially with bone metastasis).

Dosing: *Choline salicylate*

Pain and fever: PO 435–870 mg or 2.5–5.0 mL (10–15 mg/kg or 0.05–0.1 mL/kg) every 4 hours.

Inflammatory disease: PO 4.8–7.2 grams or 28–41 mL (100–140 mg/kg or 0.6–0.8 mL/kg) daily in divided doses.

Choline salicylate and magnesium salicylate

Pain and fever, inflammatory disease: PO 1.0–1.5 grams (25 mg/kg twice daily).

Dosage of combination preparations is expressed in terms of salicylate content. The oral solution may be mixed with fruit juice, carbonated beverage, or water but should not be mixed with antacid.

Dosage should be adjusted according to the patient's response, tolerance, and serum salicylate levels. Administer analgesic regularly (not as needed). Addition of opioid analgesics, antidepressant agents, and use of nondrug therapies such as transcutaneous electrical nerve stimulation (TENS) may enhance analgesia (see pages xxvi–xliv for drug combinations). In rheumatoid arthritis or juvenile rheumatoid arthritis, second-line rheumatoid agents may include leflunomide (Arava), etanercept (Enbrel), antimalarials, or methotrexate. In geriatric patients and patients with decreased renal or hepatic function, decrease doses by one-third to one-half. The incidence of choline salicylate–induced gastropathy may be decreased by concomitant administration of antacids or sucralfate (PO 1 g four times daily). Misoprostol (PO 100–200 µg four times daily) may be used to prevent gastric ulcers in high-risk patients.

Elimination: Hepatic, renal.

Preparations

Choline salicylate **(Arthropan):** Oral solution: 870 mg/ 5 mL.

Choline salicylate with magnesium salicylate **(Trisilate)**
   Oral solution: Salicylate content 500 mg/5 mL (choline salicylate 293 mg/5 mL and magnesium salicylate 362 mg/5 mL).
   Tablets: Salicylate content 500 mg (choline salicylate 293 mg and magnesium salicylate 362 mg).
   Tablets, film coated: Salicylate content 750 mg (choline salicylate 440 mg and magnesium salicylate 544 mg); salicylate content 1000 mg (choline salicylate 587 mg and magnesium salicylate 725 mg).

Pharmacology

Choline salicylate, a nonsteroidal anti-inflammatory drug (NSAID), is a salt of salicylic acid. It is structurally and pharmacologically similar to the other salicylate salts (e.g., magnesium salicylate, sodium salicylate). The analgesic and anti-inflammatory activity of choline salicylate may be mediated by inhibition of the biosynthesis and release of prostaglandins that sensitize C fibers' nociceptors to mechanical stimuli and chemical mediators (e.g., bradykinin, histamine), and that may interfere with the endogenous descending pathways that inhibit pain transmission. Choline salicylate irreversibly acetylates and inactivates cyclooxygenase (prostaglandin synthetase), an enzyme that catalyzes the formation of prostaglandin precursors (endoperoxides) from arachidonic acid. The antipyretic activity of choline salicylate may occur secondary to inhibition of pyrogen-induced release of prostaglandins in the central nervous system (including the hypothalamus) and possibly to centrally mediated peripheral vasodilatation.

The analgesic, anti-inflammatory, and antipyretic effects of choline salicylate are comparable with those of aspirin. Unlike aspirin, choline salicylate (and other salicylate salts) do not inhibit platelet aggregation and should not be substituted for aspirin in the prophylaxis of thrombosis. Choline salicylate is better tolerated than aspirin and associated with less gastric mucosal abnormalities. The drug is particularly useful in patients with GI intolerance to aspirin or in patients in whom interference with normal platelet function by aspirin or other NSAIDs is undesirable. Choline salicylate (like other NSAIDs) exhibits a ceiling effect for analgesia. Exceeding recommended doses results in increased toxicity without improvement in analgesia. Inhibition of prostaglandin synthesis may result in decreased uterine tone and contractility and prolonged gestation in the parturient and premature closure of the ductus arteriosus in the fetus.

Pharmacokinetics

Onset of Action: PO, analgesic effect 5–30 minutes.
Peak Effect: PO, analgesic effect 0.5–2 hours.
Duration of Action: PO, analgesic effect 3–7 hours.

Interactions

Incidence of GI side effects increased with concomitant NSAIDs, alcohol ingestion; enhances toxicity of lithium, methotrexate, valproic acid; serum levels of choline salicylate increased by carbonic anhydrous inhibitors; decreases diuretic effects of spirinolactone; decreased serum concentration of choline salicylate with con-comitant corticosteroids; enhances hypoglycemic effects of sulfonylureas; decreases antihypertensive effects of β-adrenergic blockers, ACE inhibitors; enhances hy-potensive effects of nitroglycerin; urinary excretion of choline salicylate increased by antacids and urinary alkalinizers; absorption delayed by food, milk, and concomitant administration of activated charcoal; prostaglandin-mediated natriuretic effects of spirinolac-tone and furosemide antagonized by choline salicylate.

Toxicity

Toxic Range: Salicylic acid >250 μg/mL (mild sali-cylism); salicylic acid >400–500 μg/mL (severe toxicity).
Manifestations: *Chronic:* Tinnitus, hearing loss, dimness of vision, headache, hyperventilation, GI ulcer-ation, dyspepsia, dizziness, mental confusion, drowsi-ness, sweating, thirst, nausea and vomiting, diarrhea, tachycardia. *Acute:* In addition to the previously listed symptoms, acid-base and electrolyte disturbance, de-hydration, hyperpyrexia, oliguria, acute renal failure, hyperthermia, restlessness, irritability, vertigo, asterixis,

tremor, diplopia, delirium, mania, hallucinations, EEG abnormalities, seizures, lethargy, coma.

Antidote: None.

Management: Discontinue or reduce medication. Correct fluid, electrolyte, and acid-base disturbances. Support ventilation and circulation (patent airway, oxygen, IV fluids, vasopressors). Airway-protected, ipecac syrup–induced emesis (30 mL or 0.5 mL/kg ipecac syrup followed by 200 mL or 4 mL/kg of water or clear fluid) or gastric lavage (with drug ingestion) followed by administration of activated charcoal (PO 50–100 g or 1–2 g/kg). Forced alkaline diuresis with IV sodium bicarbonate (IV furosemide if necessary) after correction of dehydration. Hemodialysis or hemoperfusion. Symptomatic treatment.

Guidelines/Precautions

1. Avoid the use of choline salicylate in children or teenagers with influenza or chickenpox. There is an increased risk of developing Reye's syndrome, an acute life-threatening condition characterized by vomiting, lethargy, delirium, and coma.
2. Discontinue use of the drug if dizziness, tinnitus, or hearing loss occurs. Tinnitus may herald the approach of salicylate levels to the upper limit of the therapeutic range. The temporary hearing loss remits gradually upon discontinuation of choline salicylate.
3. Salicylate salts should not be used for self-medication of fever longer than 3 days in adults or children, or for self-medication of pain for longer than 10 days in adults or 5 days in children unless directed by a physician.

4. Use with caution in patients with hepatic/renal dysfunction, active GI lesions (e.g., erosive gastritis, peptic ulcer), or a history of recurrent GI lesions. Choline salicylate may precipitate renal failure in patients with impaired renal function, heart failure, or liver dysfunction.
5. Electrolyte-containing salicylate salts (e.g., sodium salicylate or magnesium salicylate) should be used with caution in patients for whom a high sodium or magnesium intake would be harmful (e.g., patients with congestive heart failure and acute renal failure, respectively).
6. Patient response to NSAIDs is variable. Patients who do not respond to or cannot tolerate choline salicylate may be successfully treated with another NSAID.
7. Contraindicated in patients with previously demonstrated hypersensitivity to choline salicylate, or with the complete or partial syndrome of nasal polyps, angioedema, or bronchospastic reactivity to aspirin or other NSAIDs.
8. The antipyretic and anti-inflammatory effects of choline salicylate may mask signs and symptoms of infection or other disease.
9. Monitor stool for blood every 14 days, and monitor BUN, serum creatinine, and urinalysis every 1–2 months when administering choline salicylate at chronic high doses.

Principal Adverse Reactions

Cardiovascular: Vasodilatation, pallor, angina.
Pulmonary: Dyspnea, asthma.
CNS: Drowsiness, dizziness, headache, sweating, depression, euphoria.

Gastrointestinal: Ulceration, bleeding, dyspepsia, nausea, vomiting, diarrhea, hepatic dysfunction.

Genitourinary: Dysuria, interstitial nephritis, renal papillary necrosis.

Dermatologic: Pruritus, urticaria.

Hematologic: Leukopenia, thrombocytopenia, purpura, decreased plasma iron concentration, shortened erythrocyte survival time, prolongation of bleeding time.

CIMETIDINE

Class: Histamine H_2 Blocker

Use(s): Treatment of peptic ulcer, pathologic hypersecretory states; prophylaxis against acid pulmonary aspiration, stress ulcers, upper GI bleeding in critically ill patients.

Dosing: PO: 300 mg (7.5 mg/kg) every 6–8 hours; alternately, 400–1600 mg at bedtime.

Slow IV/IM: 300 mg (7.5 mg/kg) every 6–8 hours. Dilute IV dose in 20 mL D5W or normal saline (15 mg/mL) and infuse over 2 minutes.

Infusion: 50 mg/hr.

Elimination: Renal, hepatic.

Preparations

Cimetidine hydrochloride **(Tagamet)**
  Tablets: 200 mg, 300 mg, 400 mg, 800 mg.
  Oral solution: 60 mg/mL.
  Injection: 150 mg/mL.

Dilution for Infusion: 50 mg in 50 mL D5W or normal saline (concentration 5 mg/mL; rate 10 mL/hr).

Pharmacology

Cimetidine is a competitive histamine H_2 receptor antagonist that blocks the effects of histamine, pentagastrin, and acetylcholine on gastric acid secretion. It has no significant effect on gastric emptying time, volume, lower esophageal sphincter tone, or pancreatic secretions. Like ranitidine, it will not reduce the pH of gastric fluid already present in the stomach, but it will increase the pH of fluid produced thereafter.

Pharmacokinetics

Onset: PO/IV, <45 minutes.
Peak Effect: PO/IV, 60–90 minutes.
Duration of Action: PO, 6–8 hours; IV, 4–4.5 hours.

Interactions

May inhibit metabolism of benzodiazepines, caffeine, calcium channel blockers, carbamazepine, chloroquine, labetalol, lidocaine, metoprolol, metronidazole, pentoxifylline, phenytoin, propranolol, quinidine, quinine, sulfonylureas, theophyllines, triamterene, tricyclic antidepressants, coumarin anticoagulants; decreases renal tubular secretion of procainamide; may decrease serum concentrations of digoxin; may decrease effects of tocainide; increases the neuromuscular blocking effects of succinylcholine and nondepolarizing muscle relaxants; absorption of cimetidine may be decreased by antacids, anticholinergics, metoclopramide.

Toxicity

Toxic Range: Not routinely monitored.
Manifestations: Tachycardia, respiratory failure, headache, delirium, psychosis.

Antidote: No specific antidote.

Management: Discontinue or reduce medication. Support ventilation and circulation (patent airway, oxygen, IV fluids). Treat tachycardia with a β-blocker (e.g., esmolol IV 10–40 mg or propranolol IV 0.5–3 mg). Remove ingested drug by induced emesis. Symptomatic treatment.

Guidelines/Precautions

1. Rapid IV administration may produce hypotension, bradycardia, or heart block.
2. Use with caution in elderly patients because it may produce central nervous system dysfunction (e.g., confusion, agitation, seizures).
3. May increase airway resistance in patients with bronchial asthma, reflecting loss of H_2 receptor–mediated bronchodilatation, leaving unopposed H_1 receptor–mediated bronchoconstriction.

Principal Adverse Reactions

Cardiovascular: Bradycardia, arrhythmias.

CNS: Dizziness, somnolence, confusion, disorientation, seizures.

Gastrointestinal: Diarrhea.

Dermatologic: Rash.

Musculoskeletal: Arthralgia.

Endocrinologic: Gynecomastia.

Hematologic: Agranulocytosis, aplastic anemia, thrombocytopenia.

Renal: Minor reversible elevations of serum creatinine concentration.

CLONAZEPAM

Class: Benzodiazepine

Use(s): Anticonvulsant, adjunct treatment of neuro-pathic pain (e.g., phantom limb), reflex sympathetic dystrophy (chronic regional pain syndrome), trigeminal and other cranial neuralgias, migraine or cluster headache; treatment of panic disorder and restless legs syndrome; treatment of myoclonus.

Dosing: *Seizure control*

Initial: PO 1.5 mg (0.01–0.03 mg/kg) daily in two or three divided doses.

Maintenance: PO 1.5–20.0 mg daily in two or three divided doses. Doses should be titrated upward in increments of 0.5–1.0 mg every third day until seizure control is achieved with minimal adverse effects.

Neuropathic pain/panic disorder/myoclonus:
PO 0.25 mg twice daily, increasing to 1 mg/day after 3 days in most patients. Doses should be titrated upwards in incre-ments of 0.5–1.0 mg every third day.

Maximum daily dose is 4 mg.

The brand Clonopin is superior to the generic form. For predictable therapeutic efficacy, do not prescribe generic formulation of anticonvulsant drugs.

Elimination: Hepatic, renal.

Preparations

Clonazepam **(Clonopin):** Tablets: 0.5 mg, 1 mg, 2 mg.

Pharmacology

This benzodiazepine produces a dose-related sedation, relief of anxiety, and skeletal muscle relaxation. Like other benzodiazepines, the action of the drug is mediated in the brain by γ-aminobutyric acid (GABA), an inhibitory neurotransmitter. Clonazepam, more than any other benzodiazepine, is used alone or with other drugs as an anticonvulsant. In chronic pain syndromes, the pain threshold may be increased by relief of anxiety and agitation. Clonazepam does not have intrinsic analgesic activity and should be used in combination with analgesics (e.g., opioids, NSAIDs, antidepressant agents). As an adjunct, clonazepam is effective in the relief of acute muscle spasm, lancinating or burning neuropathic pain, and concomitant chronic pain and anxiety. Clonazepam relieves myoclonic activity associated with high-dose opioid therapy. Clonazepam alone or in combination with baclofen may relieve the syndrome of painful legs and involuntary movement of the toes that may result from ephatic transmission in damaged nerve roots secondary to spinal cord or cauda equina trauma, lumbar radiculopathy, injury to the feet, peripheral neuropathy, or drug therapy. Clonazepam produces minimal depressant effects on ventilation and circulation in the absence of other CNS depressant drugs. The drug is intermediate in speed of onset compared with other benzodiazepines.

Pharmacokinetics

Onset of Action: PO, 20–30 minutes.
Peak Effect: PO, 1–2 hours.
Duration of Action: PO, 6–10 hours.

Interactions

CNS and circulatory depressant effects potentiated by alcohol, narcotics, sedatives, barbiturates, phenothiazines, MAO inhibitors, and volatile anesthetics; decreases requirements for volatile anesthetics; effects antagonized by flumazenil.

Toxicity

Toxic Range: Not routinely monitored.
Manifestations: Respiratory depression, apnea, hypotension, confusion, coma, seizures.
Antidote: Flumazenil IV 0.2–2.0 mg.
Management: Discontinue or reduce medication. Support ventilation and circulation (patent airway, oxygen, IV fluids, vasopressors). Administer antidote. Symptomatic treatment. Airway-protected, ipecac syrup–induced emesis (30 mL or 0.5 mL/kg ipecac syrup followed by 200 mL or 4 mL/kg of water or clear fluid) or gastric lavage (with drug ingestion) followed by administration of activated charcoal (PO 50–100 g or 0.5–1.0 g/kg). Hemodialysis is not useful. Treat withdrawal hyperactivity with low-dose barbiturate.

Guidelines/Precautions

1. Intra-arterial injection may produce arteriospasm resulting in gangrene. Treat with local infiltration of phentolamine (5–10 mg in 10 mL normal saline) and, if necessary, sympathetic block.
2. Use with caution in elderly patients because excessive sedation and hypoventilation may occur.
3. The drug is not for use in children younger than 12 years.

4. Patients should be warned that clonazepam may impair their ability to perform activities requiring mental alertness or physical coordination (e.g., operating heavy machinery, driving a motor vehicle). Patients should be advised that clonazepam may produce psychological and physical dependence and they should consult with their physician before increasing or abruptly discontinuing the drug.

5. Contraindicated in patients with known hypersensitivity to benzodiazepines or any ingredients in the parenteral formulation (i.e., polyethylene glycol, propylene glycol, or benzyl alcohol) and in patients with acute close-angle glaucoma.

6. Clonazepam is subject to control under the Federal Controlled Substances Act of 1970 as a Schedule IV (C-IV) drug.

7. The abrupt withdrawal of clonazepam, particularly in patients on long-term, high-dose therapy, may precipitate status epilepticus. Therefore, when discontinuing clonazepam, gradual withdrawal is essential.

Principal Adverse Reactions

Cardiovascular: Hypotension, hypertension, bradycardia, tachycardia.
Pulmonary: Respiratory depression.
CNS: Sedation, dizziness, weakness, depression, agitation, amnesia.
Psychological: Hysteria, psychosis.
Gastrointestinal: Change in appetite.
Other: Visual disturbances, urticaria, pruritus.

CLONIDINE HYDROCHLORIDE

Class: α_2-Agonist

Use(s): Supplemental relief (in combination with opioids) of pain and muscle spasm in fibromyalgia, and back, chronic, cancer, and neuropathic pain; treatment of hypertension; migraine prophylaxis; treatment of opioid/alcohol withdrawal states; epidural/spinal analgesia; prolongation of duration of action of local anesthetics.

Dosing: *Premedication:* PO 0.1–0.3 mg (3–5 μg/kg).

Antihypertensive: Initial dose, PO 0.05–0.1 mg twice daily (morning and bedtime). Maintenance dose, PO 0.05–0.2 mg two to four times daily. Use lower doses in geriatric patients.

Migraine prophylaxis: PO 0.025–0.1 mg two or three times daily (children: 0.5–2.0 μg/kg/day).

Detoxification: PO 0.1–0.3 mg three or four times daily. Titrate to patient response and tolerance.

Hypertensive crisis: IV 0.15–0.3 mg over 5 minutes.

Supplementation of analgesia

PO: 0.025–0.1 mg two to four times daily (0.05–0.4 mg/day).

Transdermal: 0.1–0.3 mg/day. Replace systems every 7 days. Dosage adjustments may be made at weekly intervals. The transdermal system provides reliable delivery of clonidine for 7 days. Therapeutic plasma levels are achieved after

2–3 days. Therapeutic levels persist for about 8 hours following removal of the systems, then decline over several days.

IV

> Bolus: 0.1–0.2 mg (2–4 μg/kg) over 5 minutes.
>
> Infusion: 0.05–0.1 mg/hr (1–2 μg/kg/hr).

Epidural analgesia

> Bolus: 100–200 μg (2–4 μg/kg). Dilute in 10 mL preservative-free normal saline or local anesthetic.
>
> Infusion: 10–40 μg/hr (0.2–0.8 μg/kg/hr). Start infusion (concentration 2 μg/mL) at 5 mL/hr and titrate to effect.

Epidural anesthesia: Bolus: 200–500 μg (4–10 μg/kg). Dilute in 10 mL preservative-free normal saline or local anesthetic.

Spinal analgesia

> Bolus: 15–100 μg (0.3–2.0 μg/kg).
>
> Infusion: 2–8 μg/hr (0.04–0.16 μg/kg/hr) or three times the bolus dose per 24 hours.

Brachial plexus block: Add 25–150 μg (0.5–3.0 μg/kg) clonidine to 40 mL local anesthetic.

Peripheral nerve block: Dilute clonidine in local anesthetic to concentration of 5 μg/mL. Maximum dose of 100–150 μg clonidine.

Caution: Significant hypotension and sedation may occur at the high-dose ranges of clonidine (100–150 μg). Treat with intravenous fluids.

Elimination: Renal, hepatic.

Preparations

Clonidine hydrochloride **(Catapres, Combipres):** Tablets: 0.1 mg, 0.2 mg, or 0.3 mg.

Clonidine hydrochloride **(Catapres TTS):** Transdermal therapeutic system releases: 0.1, 0.2, 0.3 mg/24 hours.

Clonidine hydrochloride **(Duraclon):** Injection (epidural preparation): 100 μg/mL.

The parenteral formulation for intravenous administration is not commercially available in the United States.

Dilution for Infusion: Epidural: Use commercial epidural preparation or dilute 200 μg in 100 mL (2 μg/mL) local anesthetic (e.g., 0.125% bupivacaine) or preservative-free normal saline solution (2 μg/mL) with or without epidural morphine (0.1 mg/mL). Do not use with preservative.

Pharmacology

Clonidine is a selective agonist at the α_2-adrenoceptor with a ratio of 200:1 ($\alpha_2 : \alpha_1$). It inhibits central sympathetic outflow through activation of α_2-adrenergic receptors in the medullary vasomotor center. Clonidine decreases blood pressure, heart rate, and cardiac output and produces a dose-dependent sedation. Unlike opioids, it produces minor respiratory depression with a ceiling effect; unlike benzodiazepines, it does not enhance opioid-induced respiratory depression. Direct stimulation of peripheral α_1-adrenergic receptors results in transient vasoconstriction. Rebound hypertension occurs when therapy is discontinued abruptly. Clonidine suppresses signs and symptoms of opioid withdrawal by replacing opioid-mediated inhibition with α_2-mediated inhibition of central nervous system sympathetic activity.

The analgesic activity of clonidine may be mediated by attenuation of noxious stimulus-evoked and α_2-mediated neuronal firing. Epidural/intrathecal clonidine produces analgesia by acting on α_2-adrenoceptors located in the dorsal horn neurons of the spinal cord. Local effects may include inhibition of the release of nociceptive neurotransmitters such as substance P (presynaptic first-order neurons) and decrease in the rate of depolarization (postsynaptic second-order neurons). These effects, which are separate from opiate-mediated analgesia, are not inhibited by opiate antagonists (e.g., naloxone) but are blocked by α_2-antagonist drugs (e.g., phentolamine). Epidural/spinal analgesia with clonidine may be accompanied by sensory and motor blockade. This may be due to membrane-stabilizing effects on neurons similar to that of local anesthetics. Compared with opioids, epidural clonidine is more effective in patients with neuropathic pain. As an analgesic adjunct, clonidine reduces requirements for opioids, prolongs regional block, and enhances postoperative analgesia. Clonidine (oral, transdermal, intrathecal) may be effective in the treatment of fibromyalgia and spasticity (alone or combined with baclofen), presumably by α_2-adrenergic-mediated presynaptic inhibition of spinal motor neurons. Clonidine (like tizanidine) mediates gastric mucosal protection and may reduce the incidence of NSAID-induced gastric irritation.

Pharmacokinetics

Onset of Action: PO (hypotensive effect), 30–60 minutes. IV (hypotensive effect), <5 minutes. Epidural/spinal (analgesia), <15 minutes. Transdermal (hypotensive effect), <2 days.

Peak Effect: PO (hypotensive effect), 2–4 hours. Transdermal (hypotensive effect), 2–3 days. IV (hypotensive effect), 30–60 minutes.

Duration of Action: PO (hypotensive effect), 8 hours. IV (hypotensive effect), >4 hours. Epidural/spinal (analgesia and sedation), 3–4 hours. Transdermal (hypotensive effect): 7 days.

Interactions

Potentiates effects of opioids, alcohol, barbiturates, sedatives; augments pressor response to intravenous ephedrine; decreased effects with α_2-antagonists, tricyclic antidepressants; addition of clonidine to epidural or spinal anesthetics or narcotics prolongs duration of sensory and motor block and may be accompanied by hypotension and bradycardia; addition of clonidine to local anesthetics results in prolonged anesthesia and analgesia.

Toxicity

Toxic Range: Serum levels >4.5 ng/mL.

Manifestations: Hypotension, postural hypotension, transient hypertension, sedation, tachycardia, hypoventilation, dryness of the mouth.

Antidote: No specific antidote.

Management: Discontinue or reduce medication. Remove all transdermal systems. Support ventilation and circulation (patent airway, oxygen, IV fluids, vasopressors). Remove ingested drug by induced emesis or airway-protected lavage followed by activated charcoal. Respiratory depression, hypotension, and/or coma may be treated with naloxone. Monitor blood pressure because the administration of naloxone has occasionally resulted in paradoxical hypertension. Hypotension is usually responsive to intravenous fluids and, if necessary, parenterally administered epinephrine. Reverse initial hypertension with α-adrenergic blockers such as phentolamine or tolazoline (IV 10 mg at 30-minute intervals). Symptomatic treatment.

Guidelines/Precautions

1. Sudden cessation of clonidine therapy may result in rebound hypertension, nervousness, agitation, and tremor. Discontinuation for 6 hours or more prior to surgery may result in perioperative hypertension. These reactions appear to be greater after administration of high doses or continuation of concomitant β-blocker therapy. Caution is therefore advised. These reactions may be minimized by tapered withdrawal of the drug over 2 to 4 days. If therapy is to be discontinued in a patient receiving a β-blocker and clonidine concurrently, the β-blocker should be withdrawn several days before the gradual discontinuation of clonidine.
2. Rebound hypertension following discontinuation of clonidine may be treated by administration of clonidine or intravenous phentolamine.
3. Use clonidine with caution in patients with severe coronary insufficiency, recent myocardial infarction, cerebrovascular disease, chronic renal failure, Raynaud's disease, thromboangiitis obliterans, or a history of mental depression.
4. Epidural or spinal clonidine (>10 μg/kg) may produce dose-dependent maternal and fetal bradycardia.
5. Epidural, caudal, or intrathecal injections should be

avoided when the patient has septicemia, infection at the injection site, or coagulopathy. Administration of epidural clonidine above the C4 dermatome is contraindicated because there are no adequate safety data to support such use.

6. Epidural clonidine is not recommended for obstetrical, postpartum, or perioperative pain management. It is not recommended in most patients with severe cardiovascular disease. The risk of hemodynamic instability, especially hypotension and bradycardia, from epidural clonidine may be unacceptable in these patients.

7. Clonidine transdermal system is contraindicated in patients with known hypersensitivity to clonidine or to any ingredient or component in the administration system.

8. Patients receiving epidural clonidine from a continuous infusion device should be closely monitored for the first few days to assess their response.

9. Do not add preservative to epidural clonidine solution.

Principal Adverse Reactions

Cardiovascular: Hypotension, bradycardia, rebound hypertension with drug withdrawal, congestive heart failure, atrioventricular block.

Pulmonary: Mild ventilatory depression, upper respiratory tract obstruction.

CNS: Sedation, depression, anxiety.

Genitourinary: Impotence, urinary retention.

Gastrointestinal: Nausea, vomiting, parotid pain.

Dermatologic: Rash, angioneurotic edema.

COCAINE HYDROCHLORIDE

Class: Topical Anesthetic

Use(s): Topical anesthesia and vasoconstrictor (mucous membranes only).

Dosing: Topical: 1 mg/kg (1–4% solution).
Nasal: 1–2 mL each nostril (1–4% solution).
Concentrations greater than 4% are not advisable and increase potential for systemic toxic reactions. Maximum safe dose: 1.5 mg/kg.

Elimination: Plasma cholinesterase, hepatic.

Preparations

Cocaine hydrochloride **(Cocaine)**
Solvets (soluble tablets): 135 mg with lactose.
Topical solution: 4% and 10%.
Powder: 5 g, 25 g.

Pharmacology

A naturally occurring alkaloid and a topical anesthetic, cocaine stabilizes the neuronal membrane, preventing the initiation and transmission of nerve impulses. Sympathetically mediated vasoconstriction occurs secondary to a block in the uptake of catecholamines (norepinephrine, dopamine) at adrenergic nerve endings. Small doses initially produce bradycardia and a decrease in arterial pressure by central vagal stimulation, but after moderate doses blood pressure and heart rate increase. Cocaine produces uterine vasoconstriction and may significantly decrease uterine blood flow. It stimulates the central nervous system, including the vomiting center, and produces euphoria.

Pharmacokinetics

Onset of Action: <1 minute.
Peak Effect: 2–5 minutes.
Duration of Action: 30–120 minutes.

Interactions

Causes sloughing of corneal epithelium and raises intraocular pressure; potentiates arrhythmogenic effects of sympathomimetics.

Toxicity

Toxic Range: Not routinely monitored.
Manifestations: Seizures, dizziness, cyanosis, methemoglobinemia, hypertension, tachycardia, tachypnea, hypersensitivity reactions (itching, erythema, excoriation, edema), arrhythmias, cardiac arrest.
Antidote: No specific antidote.
Management: Discontinue or reduce medication. Support ventilation and circulation (patent airway, oxygen, IV fluids). Vasopressors may be hazardous. Benzodiazepines (diazepam IV 0.05–0.2 mg/kg, midazolam IV/IM 0.025–0.1 mg/kg) or barbiturates (thiopental sodium IV 0.5–2.0 mg/kg) to control seizures. Treat tachycardia and hypertension with a cardioselective β-blocker (e.g., esmolol IV 10–40 mg), an α-adrenergic blocker (e.g., phentolamine IV 5 mg), or with a calcium channel blocker (e.g., verapamil IV 2.5–10.0 mg). Use of a nonselective β-blocker may result in paradoxical hypertension due to blocking of $β_2$-vasodilating effects and unopposed α-vasoconstricting effects of accumulated catecholamines. Treat sodium channel blockade–induced QRS prolongation with sodium bicarbonate IV 1–2 mEq/kg. Remove ingested drug by airway-protected induced emesis or gastric lavage (with

drug ingestion) followed by activated charcoal. Treat methemoglobinemia with methylene blue. Hypersensitivity reactions: Remove from further exposure and treat dermatitis.

Guidelines/Precautions

1. This drug is not for intraocular or intravenous use.
2. Cocaine sensitizes the heart to catecholamines. Concomitant use with epinephrine is dangerous and unnecessary.
3. In some patients, even small doses of 0.4 mg/kg may cause hypertension, ventricular fibrillation, and cardiac arrest.
4. Use with caution in patients with severely traumatized mucosa and sepsis in the region of proposed application.
5. The drug has a high addiction potential. Cocaine is subject to control under the Controlled Substances Act of 1970 as a Schedule II (C-II) drug.

Principal Adverse Reactions

Cardiovascular: Hypertension, bradyarrhythmia and tachyarrhythmia, ventricular fibrillation.
Pulmonary: Tachypnea, respiratory failure.
CNS: Euphoria, excitement, seizures.
Ocular: Sloughing of corneal epithelium.

CODEINE PHOSPHATE/CODEINE SULFATE

Class: Narcotic Agonist and Antitussive

Use(s): Treatment of acute, chronic, and cancer pain; treatment of coughing induced by chemical or mechanical irritation of the respiratory system.

Dosing: *Analgesia:* PO/IM/IV/SC, 15–60 mg (0.5 mg/kg) every 4 hours. Maximum daily dose 120 mg.

Antitussive: PO/IM/IV/SC, 10–20 mg (0.3 mg/kg) every 4–6 hours. Maximum daily dose 120 mg.

Administer analgesic regularly (not as needed). Due to impaired elimination, accumulation and excess sedation may occur in patients with renal or hepatic dysfunction. Analgesia may be enhanced by addition of adjuvant drugs such as nonsteriodal anti-inflammatory drugs (NSAIDs) and antidepressant agents (see pages xxvi–xliv for drug combinations) and use of nondrug therapies such as transcutaneous electrical nerve stimulation (TENS).

Elimination: Hepatic, renal.

Preparations

Codeine sulfate **(Codeine Sulfate)**
Tablets: 15 mg, 30 mg, 60 mg.
Tablets, soluble: 15 mg, 30 mg, 60 mg.
Codeine phosphate **(Codeine Phosphate)**
Tablets, soluble: 15 mg, 30 mg, 60 mg.
Oral solution: 15 mg/5 mL.
Injection: 30 mg/mL, 60 mg/mL.
Codeine phosphate and acetaminophen **(Tylenol with Codeine No. 2):** Tablets: Codeine phosphate 15 mg and acetaminophen 325 mg.
Codeine phosphate and acetaminophen **(Tylenol with Codeine No. 3):** Tablets: Codeine phosphate 30 mg and acetaminophen 325 mg.

Codeine phosphate and acetaminophen **(Tylenol with Codeine No. 4):** Tablets: Codeine phosphate 60 mg and acetaminophen 325 mg.

Codeine phosphate and acetaminophen **(Phenaphen with Codeine No. 2):** Tablets: Codeine phosphate 15 mg and acetaminophen 325 mg.

Codeine phosphate and acetaminophen **(Phenaphen with Codeine No. 3):** Tablets: Codeine phosphate 30 mg and acetaminophen 325 mg.

Codeine phosphate and acetaminophen **(Phenaphen with Codeine No. 4):** Tablets: Codeine phosphate 60 mg and acetaminophen 325 mg.

Codeine phosphate and acetaminophen **(Phenaphen 650 with Codeine):** Tablets: Codeine phosphate 30 mg and acetaminophen 650 mg.

Codeine phosphate and acetaminophen **(Tylenol with Codeine):** Elixir: Codeine phosphate 12 mg/5 mL and acetaminophen 120 mg/5 mL.

Codeine phosphate and acetaminophen **(Capital and Codeine):** Suspension: Codeine phosphate 12 mg/5 mL and acetaminophen 120 mg/5 mL.

Pharmacology

A synthetic phenanthrene derivative opiate agonist and antitussive, codeine differs from morphine by the substitution of a methyl group for the hydroxyl group on the third carbon atom. Ten percent of administered codeine is demethylated in the liver to morphine, which may be responsible for the mild analgesic effects. Codeine is often used in combination with non-narcotic analgesics (e.g., aspirin, acetaminophen) for the treatment of mild to moderate pain. Oral codeine IM 20 mg or codeine IM 13 mg is equivalent in analgesic efficacy to 6mg of oral morphine. Codeine is an effective anti-tussive and is widely used as a cough suppressant. Abuse liability is less than that of morphine and occurs rarely after oral analgesic use. Codeine produces minimal sedation, nausea, vomiting, and constipation. Codeine crosses the placental barrier and may produce depression in the neonate. The drug may appear in breast milk, but at usual doses the effects on the infant may not be clinically significant. The intravenous route is not recommended due to the increased likelihood of histamine-induced hypotension.

Pharmacokinetics

Onset of Action: PO, 15–30 minutes.
Peak Effect: PO, 30–60 minutes.
Duration of Action: PO, 3–6 hours.

Interactions

Potentiates CNS and circulatory depressant effects of other narcotic analgesics, volatile anesthetics, pheno-thiazines, sedative-hypnotics, alcohol, and tricyclic anti-depressants; analgesia is enhanced and prolonged by narcotic and non-narcotic analgesics (e.g., aspirin, acetaminophen) and α_2-agonists (e.g., clonidine).

Toxicity

Toxic Range: Not routinely monitored.
Manifestations: Somnolence, coma, respiratory arrest, apnea, cardiac arrhythmias, combined respiratory and metabolic acidosis, circulatory collapse, cardiac arrest, death.
Antidote: Naloxone IV/IM/SC 0.4–2.0mg. Repeat dose every 2 to 3 minutes to a maximum of 10–20mg.
Management: Discontinue or reduce medication.

Support ventilation and circulation (patent airway, oxygen, IV fluids, vasopressors). Administer antidote. Monitor blood gases, pH, and electrolytes. Correct acidosis and electrolyte disturbance (lactic acidosis may require sodium bicarbonate IV 1–2 mEq/kg). Symptomatic treatment. Airway-protected, ipecac syrup–induced emesis (30 mL or 0.5 mL/kg ipecac syrup followed by 200 mL or 4 mL/kg of water or clear fluid) or gastric lavage (with drug ingestion) followed by administration of activated charcoal (PO 50–100 g or 1–2 g/kg).

Guidelines/Precautions

1. Reduce dosage in elderly patients and with concomitant use of narcotics and sedative hypnotics.
2. Prescribe or supply an antiemetic (e.g., metoclopramide) for use in the event of nausea and/or vomiting.
3. Constipation may be more difficult to control than pain. Prevent and/or treat by daily administration of laxatives and stool softeners, for example, Colace (docusate sodium) 100–300 mg/day. Do not administer bulk-forming agents that contain methylcellulose, psyllium, or polycarbophil. Temporary arrest in the passage through the gastrointestinal tract may lead to fecal impaction or bowel obstruction.
4. Tolerance may develop in all patients taking narcotic analgesics for more than a couple of weeks. It may be a function of dose, frequency, and route of administration because IV and spinal infusions of narcotics are associated with rapid development of tolerance. The first sign is a decrease in duration of effective analgesia. To

delay the development of tolerance, add adjuvant drugs (e.g., NSAIDs, antidepressant agents, dextromethorphan), or switch to alternative opioids (starting at one-half the equianalgesic dose), or supplement with nondrug therapies such as TENS.

5. Physical dependence may be revealed with abrupt discontinuation of chronically administered opioids (>2 weeks). Withdrawal symptoms may manifest by anxiety, nervousness, irritability, chills alternating with hot flashes, diaphoresis, insomnia, abdominal cramps, nausea, vomiting, and myoclonus. To avoid withdrawal, doses should be reduced slowly (e.g., dose reduction of 75% every 2 days). Withdrawal should be treated symptomatically.

6. Addiction (psychological dependence) is characterized by a continued craving for a narcotic and the need to use the narcotic for effects other than for pain relief. The patient exhibits drug-seeking behavior. Most patients with psychological dependence are also physically dependent, but the reverse is rare in patients using narcotics for the management of pain.

7. Drug combinations with adjuvant drugs enhance analgesia (see pages xxvi–xliv).

8. Adjuvant drug therapies also include regional blockade, trigger-point injections (with local anesthetics and steroids), and intravenous regional anesthesia.

9. Adjuvant nondrug therapies include TENS and modalities such as ice or heat application, ultrasound, and soft tissue mobilization.

10. Patients should be warned that codeine may

impair their ability to perform hazardous tasks requiring mental alertness or physical coordination (e.g., driving a motor vehicle, operating heavy machinery).

11. The drug preparation may contain sulfites, which may cause allergic reactions or anaphylaxis in susceptible individuals.

12. Codeine is subject to control under the Federal Controlled Substances Act as a Schedule II (C-II) drug as a single entity, Schedule III (C-III) as a combination in pain medications (e.g., Tylenol with codeine), and Schedule V (C-V) when used with cough syrups (e.g., phenergan with codeine).

13. Ten percent of the population may lack the hepatic enzyme (CYP2D6) required to demethylate codeine into morphine. In these patients, codeine at any dosage will be ineffective and pain will not be relieved.

Principal Adverse Reactions

Cardiovascular: Hypotension, circulatory depression, bradycardia, syncope.

Pulmonary: Respiratory depression.

CNS: Sedation, somnolence, euphoria, dysphoria, disorientation.

Genitourinary: Urinary retention.

Gastrointestinal: Nausea, vomiting, abdominal pain, biliary tract spasm, constipation, anorexia, hepatic dysfunction.

Ocular: Miosis.

Allergic: Rash, pruritus, urticaria.

COSYNTROPIN

Class: Synthetic Hormone

Use(s): Treatment of postdural puncture headache, diagnostic agent for adrenocortical insufficiency.

Dosing: *Postdural puncture headache:* IM/SC 0.5–1.0 mg. May repeat in 24 hours.

Screening test for adrenal function: IM/IV 0.25–0.75 mg.

Reconstitute 0.25 mg cosyntropin in 1 mL of normal saline.

Elimination: Hepatic, renal.

Preparations

Cosyntropin **(Cortrosyn):** Injection: 0.25 mg. Reconstitute in 1 mL of supplied solvent (ampules of normal saline).

Pharmacology

A synthetic subunit of adrenocorticotrophic hormone (ACTH), cosyntropin is α-1-24-corticotropin. Cosyntropin exhibits the full corticosteroidogenic activity of ACTH. 0.25 mg of cosyntropin will stimulate the adrenal cortex maximally and to the same extent as 25 units of natural ACTH. In contrast to human and synthetic ACTH, which all contain 39 amino acids and exhibit similar immunologic activity, cosyntropin contains 24 amino acids and has very little immunologic activity yet retains full biologic activity. This property of cosyntropin assumes added importance in view of the known antigenicity of natural ACTH. Case reports have documented complete and permanent relief from postdural puncture headache after intravenous infusion of ACTH or IM/IV administration of cosyntropin.

Pharmacokinetics

Onset of Action: IM/IV, <30 minutes.
Peak Effect: IM/IV, 45–60 minutes.
Duration of Action: IM/IV, variable.

Interactions

May accentuate the electrolyte loss associated with diuretic therapy.

Toxicity

Toxic Range: Not routinely monitored.
Manifestations: Erythema at injection site.
Antidote: None.
Management: Discontinue or reduce medication. Symptomatic treatment.

Guidelines/Precautions

1. Cosyntropin exhibits slight immunologic activity and does not contain foreign animal protein; therefore, it is less risky to use than natural ACTH. Patients known to be sensitized to natural ACTH with markedly positive skin tests will, with few exceptions, react negatively when tested intradermally with cosyntropin. Most patients with a history of a previous hypersensitivity reaction to natural ACTH or a preexisting allergic disease will tolerate cosyntropin without incident. However, cosyntropin is not completely devoid of immunologic activity and hypersensitivity reactions are still possible, at least in susceptible patients. The physician should there-

fore be prepared prior to injection to treat any possible acute hypersensitivity reaction.
2. Cosyntropin is contraindicated in patients with a
history of a previous adverse reaction to the drug.

Principal Adverse Reactions

Cardiovascular: Hypotension, circulatory depression,
tachycardia.
Allergic: Rash, pruritus, urticaria, hypersensitivity
reactions.

DESIPRAMINE HYDROCHLORIDE

Class: Tricyclic Antidepressant

Use(s): Treatment of neurotic and endogenous depression; adjunct treatment of neuropathic pain syndromes,
including diabetic neuropathy, postherpetic neuralgia,
tic douloureux, and cancer pain; anxiety disorders;
phobias; panic disorders; enuresis; eating disorders;
attention deficit disorders.

Dosing: *Pain syndromes*
Initial: PO 50–100 mg (1–2 mg/kg) daily in
the morning or at bedtime. Titrate dose
upward every 3 to 4 weeks by increments of 25–50 mg as necessary.
Maintenance: PO 50–200 mg (1–4 mg/kg)
daily in the morning or at bedtime.
Doses should be decreased if unacceptable side effects occur. Serum levels
should be determined if there are signs
of toxicity. The higher end of the dose
range may be required in the management of painful diabetic neuropathy.

Depression

Initial: PO 75–100 mg daily in one to four divided doses.

Maintenance: PO 50–300 mg daily in one to four divided doses. Doses greater than 200 mg daily are not recommended for outpatients.

IM: 100 mg daily in divided doses. Replace with oral medication as soon as possible. Do not administer intravenously.

Doses for pain are generally smaller than those used for treatment of affective disorders. Medication should be administered on a fixed schedule and not as needed. Administration of the entire daily dose at bedtime may reduce daytime sedation. After symptoms are controlled, dosage should be gradually reduced to the lowest level that will maintain relief of symptoms. Analgesia may be enhanced by addition of opioid analgesics (see pages xxvi–xliv for drug combinations), nonsteroidal anti-inflammatory drugs (NSAIDs), and use of nondrug therapies such as transcutaneous electrical nerve stimulation (TENS). In geriatric patients and patients with decreased renal or hepatic function, decrease doses by one-third to one-half. The possibility for suicide is inherent in depression and may persist until significant remission occurs. The quantity of drug dispensed should reflect this consideration.

Elimination: Hepatic, renal.

Preparations

Desipramine hydrochloride **(Norpramin, Desipramine)**
  Tablets: 10 mg, 25 mg, 50 mg, 75 mg, 100 mg, 150 mg.
  Injection: 12.5 mg/mL.

Pharmacology

A dibenzazepine derivative and a secondary amine tricyclic antidepressant, desipramine is the active metabolite of imipramine. Antidepressant activity may be partly due to inhibition of the amine-pump uptake of norepinephrine and serotonin at the presynaptic neuron and down-regulation of β-receptor sensitivity. Desipramine has fewer side effects such as orthostatic hypotension and may be used in patients who cannot tolerate the parent drug (imipramine) or some of the other tricyclic antidepressants (e.g., amitriptyline or doxepin). Desipramine has a low incidence of anticholinergic or antihistaminic effects. It is not sedating for most patients and may even stimulate some. Thus, it may be given in the morning. Although blockade of neurotransmitter uptake may occur immediately, the initial antidepressant response may take a week. Desipramine may have a more rapid onset of action than imipramine. As with other secondary amines, patients with low norepinephrine levels respond better to desipramine compared with serotonin-deficient patients. Desipramine does not inhibit the monoamine oxidase (MAO) system.

The analgesic effects of desipramine may occur partly through the alleviation of depression, which may be responsible for increased pain suffering, but also by mechanisms that are independent of mood effects. Serotonin and norepinephrine activity may be increased in descending pain inhibitory pathways. Activation of these pathways decreases the transmission of nociceptive impulses from primary afferent neurons to first-order cells in laminae I and V of the spinal cord dorsal horn. Desipramine may also potentiate the analgesic effect of opioids by increasing their binding efficacy to opioid receptors. Desipramine has varying degrees of efficacy in different pain syndromes and may be better at relieving the burning, aching, and dyesthetic component of neuropathic pain. The drug is seldom useful in the management of lancinating, shooting paroxysmal pain.

The seizure threshold may be lowered. Therapeutic doses do not affect respiration, but toxic doses may lead to respiratory depression. The direct quinidine-like effects may manifest at toxic doses and produce cardiovascular disturbances (e.g., conduction blockade). Desipramine does not have addiction liability and its use is not associated with drug-seeking behavior. Withdrawal symptoms, including nausea, headache, and malaise, may be precipitated by acute withdrawal. Tolerance develops to the sedative and anticholinergic effects, but there are no reports of tolerance to the analgesic effects. Desipramine crosses the placenta and is excreted in breast milk. Usage in pregnant or nursing mothers should occur only if the potential benefit justifies the potential risk.

Pharmacokinetics

Onset of Action: Analgesic effect: PO, <5 days. Antidepressant effect: PO, 2–5 days.
Peak Effect: Antidepressant effect: PO, 2–3 weeks.
Duration of Action: Antidepressant effect: PO, variable.

Interactions

Increased risk of hyperthermia with concomitant administration of anticholinergics (e.g., atropine), phenothiazines, and thyroid medications; serum levels and toxic effects of desipramine increased by concomitant methylphenidate, fluoxetine, cimetidine, phenothiazines, and haloperidol; ventilatory and circulatory depressant effects of CNS depressant drugs and alcohol potentiated by desipramine; increases the pressor and cardiac effects of sympathomimetics (e.g., isoproterenol, phenylephrine, norepinephrine, epinephrine, amphetamine); decreases serum levels and pharmacologic effects of levodopa and phenylbutazone; increases serum levels and toxic effects of dicumarol; onset of therapeutic effects shortened and adverse cardiac effects of desipramine increased with concomitant administration of levothyroxine and liothyronine; fatal hyperpyretic crisis or seizures with concomitant use of MAO inhibitors; uptake-dependent efficacy of IV regional bretylium decreased by desipramine.

Toxicity

Toxic Range: Not routinely monitored. Blood and urine levels may not correlate with the degree of intoxication and are not reliable guides for clinical management.

Manifestations: *Chronic:* Dreams and sleep disturbances, akathisia, anxiety, chills, coryza, malaise, myalgia, headache, dizziness, nausea and vomiting. *Acute:* In addition to the previously listed symptoms, CNS stimulation with excitement, delirium, hallucinations, hyperreflexia, myoclonus, choreiform movements, parkinsonian symptoms, seizures, and hyperpyrexia, then CNS depression with drowsiness, areflexia, hypothermia, respiratory depression, cyanosis, hypotension, coma; peripheral anticholinergic symptoms, including urinary retention, dry mucous membranes, mydriasis, constipation, adynamic ileus; cardiac irregularities, including tachycardia, QRS prolongation; metabolic and/or respiratory acidosis; polyradiculoneuropathy; renal failure; vomiting; ataxia; dysarthria; bullous cutaneous lesions; pulmonary consolidation.

Antidote: None.

Management: Discontinue or reduce medication. Correct fluid, electrolyte, and acid-base disturbances. Airway-protected, ipecac syrup–induced emesis (30 mL or 0.5 mL/kg ipecac syrup) or gastric lavage (with drug ingestion) followed by administration of activated charcoal (PO 50–100 g or 1–2 g/kg). These purging actions should be performed even if several hours have elapsed after ingestion because the anticholinergic effects may delay gastric emptying and the drug may also be secreted into the stomach. Control seizures: IV benzodiazepines are the first choice because IV barbiturates may enhance respiratory depression; however, IV barbiturates or phenytoin may be useful in refractory seizures. Support ventilation and circulation (patent airway, oxygen, IV fluids, vasopressors). Continuous EKG monitoring. Treat cardiac arrhythmias with IV lidocaine or propranolol. Digoxin, quinidine, procainamide, and diisopyramide should be avoided because they may further depress myocardial conduction and/or contractility. Temporary pacemakers may be necessary in patients with advanced atrioventricular block, severe bradycardia, and/or life-threatening ventricular arrhythmias unresponsive to drug therapy. Control hyperpyrexia with ice packs and cooling sponge baths. Physostigmine (slow IV 1–3 mg) may be used in the treatment of life-threatening anticholinergic toxicity. Routine use of physostigmine is not advisable due to its serious adverse effects (e.g., seizures, bronchospasm, and severe bradyarrhythmias). Hemodialysis or peritoneal dialysis is ineffective because the drug is highly protein bound. Symptomatic treatment. Consider the possibility of multiple drug involvement. Counseling prior to and after discharge for patients who attempted suicide.

Guidelines/Precautions

1. To avoid withdrawal symptoms, the medication should be tapered down over a couple of weeks and not discontinued abruptly.
2. Use with caution in patients with cardiovascular disease, thyroid disease, seizure disorders, and in those in whom excessive anticholinergic activity may be harmful (e.g., patients with benign prostatic hypertrophy, a history of urinary retention, or increased intraocular pressure). The drug should be used in close-angle glaucoma only when the glaucoma is adequately controlled by drugs and closely monitored.
3. Contraindicated in patients receiving MAO inhibitors (concurrently or within the previous 2 weeks), patients in the acute recovery phase following myocardial infarction, and those with demonstrated hypersensitivity to desipramine. Cross-sensitivity with other tricyclic antidepressants may occur.
4. The drug may cause exacerbation of psychosis in schizophrenic patients.
5. Patients should be warned of the possibility of

drowsiness that may impair performance of potentially hazardous tasks such as driving an automobile or operating machinery. Persisting daytime drowsiness may be decreased by administering a lower dose, administering the dose earlier in the evening, or substituting a less sedating alternative.

Principal Adverse Reactions

Cardiovascular: Postural hypotension, arrhythmias, conduction disturbances, hypertension, sudden death.

Pulmonary: Respiratory depression.

CNS: Confusion, disorientation, extrapyramidal symptoms.

Gastrointestinal: Hepatic dysfunction, jaundice, nausea, vomiting, constipation, decrease in lower esophageal sphincter tone.

Genitourinary: Urinary retention, paradoxical nocturia, urinary frequency.

Ocular: Blurred vision, mydriasis, increased intraocular pressure.

Dermatologic: Pruritus, urticaria, petechiae, photosensitivity.

Hematologic: Leukopenia, thrombocytopenia, eosinophilia, agranulocytosis, purpura.

Endocrinologic: Increased or decreased libido, impotence, gynecomastia, SIADH.

Other: Hyperthermia.

DEXAMETHASONE

Class: Corticosteroid

Use(s): Treatment of refractory bone pain; treatment of aching, burning, lancinating neuropathic pain, severe migraine headache, malignant spinal cord compression, and pain caused by malignant lesions of the brachial and lumbosacral plexus; treatment of inflammatory diseases, cerebral edema, aspiration pneumonitis, bronchial asthma, myofascial pain with trigger points, allergic reactions; prevention of rejection in organ transplantation; replacement therapy for adrenocortical insufficiency.

Dosing: *Bone pain, neuropathic pain, plexus pain*

Initial: Dexamethasone phosphate IV 16 mg stat or dexamethasone PO 20–100 mg stat.

Maintenance: Dexamethasone PO/IV 4–8 mg every 6 hours for 1–2 weeks, then PO 1–2 mg twice daily.

Status migrainosus

Initial: Dexamethasone phosphate IV/IM 10–20 mg stat with or without an antiemetic (e.g., prochlorperazine IV 3.5 mg).

Maintenance: Dexamethasone PO/IV/IM 4–8 mg daily as needed for 1–2 weeks.

Acute epidural spinal cord compression: Dexamethasone phosphate IV 100 mg stat then IV/PO 96 mg/day in divided doses. Taper dose and maintain to minimum needed to sustain relief.

Inflammatory diseases

Dexamethasone phosphate: Intra-articular or intratissue 1–16 mg. May repeat at 1–3 weeks.

Dexamethasone acetate: IM, intra-articular, or intratissue 4–16 mg. May repeat at 1–3 weeks.

Dexamethasone phosphate: IV/IM 0.5–25 mg/day.

Cerebral edema: Dexamethasone phosphate IV 10 mg, then IM 4 mg every 6 hours or PO 1–3 mg three times daily. Taper off over 5–7 days.

Recurrent or inoperable brain tumors (relief of increased intracranial pressure): Dexamethasone phosphate IV/IM 2 mg two or three times daily.

Myofascial pain (with trigger point): Dexamethasone phosphate, intratissue 1–4 mg (dilute in 10 mL local anesthetic). May repeat at 1–3 weeks.

Bronchospasm: Dexamethasone phosphate, inhalation 300 µg (3 inhalations) three or four times daily.

Taper off dexamethasone dose if used for more than a few days. Avoid concomitant use of nonsteroidal anti-inflammatory drugs (NSAIDs).

Elimination: Hepatic.

Preparations

Dexamethasone **(Decadron, Hexadrol, Dexamethasone):** Oral solution: 0.1 mg/mL.

Dexamethasone **(Dexamethasone Intensol):** Oral solution, concentrate: 1 mg/mL.

Dexamethasone **(Decadron, Dexone, Hexadrol):** Tablets: 0.25 mg, 0.5 mg, 0.75 mg, 1.5 mg, 4 mg, 6 mg.

Dexamethasone acetate **(Decadron-L.A., Dalalone L.A., Decaject-L.A., Dekasol-L.A., Dexasone-L.A.,**

Dexone L.A., Solurex L.A., Dalalone D.P.): Parenteral suspension (IM use only): 8 mg/mL, 16 mg/mL.

Dexamethasone sodium phosphate **(Decadrol, Decadron Phosphate, Dalalone, Decaject, Dekasol, Dexacene-4, Dexasone, Hexadrol Phosphate):** Injection (IV/IM): 4 mg/mL, 10 mg/mL, 20 mg/mL.

Dexamethasone sodium phosphate **(Dexamethasone Sodium Phosphate, Hexadrol Phosphate, Decadron Phosphate):** Injection (IV use only): 20 mg/mL, 24 mg/mL.

Dexamethasone sodium phosphate and lidocaine hydrochloride **(Decadron Phosphate with Xylocaine):** Injection: Dexamethasone sodium phosphate 4 mg/mL and lidocaine hydrochloride 10 mg/mL.

Dexamethasone sodium phosphate **(Decadron Respihaler):** Aerosol: 100 μg/metered spray.

Pharmacology

Dexamethasone is a fluorinated derivative of prednisolone with potent anti-inflammatory effect. A dose of 0.75 mg is equivalent to 4 mg methylprednisolone, 5 mg prednisone, and 20 mg cortisol. Dexamethasone may decrease the number and activity of inflammatory cells, enhance the effects of β-adrenergic drugs on cyclic AMP production, and inhibit bronchoconstrictor mechanisms. At equipotent doses, dexamethasone lacks the sodium-retaining property of hydrocortisone. It may suppress the hypothalamic-pituitary-adrenal (HPA) axis. Dexamethasone is useful in the management of acute and chronic cancer pain. In metastatic bone pain, dexamethasone may interfere with the formation of prostaglandin E by inhibiting tumor-secreted phospholipase A_2, which catalyzes the release of arachidonic acid from plasma membranes. Dexamethasone may be oncolytic for certain tumors (e.g., lymphoma) and may ameliorate painful nerve or spinal cord compression by reducing edema in tumor and nerve tissue. Dexamethasone is effective in the treatment of malignant spinal cord compression. Short-term therapy (1–2 weeks) may be useful in the management of pain caused by malignant lesions of the brachial or lumbosacral plexus. In patients with severe headache and increased intracranial pressure, dexamethasone may ameliorate the pain and other neurologic symptoms. In moribund patients, dexamethasone may provide a sense of well-being, increase appetite, and relieve tumor-related pain.

Pharmacokinetics

Onset of Action: Anti-inflammatory effects: IV/IM, few minutes.
Peak Effect: Anti-inflammatory effects: IV/IM, 12–24 hours.
Duration of Action: Anti-inflammatory effects/HPA suppression: IV/IM, 36–54 hours.

Interactions

Clearance enhanced by phenytoin, phenobarbital, rifampin, ephedrine; altered response to coumarin anticoagulants; increases requirements of insulin; interacts with anticholinesterase agents (e.g., neostigmine) to produce severe weakness in patients with myasthenia gravis; potassium-wasting effects enhanced with potassium-depleting diuretics (e.g., thiazides, furosemide); diminishes response to toxoids and live or inactivated vaccines; increased risks of GI bleeding with concomitant NSAIDs.

Toxicity

Toxic Range: Not defined.

Manifestations: *Withdrawal after long-term use:* Acute adrenal insufficiency, fever, hypotension, dyspnea, dizziness, fainting, hypoglycemia. *Prolonged administration:* Cushingoid changes, moon face, central obesity, hypertension, osteoporosis, diabetes, peptic ulcer, increased susceptibility to infection, electrolyte and fluid imbalance.

Antidote: No specific antidote.

Management: Taper off or gradually reduce medication (alternate-day medication). Supplement medication during times of stress. Support ventilation and circulation (patent airway, oxygen, IV fluids, vasoactive drugs). Symptomatic treatment.

Guidelines/Precautions

1. Adrenocortical insufficiency may occur with rapid withdrawal of dexamethasone.
2. Use with caution in patients with hypertension, congestive heart failure, thromboembolytic tendencies, hypothyroidism, cirrhosis, myasthenia gravis, peptic ulcer, diverticulitis, nonspecific ulcerative colitis, fresh intestinal anastomosis, psychosis, seizure disorders, systemic fungal, or viral infections.
3. Administration of live virus vaccines (e.g., smallpox) is contraindicated in patients receiving immunosuppressive doses.
4. Avoid rapid withdrawal, which may exacerbate

pain independent of progression of systemic cancer (pseudorheumatoid syndrome).

Principal Adverse Reactions

Cardiovascular: Arrhythmias, hypertension, congestive heart failure in susceptible patients.

CNS: Seizures, increased intracranial pressure, steroid psychosis.

Dermatologic: Impaired wound healing, petechiae, erythema.

Ocular: Increased intraocular pressure, subcapsular cataracts.

Metabolic: Fluid retention, sodium retention, potassium depletion.

Endocrinologic: Secondary adrenocortical and pituitary unresponsiveness during stress; growth suppression; increased requirements for insulin.

Musculoskeletal: Myopathy, weakness, osteoporosis.

Other: Thromboembolism; diminished response to toxoids and live or inactivated vaccines; increased susceptibility to and masked symptoms of infection.

DEXTROMETHORPHAN

Class: NMDA Receptor Antagonist

Use(s): Supplementation of opioid analgesia, prevention of development of opioid tolerance, treatment of refractory somatic and neuropathic benign and malignant pain syndromes.

Dosing: PO 10–240 mg/day in divided doses; for example, 15 mg every 6 hours or 30 mg three times daily.

Dextromethorphan may be prepared in

combination with an opioid (e.g., morphine) by a compounding pharmacist. Many preparations of cough syrup contain dextromethorphan in combination with antihistamines, decongestants, and expectorants. These preparations are not recommended for use in chronic pain unless there is an indication for the other constituents of the combined preparations.

Elimination: Hepatic, renal.

Preparations

Dextromethorphan **(Diabe-Tuss DM):** Cough syrup: Dextromethorphan hydrobromide 15 mg/5 mL.

Dextromethorphan **(Delsym):** Cough syrup: Dextromethorphan polistirex (equivalent to dextromethorphan hydrobromide) 30 mg/5 mL.

Dextromethorphan **(Drixoral Cough Liquid Caps):** Oral capsules, liquid filled: Dextromethorphan hydrobromide 30 mg.

Dextromethorphan, brompheniramine, and pseudoephedrine **(Bromfed-DM, Dimetane DX):** Cough syrup: Dextromethorphan hydrobromide 10 mg/5 mL, brompheniramine maleate 2 mg/5 mL, and pseudoephedrine hydrochloride 30 mg/5 mL.

Dextromethorphan and promethazine hydrochloride **(Bromfed-DM, Dimetane DX):** Cough syrup: Dextromethorphan hydrobromide 15 mg/5 mL and phenergan hydrochloride 6.25 mg/5 mL.

Dextromethorphan and guaifenesin **(Duratuss DM):** Cough syrup: Dextromethorphan hydrobromide 20 mg/5 mL and guaifenesin 200 mg/5 mL.

Pharmacology

Dextromethorphan is the methyl ether analogue of levorphanol. The only morphine-like characteristic dextromethorphan retains is its antitussive property. The drug temporarily controls and suppresses the cough reflex by a direct action on the cough center. Dextromethorphan is a noncompetitive N-methyl D-aspartate (NMDA) receptor antagonist. The drug attenuates intracellular Ca^{2+} influx through both NMDA receptor–gated channels as well as voltage-gated Ca^{2+} channels (activated by high concentrations of extracellular K^+). Opioid tolerance requires a functional NMDA receptor, and blockade of this receptor attenuates or reverses the development of opioid tolerance. The opioid-sparing activity may enable a decrease of up to 50% in the dose of opioid required to maintain pain control with minimal side effects. Dextromethorphan suppresses NMDA-provoked seizures and NMDA-induced neuronal firing of the spinal cord. The drug also provides protection against glutamate-induced neurotoxicity. Chronic pain can lead to central sensitization—a wind-up state of abnormal neuronal excitability in the spinal cord—secondary to spinal glutamate release and NMDA-induced neuronal firing. Central sensitization can be prevented from developing by administration of an NMDA receptor antagonist. Systemic dextromethorphan suppresses the development of wind-up as assessed by the electrophysiologic responses of deep multireceptive dorsal horn neurons. Dextromethorphan binds to and blocks the NMDA receptor in a dose-dependent manner. Dextromethorphan has been used as an antitussive (alone or in com-

bination with antihistamines, decongestants, and expectorants) and has a long history of clinical safety.
Dextromethorphan may be prepared in combination
with an opioid (e.g., morphine) by a compounding
pharmacist.

Pharmacokinetics

Onset of Action: PO, 15–20 minutes.
Peak Effect: PO, variable.
Duration of Action: PO, variable.

Interactions

Serious toxicity (serotonin syndrome) with monoamine
oxidase (MAO) inhibitors; additive CNS depression
with coadministration of alcohol, antihistamines, psy-
chotropics, or other CNS depressants.

Toxicity

Toxic Range: Not defined.
Manifestations: Central excitement, mental confusion,
respiratory depression (with very high doses).
Antidote: No specific antidote.
Management: Empty stomach (emesis, gastric lavage).
Support ventilation and circulation (patent airway,
oxygen, IV fluids). Symptomatic treatment.

Guidelines/Precautions

1. Do not use dextromethorphan preparations in
   patients receiving MAO inhibitors, or prior to 14
   days after stopping the MAO inhibitor.

Principal Adverse Reactions

CNS: Dizziness, drowsiness.
Gastrointestinal: Nausea.

DIAZEPAM

Class: Benzodiazepine

Use(s): Sedation, relief of anxiety, anticonvulsant, treatment of painful leg spasms in multiple sclerosis, treatment of skeletal muscle spasticity (e.g., secondary to trauma, inflammation, upper motor neuron disease), treatment of acute alcohol withdrawal and panic attacks, adjunct treatment of trigeminal neuralgia.

Dosing: *Sedation:* PO/rectal, 5–10 mg at bedtime.
Antispasmodic: PO 5–10 mg three times daily.
Anticonvulsant
  IV: 0.05–0.2 mg/kg every 10–15 minutes. Maximum dose 30 mg.
  PO/Rectal: 2–10 mg two to four times daily.
  PO, extended release: 15–30 mg once daily.
Withdrawal
  IV: 5–10 mg (0.15–0.2 mg/kg) every 3–4 hours.
  PO: 5–10 mg three or four times daily.
  PO, extended release: 15–30 mg once daily.

Elimination: Hepatic.

Preparations

Diazepam **(Valium):** Tablets: 2 mg, 5 mg, 10 mg.
Diazepam **(Diazepam Solution):** Oral solution: 1 mg/mL.
Diazepam **(Diazepam Solution):** Solution concentrate: 5 mg/mL.
Diazepam **(Valium, Zetran):** Injection: 5 mg/mL.

Pharmacology

This benzodiazepine derivative acts on the limbic system, thalamus, and hypothalamus, inducing calming effects. Diazepam exerts antianxiety and skeletal muscle relaxing effects by increasing the availability of the glycine inhibitory neurotransmitter, whereas the sedative action reflects the ability of benzodiazepines to facilitate actions of the inhibitory neurotransmitter γ-aminobutyric acid (GABA). In chronic pain syndromes, relief of anxiety and agitation may increase the pain threshold. Reduction of muscle spasticity may lead to reduction in pain. Diazepam does not have intrinsic analgesic activity and should be used in combination with analgesics (e.g., opioids, NSAIDs, antidepressant agents). Diazepam has minimal effects on ventilation and circulation in the absence of other CNS depressant drugs. Intravenous diazepam is considered the drug of choice for termination of status epilepticus or acute seizure episodes resulting from drug overdose and poisons. Due to the short-lived effect, other agents should be used for long-term seizure control.

Pharmacokinetics

Onset of Action: IV, <2 minutes. Rectal, <10 minutes. PO, 15 minutes to 1 hour (shorter in children).
Peak Effect: IV, 3–4 minutes. PO, 1 hour.
Duration of Action: IV, 15 minutes to 1 hour. PO, 2–6 hours.

Interactions

Sedative and circulatory depressant effect potentiated by opioids, alcohol, and other CNS depressants; elimination reduced by cimetidine; reduces requirements for volatile anesthetics; thrombophlebitis with intravenous administration; decreased clearance and dosage requirements in old age; effects antagonized by flumazenil; may cause neonatal hypothermia; interacts with plastic containers and administration sets, significantly decreasing bioavailability.

Toxicity

Toxic Range: Not routinely monitored.

Manifestations: Respiratory depression, apnea, hypotension, confusion, coma, seizures.

Antidote: Flumazenil IV 0.2–2.0 mg.

Management: Discontinue or reduce medication. Support ventilation and circulation (patent airway, oxygen, IV fluids, vasopressors). Administer antidote (flumazenil IV 0.2–2.0 mg). Symptomatic treatment. Airway-protected, ipecac syrup–induced emesis (30 mL or 0.5 mL/kg ipecac syrup followed by 200 mL or 4 mL/kg of water or clear fluid) or gastric lavage (with drug ingestion) followed by administration of activated charcoal (PO 50–100 g or 0.5–1.0 g/kg). Hemodialysis is not useful. Treat withdrawal hyperactivity with low-dose barbiturate.

Guidelines/Precautions

1. Diazepam is contraindicated in acute narrow-angle or open-angle glaucoma unless patients are receiving appropriate therapy. The drug is also contraindicated in patients with known hypersensitivity to benzodiazepines or any ingredients in the parenteral formulation (i.e., polyethylene glycol, propylene glycol, or benzyl alcohol).
2. Reduce dose in elderly patients, in patients with

limited pulmonary reserve, and with concomitant use of narcotics and other sedatives.
3. Use slow injection through large veins to reduce thrombophlebitis.
4. Return of drowsiness may occur 6–8 hours after dose due to enterohepatic recirculation.
5. IM route is painful and results in slow, erratic absorption.
6. Do not mix or dilute with other solutions or drugs.
7. Patients should be warned that diazepam may impair their ability to perform activities requiring mental alertness or physical coordination (e.g., operating heavy machinery, driving a motor vehicle).
8. Diazepam is subject to control under the Federal Controlled Substances Act of 1970 as a Schedule IV (C-IV) drug.

Principal Adverse Reactions

Cardiovascular: Bradycardia, hypotension.
Pulmonary: Respiratory depression.
CNS: Drowsiness, ataxia, confusion, depression, paradoxical excitement.
Genitourinary: Incontinence.
Dermatologic: Skin rash.
Other: Venous thrombosis and phlebitis at site of injection, dry mouth.

DICLOFENAC SODIUM

Class: Nonsteroidal Anti-inflammatory Drug

Use(s): Symptomatic treatment of mild to moderate inflammatory and degenerative arthritis, primary dysmenorrhea, postoperative and posttraumatic pain, chronic pain, and cancer pain (especially with bone metastasis).

Dosing: *Pain and inflammatory disease:*

> PO: 50 mg two to four times daily.
>
> PO, delayed release: 75 mg twice daily.
>
> PO, extended release: 100 mg once or twice daily.
>
> Maximum dose: 200 mg daily.
>
> Arthrotec 50: PO 1 tablet three to four times daily.
>
> Arthrotec 75: PO 1 tablet twice daily.
>
> Administer analgesic regularly (not as needed). Addition of opioid analgesics, antidepressant agents, and use of nondrug therapies such as transcutaneous electrical nerve stimulation (TENS) may enhance analgesia (see pages xxvi–xliv for drug combinations). In rheumatoid arthritis or juvenile rheumatoid arthritis, second-line rheumatoid agents may include leflunomide (Arava), etanercept (Enbrel), antimalarials or methotrexate. The incidence of diclofenac-induced gastropathy may be decreased by administration with meals, milk, antacids, or sucralfate (PO 1 g four times daily). Misoprostol (PO 100–200 µg four times daily) may be used to prevent gastric ulcers in high-risk patients.

Elimination: Hepatic, renal.

Preparations

Diclofenac potassium immediate release **(Cataflam):** Tablets: 50 mg.

Diclofenac sodium **(Voltaren):** Tablets: 25 mg, 50 mg, 75 mg.

Diclofenac sodium extended release **(Voltaren XR):** Tablets 100 mg.

Diclofenac sodium and misoprostol **(Arthrotec 50):** Tablets: Diclofenac 50 mg and misoprostol 200 µg.

Diclofenac sodium and misoprostol **(Arthrotec 75):** Tablets: Diclofenac 75 mg and misoprostol 200 µg.

Parenteral formulations are not available for general clinical use in the United States.

Pharmacology

A phenylacetic acid derivative and nonsteroidal anti-inflammatory drug (NSAID), diclofenac is structurally and pharmacologically related to mefenamic acid and meclofenamate sodium. As with other NSAIDs, the analgesic and anti-inflammatory activities of diclofenac are partly due to the inhibition of prostaglandin synthesis and/or release secondary to the inhibition of cyclooxygenase. Cyclooxygenase catalyzes the formation of prostaglandin precursors (endoperoxides) from arachidonic acid. High concentrations of diclofenac may inhibit formation of other arachidonic acid metabolites, including leukotrienes and 5-hydroxyeicosatetraenoic acid (5-HETE). Diclofenac may inhibit the migration of leukocytes, especially polymorphonuclear leukocytes, into inflammatory sites. The drug may also inhibit lysosomal enzyme release, superoxide production, and chemotaxis of polymorphonuclear leukocytes. The antipyretic activity of diclofenac may occur secondary to inhibition of pyrogen-induced release of prostaglandins in the central nervous system (including the hypothalamus) and possibly to centrally mediated peripheral vasodilatation.

Diclofenac has an analgesic potency similar to that of indomethacin, sulindac, or codeine and about 5 to 15 times that of naproxen and aspirin. Diclofenac (and other NSAIDs) exhibits a ceiling effect for analgesia. Exceeding recommended doses results in increased toxicity without improvement in analgesia. Diclofenac may cause gastric mucosal damage that may result in ulceration and/or bleeding. Inhibition of prostaglandin synthesis may result in decreased uterine tone and contractility and prolonged gestation in the parturient and premature closure of the ductus arteriosus in the fetus. Diclofenac inhibits platelet aggregation and prolongs bleeding time. The drug has no uricosuric activity.

Pharmacokinetics

Onset of Action: PO, analgesic effect 15–30 minutes.
Peak Effect: PO, analgesic effect 1–3 hours
Duration of Action: PO, analgesic effect 4–6 hours.

Interactions

Risks of bleeding increased with concomitant NSAIDs, anticoagulant or heparin therapy, alcohol ingestion; decreases antihypertensive effects of β-adrenergic blocking agents; serum levels of diclofenac decreased by concomitant aspirin, phenobarbital; GI absorption of diclofenac delayed by food and milk; prostaglandin-mediated natriuretic effects of loop diuretics antagonized by diclofenac; renal elimination decreased and serum levels and toxic effects of cyclosporine, digoxin, methotrexate, and lithium increased by concomitant diclofenac.

Toxicity

Toxic Range: Not routinely monitored.

Manifestations: *Acute:* Coma, hypotension, metabolic acidosis, respiratory depression, acute renal failure, hypotonia, tachycardia.

Antidote: None.

Management: Discontinue or reduce medication. Correct fluid, electrolyte, and acid-base disturbances. Support ventilation and circulation (patent airway, oxygen, IV fluids, vasopressors). Airway-protected, ipecac syrup–induced emesis (30 mL or 0.5 mL/kg ipecac syrup followed by 200 mL or 4 mL/kg of water or clear fluid) or gastric lavage (with drug ingestion) followed by administration of activated charcoal (PO 50–100 g or 1–2 g/kg). Forced alkaline diuresis with IV sodium bicarbonate (IV furosemide if necessary) after correction of dehydration. Monitor fluid and electrolyte balance. Symptomatic treatment.

Guidelines/Precautions

1. Use with caution in patients with active GI lesions (e.g., erosive gastritis, peptic ulcer), a history of recurrent GI lesions, hepatic or renal dysfunction, preexisting hypoprothrombinemia, or vitamin K deficiency.
2. Carefully observe patients with coagulation disorders and those receiving drug therapy that interferes with hemostasis.
3. Use with caution in pregnancy and only when the perceived benefits outweigh the potential risks.
4. Patient response to NSAIDs is variable. Patients who do not respond to or cannot tolerate diclofenac may be successfully treated with another NSAID.

5. Diclofenac and salicylates should not be administered concomitantly because there may not be any therapeutic advantage and the incidence of adverse GI side effects may be increased.

6. Contraindicated in patients with previously demonstrated hypersensitivity to diclofenac or with the complete or partial syndrome of nasal polyps, angioedema, or bronchospastic reactivity to aspirin or other NSAIDs.

7. Signs and symptoms of infection or other diseases may be masked by the antipyretic and anti-inflammatory effects of diclofenac.

8. Monitor stool for blood every 14 days, and monitor BUN, serum creatinine, and urinalysis every 1–2 months when administering diclofenac at chronic high doses.

Principal Adverse Reactions

Cardiovascular: Peripheral edema, fluid retention, hypertension, palpitation.

Pulmonary: Dyspnea, bronchospasm.

CNS: Drowsiness, dizziness, headache, anxiety, confusion.

Gastrointestinal: Ulceration, bleeding, dyspepsia, nausea, vomiting, diarrhea, hepatic dysfunction.

Genitourinary: Renal dysfunction, acute renal failure, azotemia, cystitis, hematuria.

Dermatologic: Pruritus, urticaria.

Hematologic: Prolongation of bleeding time, leukopenia, thrombocytopenia, aplastic anemia, hemolytic anemia.

Other: Tinnitus, blurred vision.

DIFLUNISAL

Class: Nonsteroidal Anti-inflammatory Drug

Use(s): Symptomatic treatment of mild to moderate pain, inflammatory conditions (e.g., rheumatic fever, rheumatoid arthritis, osteoarthritis), chronic pain, cancer pain (especially with bone metastasis).

Dosing: *Pain and inflammatory disease:* PO 1 g (20 mg/kg) then 500 mg (10 mg/kg) two or three times daily. Dosage should be adjusted according to the patient's response and tolerance.

Administer analgesic regularly (not as needed). Addition of opioid analgesics, antidepressant agents, and use of nondrug therapies such as transcutaneous electrical nerve stimulation (TENS) may enhance analgesia (see pages xxvi–xliv for drug combinations). In rheumatoid arthritis or juvenile rheumatoid arthritis, second-line rheumatoid agents may include leflunomide (Arava), etanercept (Enbrel), antimalarials, or methotrexate. In geriatric patients and patients with decreased renal or hepatic function, decrease doses by one-third to one-half. The incidence of diflunisal-induced gastropathy may be decreased by concomitant administration of antacids or sucralfate (PO 1 g four times daily). Misoprostol (PO 100–200 µg four times daily) may be used to prevent gastric ulcers in high-risk patients.

Elimination: Hepatic, renal.

Preparations

Diflunisal **(Dolobid):** Tablets, film coated: 250 mg, 500 mg.

Pharmacology

Diflunisal, a nonsteroidal anti-inflammatory drug (NSAID), is a difluorophenyl derivative of salicylic acid. Although it is structurally and pharmacologically similar to the salicylates, it does not undergo hydrolysis in vivo to salicylic acid and thus is not considered a true salicylate. The analgesic and anti-inflammatory activity of diflunisal may be mediated by inhibition of the biosynthesis and release of prostaglandins that sensitize C fibers' nociceptors to mechanical stimuli and chemical mediators (e.g., bradykinin, histamine) and that may interfere with the endogenous descending pathways that inhibit pain transmission. Diflunisal irreversibly acetylates and inactivates cyclooxygenase (prostaglandin synthetase), an enzyme that catalyzes the formation of prostaglandin precursors (endoperoxides) from arachidonic acid. The antipyretic activity of diflunisal may occur secondary to inhibition of pyrogen-induced release of prostaglandins in the central nervous system (including the hypothalamus) and possibly to centrally mediated peripheral vasodilatation.

The analgesic, anti-inflammatory, and antipyretic effects of diflunisal are 3.5 to 13 times those of aspirin on a weight basis. Diflunisal may cause gastric mucosal damage that may result in ulceration and/or bleeding. This may be due to inhibition of synthesis of prostaglandins (e.g., prostacyclin, prostaglandins of the E series) that have cytoprotective effects on GI mucosa. The drug may exhibit dose-dependent inhibition of platelet aggregation and prolongation of bleeding time. In contrast to the prolonged effects of aspirin, platelet aggregation returns to normal within 24 hours. Diflunisal (like other NSAIDs) exhibits a ceiling effect for analgesia. Exceeding recommended doses results in increased toxicity without improvement in analgesia. Inhibition of prostaglandin synthesis may result in decreased uterine tone and contractility and prolonged gestation in the parturient and premature closure of the ductus arteriosus in the fetus.

Pharmacokinetics

Onset of Action: PO, analgesic effect <60 minutes.
Peak Effect: PO, analgesic effect 2–3 hours.
Duration of Action: PO, analgesic effect 3–7 hours.

Interactions

Incidence of GI side effects and risk of bleeding increased with concomitant NSAIDs, anticoagulant or heparin therapy, alcohol ingestion; enhances toxicity of lithium, methotrexate, valproic acid; serum levels of diflunisal increased by carbonic anhydrous inhibitors; decreases diuretic effects of spirinolactone; decreased serum concentration of diflunisal with concomitant corticosteroids, aspirin; increased serum concentration of diflunisal with concomitant acetaminophen; enhances hypoglycemic effects of sulfonylureas; increases renal toxic effects of cyclosporine; decreases antihypertensive effects of β-adrenergic blockers, ACE inhibitors; enhances hypotensive effects of nitroglycerin; urinary excretion of diflunisal increased by antacids and urinary alkalinizers; absorption delayed by food, milk, and concomitant administration of activated charcoal, antacids;

prostaglandin-mediated natriuretic effects of spirinolac-tone and furosemide antagonized by diflunisal.

Toxicity

Toxic Range: Not routinely monitored.

Manifestations: GI ulceration, dyspepsia, nausea, vomiting, hyperventilation, sweating, tachycardia, tin-nitus.

Antidote: None.

Management: Discontinue or reduce medication. Correct fluid, electrolyte, and acid-base disturbances. Support ventilation and circulation (patent airway, oxygen, IV fluids, vasopressors). Airway-protected, ipecac syrup–induced emesis (30 mL or 0.5 mL/kg ipecac syrup followed by 200 mL or 4 mL/kg of water or clear fluid) or gastric lavage (with drug ingestion) followed by administration of activated charcoal (PO 50–100 g or 1–2 g/kg). Symptomatic treatment.

Guidelines/Precautions

1. Discontinue use of the drug if dizziness, tinnitus, or hearing loss occurs. Tinnitus may herald the approach of salicylate levels to the upper limit of the therapeutic range. The temporary hearing loss remits gradually upon discontinuation of diflunisal.
2. Salicylate salts should not be used for self-medication of fever for longer than 3 days in adults or children, or for self-medication of pain for longer than 10 days in adults or 5 days in children unless directed by a physician.
3. Use with caution in patients with active GI lesions (e.g., erosive gastritis, peptic ulcer), a history of recurrent GI lesions, hepatic or renal dysfunction,

preexisting hypoprothrombinemia, or vitamin K deficiency. Diflunisal may precipitate renal failure in patients with impaired renal function, heart failure, or liver dysfunction.

4. Patient response to NSAIDs is variable. Patients who do not respond to or cannot tolerate diflunisal may be successfully treated with another NSAID.

5. Diflunisal and salicylates should not be administered concomitantly because there may not be any therapeutic advantage and the incidence of adverse GI side effects may be increased.

6. Contraindicated in patients with previously demonstrated hypersensitivity to diflunisal, or with the complete or partial syndrome of nasal polyps, angioedema, or bronchospastic reactivity to aspirin or other NSAIDs.

7. Signs and symptoms of infection or other diseases may be masked by the antipyretic and anti-inflammatory effects of diflunisal.

8. Monitor stool for blood every 14 days, and monitor BUN, serum creatinine, and urinalysis every 1–2 months when administering diflunisal at chronic high doses.

Principal Adverse Reactions

Cardiovascular: Vasodilatation, pallor, angina.

Pulmonary: Dyspnea, asthma.

CNS: Drowsiness, dizziness, headache, sweating, depression, euphoria.

Gastrointestinal: Ulceration, bleeding, dyspepsia, nausea, vomiting, diarrhea, hepatic dysfunction.

Genitourinary: Dysuria, interstitial nephritis, renal papillary necrosis.

Dermatologic: Pruritus, urticaria.

Hematologic: Leukopenia, thrombocytopenia, purpura, decreased plasma iron concentration, shortened erythrocyte survival time.

DIHYDROERGOTAMINE MESYLATE

Class: Serotonin Agonist

Use(s): Acute treatment of migraine attacks with or without auras.

Dosing: SC/Deep IM: 1 mg. Dose may be repeated at 1-hour intervals to a total dose of 3 mg.

IV: 1 mg. Dose may be repeated at 1-hour intervals to a total dose of 2 mg.

Administer at the first sign of attack. Delayed administration results in increased dosage requirements and a longer onset of action. The intravenous route should be used when a more rapid effect is desired. To reduce the incidence of severe side effects, administer an antiemetic (e.g., metoclopramide or a phenothiazine) at least 1 hour before the first intravenous dose. Maximum weekly dose IM or IV should not exceed 6 mg. Visually inspect parenteral products for particulate matter and discoloration prior to administration whenever solution and container permit. Do not use if solution is discolored.

Intranasal: Administer one spray (0.5 mg) in each nostril. Dose may be repeated in 15 minutes if needed. There is no additional benefit from an acute dose greater than 2 mg for a single migraine episode. The safety of doses greater than 3 mg in a 24-hour period and 4 mg in a 7-day period has not been established. When spraying, the head should not be tilted back and the patient should not inhale through the nose. The nasal sprayer should be assembled immediately prior to use. To assemble, 1) tap the top of the ampule until all the medication is the bottom; 2) place ampule upright and straight in the well of the assembly case with the breaker cap pointing up; 3) push down the assembly vase lid slowly but firmly until you hear the ampule snap open; 4) without removing the ampule from the well, push nasal sprayer onto ampule until it clicks. Prior to administration, the pump must be primed (squeeze four times). Once the nasal spray applicator has been prepared, it should be discarded (with any remaining drug in opened ampule) after 8 hours.

Elimination: Hepatic, renal.

Preparations

Dihydroergotamine mesylate **(DHE 45 Injection):** Injection: 2 mg/mL.

Dihydroergotamine mesylate **(Migranal):** Nasal spray: Available in 1-mL glass amber ampules, each containing 4 mg of dihydroergotamine mesylate (4 mg/mL). Each individual kit contains four unit dose trays; each tray contains one ampule, a nasal spray applicator, and a breaker cap on the ampule.

Pharmacology

An ergot alkaloid, dihydroergotamine (DHE) binds with high affinity to all known 5-hydroxytryptamine-1 (5-HT1) receptors as well as other biogenic amine receptors such as 5-HT2 (subtypes A and C), α_1- and α_2-adrenergic receptors, and DA_2 dopaminergic receptors. The therapeutic effect of DHE in the treatment of migraine is thought to be primarily due to agonist activity at 5-HT1 subtype D receptors. The efficacy of sumatriptan, a selective serotonin agonist in the treatment of migraine, is attributed to agonist activity at 5-HT1 receptors (subtypes B and D). Activation of 5-HT1 receptors (subtypes B and D) located on intracranial blood vessels may cause vasoconstriction of large intracranial conductance arteries and closure of arteriovenous anastomosis, which correlates with the relief of migraine headache. Activation of 5-HT1 receptors on sensory nerve endings of the trigeminal system may also inhibit the release of proinflammatory neuropeptides (e.g., substance P and calcitonin gene-related peptide [CGRP] from the trigeminal nerve). Substance P and CGRP may be involved in the generation of pain during a migraine episode. In the periphery, DHE causes vasoconstriction by stimulating α-adrenergic receptors. Although it is also a competitive α-adrenergic blocker at high doses, this effect is somewhat masked by the drug's α-adrenergic agonist activity. With therapeutic doses, DHE also inhibits reuptake of norepinephrine, thereby increasing vasoconstriction. Effects of DHE on blood pressure are unpredictable, but the drug vasoconstricts capacitance vessels more than resistance vessels; therefore, it decreases venous return and decreases venous stasis and pooling. DHE has less vasoconstrictor activity than ergotamine. The oxytocic activity of DHE is less than that of ergotamine and much less than that of ergonovine or methylergonovine.

Pharmacokinetics

Onset: SC/IM, 15–30 minutes. Intranasal, <30 minutes. IV, <5 minutes.
Peak Effect: SC/IM/Intranasal, 30–60 minutes.
Duration of Action: IM, 3–4 hours.

Interactions

Additive adverse cardiovascular effects may occur with concomitant use of ergot compounds, vasoconstrictor agents (e.g., norepinephrine, dopamine); DHE decreases the effectiveness of antihypertensive agents, antianginal agents (e.g., nitrates, calcium channel blockers); excessive peripheral vasoconstriction may occur with concomitant use of β-blockers; ergot toxicity (severe peripheral vasospasm with possible ischemia, cyanosis, numbness) may occur with concomitant use of macrolide antibiotics (e.g., erythromycin, clarithromycin); additive vasospasm with concomitant use of other ergot alkaloids and sumatriptan; increased risk of injection site reactions with IM injection of DHE combined with heparin.

Toxicity

Toxic Range: Not routinely monitored.
Manifestations: Ergotism—numbness, tingling, pain, cyanosis of the extremities; diminished or absent peripheral pulses; hypertension; coronary vasospasm; palpitations; arrhythmias; nausea, vomiting; pain;

seizures; respiratory depression; confusion; delirium; convulsions; coma.

Antidote: No specific antidote.

Management: Discontinue or reduce medication. Local application of warmth to the affected area. Administration of vasodilators (e.g., sodium nitroprusside or phentolamine). Nursing care to prevent tissue damage. Support ventilation and circulation (patent airway, oxygen, IV fluids, vasodilators). Monitoring should continue while symptoms and signs persist and for at least 10 hours thereafter. Symptomatic treatment.

Guidelines/Precautions

1. DHE is contraindicated in peripheral vascular disease, ischemic heart disease, Prinzmetal's angina, sepsis, history of myocardial infarction, or uncontrolled hypertension. DHE should not be given to patients in whom unrecognized coronary disease is predicted by the presence of risk factors (e.g., hypertension, hypercholesterolemia, current tobacco smoking, obesity, diabetes mellitus, strong family history of ischemic heart disease, postmenopausal females, or males older than 40 years) unless a cardiovascular evaluation provides sufficient evidence that the patient is reasonably free of ischemic heart disease.

2. Use with caution in patients with impaired renal or hepatic function. Do not use in patients with severe hepatic or renal impairment.

3. DHE is contraindicated in patients with known ergot alkaloid hypersensitivity.

4. DHE should not be used in breast-feeding women. The drug is excreted into breast milk and may

cause vomiting, diarrhea, weak pulse, and unstable blood pressure in nursing infants.

5. Parenteral administration should be avoided in patients with ischemic heart disease or Prinzmetal's angina. DHE should not be used within 24 hours of administration of an ergot compound.

6. DHE should not be administered in patients with basilar or hemiplegic migraine.

7. Use with caution in children. Safe and effective use has not been established, but children older than 6 years have been successfully treated for severe migraine headaches. DHE use in children should be reserved for cases where less toxic medications have failed to provide relief.

8. Do not combine DHE with heparin for intramuscular injections. There is increased risk of injection site reactions.

Principal Adverse Reactions

Cardiovascular: Hypertension, angina, arrhythmias, peripheral vasoconstriction, palpitations.

CNS: Dizziness, cerebrovascular accident.

Pulmonary: Dyspnea, bronchospasm, nasal congestion, burning sensation, dryness, discharge, pleural and retroperitoneal fibrosis (after long-term use).

Gastrointestinal: Bad taste, epistaxis.

Other: Edema; pruritus; weakness in the legs; injection site reaction, including hematomas, mild pain, burning.

DOCUSATE

Class: Stool Softener

Use(s): Prophylaxis and treatment of constipation (e.g., with chronic administration of opioids).

Dosing: PO 50–200 mg (1–4 mg/kg) daily at bedtime or in two divided doses (maximum 360 mg daily). The sodium salt of docusate may be administered rectally. Oral liquids (not syrups) of docusate sodium should be diluted with 120 mL of milk, fruit juice, or infant formula to mask their bitter taste. The oral dosage varies widely according to the severity of the condition and the response of the patient and should be adjusted to individual response.

Constipation may be minimized by a high fiber content diet, adequate fluid intake, prompt response to the defecation reflex, and exercise.

Elimination: Gastrointestinal.

Preparations

Docusate sodium **(Colace, Docusate Sodium, Dio-succin, Dionex, Disonate, DOS, D-S-S, Duosol, Modane Soft, Disonate, Doxinate, Dioeze):** Capsules: 50 mg, 100 mg, 240 mg, 250 mg.

Docusate sodium **(Colace Liquid, Diocto Liquid, Dis-onate Liquid, Doxinate Solution):** Oral solution: 10 mg/mL, 50 mg/mL.

Docusate sodium **(Di-Sosul, Regutol):** Tablets: 50 mg, 100 mg.

Docusate sodium **(Therevac S.B. Enema):** Rectal suspension: 283 mg/4 mL.

Docusate sodium **(Ex-Lax Stimulant Free):** Tablets: Docusate sodium 100 mg.

Docusate sodium and senna concentrate **(Gentlax S, Senokot S):** Tablets: Docusate sodium 50 mg and standardized senna concentrate (senosides 8.6 mg).

Docusate sodium and bisacodyl **(Modane Plus):** Capsules: Docusate sodium 100 mg and bisacodyl 5 mg.

Docusate sodium **(Correctol Stool Softener):** Soft gel: Docusate sodium 100 mg.

Docusate sodium and bisacodyl **(Phillips Liquigels):** Capsules: Docusate sodium 100 mg and bisacodyl 5 mg.

Docusate sodium and casanthranol **(Peri-Colace):** Capsules: Docusate sodium 100 mg and casanthranol 30 mg.

Docusate sodium and casanthranol **(Doxidan Liquigels):** Capsules, liquid filled: Docusate sodium 100 mg and casanthranol 30 mg.

Docusate sodium and casanthranol **(Peri-Colace Syrup, Diocto-C Syrup, D.S.S. with Casanthranol Syrup, Peri-DOS Syrup):** Oral solution: Docusate sodium 20 mg/5 mL and casanthranol 10 mg/5 mL.

Docusate sodium and carboxymethylcellulose sodium **(Disoplex):** Capsules: Docusate sodium 100 mg and carboxymethylcellulose 400 mg.

Docusate sodium, carboxymethylcellulose sodium, and casanthranol **(Disolan Forte):** Capsules: Docusate sodium 100 mg, carboxymethylcellulose 400 mg, and casanthranol 30 mg.

Docusate sodium and casanthranol **(Disanthrol, D-S-S Plus, Peri-Colace, Peri-DOS):** Capsules: Docusate sodium 100 mg and casanthranol 30 mg.

Docusate sodium and benzocaine **(Therevac Plus Enema):** Rectal suspension: Docusate sodium 283 mg/4 mL and benzocaine 20 mg/4 mL.

Docusate calcium **(Surfak, DC 240, Dioctocal, Pro-Cal-Sof):** Capsules: 50 mg, 240 mg.

Docusate potassium **(Dialose, Diocto-K, Docusate**

Potassium, DSMC, Kasof): Capsules: 100 mg, 240 mg.

Docusate potassium and casanthranol **(Dialose Plus, Diocto-K Plus, Dioctolose Plus, Docusate Potassium with Casanthranol, DSMC Plus, Perestan):** Capsules: Docusate potassium 100 mg and casanthranol 30 mg.

Pharmacology

The calcium, potassium, and sodium salts of docusate are anionic surface-active agents that have emulsifying and wetting properties. Fecal material is softened and defecation made easier secondary to a decrease in surface tension at the fecal oil-water interface, permitting water and lipids to penetrate. The laxative effects of docusate may also partly be due to cAMP-mediated stimulation of water and electrolyte secretion in the colon.

Pharmacokinetics

Onset: Stool softening, 1–3 days.
Peak Effect: Variable.
Duration of Action: Variable.

Interactions

Increased absorption of orally administered drugs; increase in extent of absorption of mineral oil and rate of absorption of phenolphthalein; coadministration with aspirin may result in increased intestinal mucosal damage.

Toxicity

Toxic Range: Not routinely monitored.

Manifestations: Diarrhea, abdominal pain.
Antidote: No specific antidote.
Management: Discontinue or reduce medication. Replace fluid or electrolyte deficits. Symptomatic treatment.

Guidelines/Precautions

1. Do not administer concurrently with mineral oil or oral drugs with low therapeutic indices.
2. Use at the lowest effective dose level.

Principal Adverse Reactions

Gastrointestinal: Diarrhea, cramping abdominal pain.
Other: Rash.

DOXEPIN HYDROCHLORIDE

Class: Tricyclic Antidepressant

Use(s): Treatment of neurotic and endogenous depression; migraine prophylaxis; adjunct treatment of sympathetic mediated pain; neuropathic pain syndromes, including diabetic neuropathy, postherpetic neuralgia, tic douloureux, and cancer pain; anxiety disorders; phobias; panic disorders; enuresis; eating disorders.

Dosing: *Pain syndromes*
　　　　　Initial: PO 25–50 mg (0.5–1.0 mg/kg) daily at bedtime. Titrate dose upward every 3 to 4 weeks by increments of 25–50 mg as necessary.
　　　　　Maintenance: PO 25–150 mg (0.5–3.0 mg/

kg) daily at bedtime. Doses should be decreased if unacceptable side effects occur. Serum levels should be determined if there are signs of toxicity. The higher end of the dose range may be required in the management of painful diabetic neuropathy.

Migraine prophylaxis and tension headache: PO 25–50 mg (0.5–1.0 mg/kg) daily.

Sympathetic mediated pain and postherpetic neuralgia: Topical: Apply cream four times daily and at bedtime. Safety and efficacy data not available for use greater than 8 days. Chronic use beyond 8 days may result in higher systemic levels. Drowsiness may occur when applied to more than 10% body surface area.

Depression

Initial: PO 30–150 mg daily in one to three divided doses.

Maintenance: PO 25–300 mg daily in one to four divided doses. Doses greater than 150 mg daily are not recommended for outpatients.

Oral concentrates may be diluted with fruit juices (orange, lemonade, tomato, Gatorade), but are incompatible with many carbonated beverages. For patients on methadone, doxepin solution and methadone syrup may be mixed together in the previously mentioned juices or water but not with grape juice.

Doses for pain are generally smaller than those used for treatment of affective disorders. Medication should be administered on a fixed schedule and not as needed. Administration of the entire daily dose at bedtime may reduce daytime sedation. After symptoms are controlled, dosage should be gradually reduced to the lowest level that will maintain relief of symptoms. Analgesia may be enhanced by addition of opioid analgesics (see pages xxvi–xliv for drug combinations) and nonsteroidal anti-inflammatory drugs (NSAIDs) and use of nondrug therapies such as transcutaneous electrical nerve stimulation (TENS). In geriatric patients and patients with decreased renal or hepatic function, decrease doses by one-third to one-half. The possibility for suicide is inherent in depression and may persist until significant remission occurs. The quantity of drug dispensed should reflect this consideration.

Elimination: Hepatic, renal.

Preparations

Doxepin hydrochloride **(Sinequan):**
Capsules: 10 mg, 25 mg, 50 mg, 75 mg, 100 mg, 150 mg.
Oral concentrate (solution): 10 mg/mL.
Doxepin hydrochloride **(Zonalon):** Cream: 5%.

Pharmacology

A dibenzoxepine derivative and a tertiary amine tricyclic antidepressant, doxepin differs structurally from amitriptyline by the substitution of oxygen for the carbon atom in the center ring. Antidepressant activity is equipotent to amitriptyline and may be partly due to inhibition of the amine-pump uptake of neurotransmitters (e.g., norepinephrine and serotonin) at the presynaptic neuron and down-regulation of β-receptor sensitivity. Doxepin has sedating, antihistaminic, and anxiolytic effects. Compared with amitriptyline, doxepin may have less anticholinergic effects. Orthostatic hypotension may occur secondary to adrenergic blockade. Although blockade of neurotransmitter uptake may occur immediately, antidepressant response may take days to weeks. Doxepin does not inhibit the monoamine oxidase (MAO) system.

The analgesic effects of doxepin may occur partly through the alleviation of depression, which may be responsible for increased pain suffering, but also by mechanisms that are independent of mood effects. Serotonin and norepinephrine activity may be increased in descending pain inhibitory pathways. Activation of these pathways decreases the transmission of nociceptive impulses from primary afferent neurons to first-order cells in laminae I and V of the spinal cord dorsal horn. Doxepin may also potentiate the analgesic effect of opioids by increasing their binding efficacy to opioid receptors. Doxepin has varying degrees of efficacy in different pain syndromes and may be better at relieving the burning, aching, and dyesthetic component of neuropathic pain. The drug is seldom useful in the management of lancinating, shooting paroxysmal pain. The topical preparation has antipruritic effects, possibly due to the sedating and potent H_1 and H_2 receptor blocking activity. The cream may also be effective in relieving various neuropathic pain syndromes (e.g., postherpetic neuralgia, sympathetic mediated pain). At full antidepressant dosages, doxepin (and other tricyclic antidepressants) are especially effective in chronic low back pain with associated major depression. Patients with uncomplicated low back pain (i.e., without major depression) do not respond as well. The antimigraine activity of doxepin is relatively independent of its antidepressant effects. Low doses of doxepin are more effective for chronic tension headache compared with barbiturates and benzodiazepines.

Doxepin may produce abnormal EEG patterns and lower the seizure threshold. Therapeutic doses do not affect respiration, but toxic doses may lead to respiratory depression. The direct quinidine-like effects may manifest at toxic doses and produce cardiovascular disturbances (e.g., conduction blockade). Doxepin does not have addiction liability and its use is not associated with drug-seeking behavior. Withdrawal symptoms may be precipitated by acute withdrawal. Tolerance develops to the sedative and anticholinergic effects, but there are no reports of tolerance to the analgesic effects. Doxepin crosses the placenta. It is excreted in breast milk and has a potential for serious adverse effects in nursing infants.

Pharmacokinetics

Onset of Action: Analgesic effect: PO, <5 days. Antidepressant effect: PO, 1–2 weeks.
Peak Effect: Antidepressant effect: PO, 2–4 weeks.
Duration of Action: Antidepressant effect: PO, variable.

Interactions

Increased risk of hyperthermia with concomitant administration of anticholinergics (e.g., atropine), phenothiazines, or thyroid medications; serum levels and toxic effects of doxepin increased by concomitant methylphenidate, fluoxetine, cimetidine, phenothiazines, and haloperidol; ventilatory and circulatory depressant effects of CNS depressant drugs and alcohol potentiated by doxepin; increases the pressor and cardiac effects of sympathomimetics (e.g., isoproterenol, phenylephrine, norepinephrine, epinephrine, amphetamine); decreases serum levels and pharmacologic effects of levodopa and phenylbutazone; increases serum levels and toxic effects of dicumarol; onset of therapeutic effects shortened and adverse cardiac effects of doxepin increased with concomitant administration of levothyroxine and liothyronine; fatal hyperpyretic crisis or seizures with concomitant use of MAO inhibitors; uptake-dependent efficacy of IV regional bretylium decreased by doxepin.

Toxicity

Toxic Range: Not routinely monitored. Blood and urine levels may not correlate with the degree of intoxication and are not reliable guides for clinical management.

Manifestations: *Chronic:* Dream and sleep disturbances, akathisia, anxiety, chills, coryza, malaise, myalgia, headache, dizziness, nausea and vomiting. *Acute:* In addition to the previously listed symptoms, CNS stimulation with excitement, delirium, hallucinations, hyperreflexia, myoclonus, choreiform movements, parkinsonian symptoms, seizures, hyperpyrexia, then CNS depression with drowsiness, areflexia, hypothermia, respiratory depression, cyanosis, hypotension, coma; peripheral anticholinergic symptoms, including urinary retention, dry mucous membranes, mydriasis, constipation, adynamic ileus; cardiac irregularities, including tachycardia, QRS prolongation; metabolic and/or respiratory acidosis; polyradiculoneuropathy; renal failure; vomiting; ataxia; dysarthria; bullous cutaneous lesions; pulmonary consolidation.

Antidote: None.

Management: Discontinue or reduce medication. Correct fluid, electrolyte and acid-base disturbances. Airway-protected, ipecac syrup–induced emesis (30 mL or 0.5 mL/kg ipecac syrup) or gastric lavage (with drug ingestion) followed by administration of activated charcoal (PO 50–100 g or 1–2 g/kg). These purging actions should be performed even if several hours have elapsed after ingestion because the anticholinergic effects may delay gastric emptying and the drug may also be secreted into the stomach. Control seizures: IV benzodiazepines are the first choice because IV barbiturates may enhance respiratory depression; however, IV barbiturates or phenytoin may be useful in refractory seizures. Support ventilation and circulation (patent airway, oxygen, IV fluids, vasopressors). Continuous EKG monitoring. Treat cardiac arrhythmias with IV lidocaine or propranolol. Digoxin, quinidine, procainamide, and diisopyramide should be avoided because they may further depress myocardial conduction and/or contractility. Temporary pacemakers may be necessary in patients with advanced atrioventricular block, severe bradycardia, and/or life-threatening ventricular arrhythmias unresponsive to drug therapy. Control hyperpyrexia with ice packs and cooling sponge baths. Physostigmine (slow IV 1–3mg) may be used in the treatment of life-threatening anticholinergic toxicity. Routine use of physostigmine is not advisable due to its serious adverse effects (e.g., seizures, bronchospasm, and severe bradyarrhythmias). Hemodialysis or peritoneal dialysis are ineffective because the drug is highly protein bound. Symptomatic treatment. Consider the possibility of multiple drug involvement. Counseling prior to and after discharge for patients who attempted suicide.

Guidelines/Precautions

1. To avoid withdrawal symptoms, the medication should be tapered down over a couple of weeks and not discontinued abruptly.
2. Use with caution in patients with cardiovascular disease, thyroid disease, or seizure disorders and in those in whom excessive anticholinergic activity may be harmful (e.g., patients with benign prostatic hypertrophy, a history of urinary retention, or increased intraocular pressure). The drug should be used in close-angle glaucoma only when the glaucoma is adequately controlled by drugs and closely monitored.
3. Contraindicated in patients receiving MAO inhibitors (concurrently or within the past 2 weeks), patients in the acute recovery phase following myocardial infarction, and those with demonstrated hypersensitivity to doxepin. Cross-sensitivity with other tricyclic antidepressants may occur.
4. Patients should be warned of the possibility of drowsiness that may impair performance of poten-

tially hazardous tasks such as driving an automobile or operating machinery. Persisting daytime drowsiness may be decreased by administering a lower dose, administering the dose earlier in the evening, or substituting a less sedating alternative.

Principal Adverse Reactions

Cardiovascular: Postural hypotension, arrhythmias, conduction disturbances, hypertension, sudden death.

Pulmonary: Respiratory depression.

CNS: Confusion, disorientation, extrapyramidal symptoms.

Gastrointestinal: Hepatic dysfunction, jaundice, nausea, vomiting, constipation, decrease in lower esophageal sphincter tone.

Genitourinary: Urinary retention, paradoxical nocturia, urinary frequency.

Ocular: Blurred vision, mydriasis, increased intraocular pressure.

Dermatologic: Pruritus, urticaria, petechiae, photosensitivity.

Hematologic: Leukopenia, thrombocytopenia, eosinophilia, agranulocytosis, purpura.

Endocrinologic: Increased or decreased libido, impotence, gynecomastia, SIADH.

Other: Hyperthermia.

EMLA (EUTECTIC MIXTURE OF LIDOCAINE AND PRILOCAINE)

Class: Topical Anesthetic

Uses: Topical anesthesia for minor and major dermal procedures.

Dosing: *Minor dermal procedures (e.g., IV cannulation):* Topical: Apply 2.5 g of EMLA cream (one-half of the 5-g tube) over 20–25 cm² of intact skin and cover with occlusive dressing for at least 45 minutes.

Neonatal circumcision: Topical: Apply 0.5–1.0 g of EMLA cream (one-tenth to one-fifth of the 5-g tube) over surgical site and cover with occlusive dressing for at least 60–80 minutes prior to surgery.

Major dermal procedures (e.g., split-thickness skin graft): Topical: Apply 2 g of EMLA cream per 10 cm² of intact skin and cover with occlusive dressing for at least 2 hours.

Maximum recommended dose: 60 g.

Maximum recommended area of application on normal intact skin:
<10 kg: 100 cm²
10–20 kg: 600 cm²
>20 kg: 2000 cm²

Maximum recommended duration of application: 4 hours.

Estimated mean absorption of lidocaine: 0.045 mg/cm²/hr.

Estimated mean absorption of prilocaine: 0.075 mg/cm²/hr.

Smaller areas of treatment are recommended in debilitated patients, small children, and patients with impaired elimination.

Elimination: Hepatic (lidocaine); hepatic and renal (prilocaine).

Preparations

Lidocaine and prilocaine **(EMLA):** Cream: Lidocaine 2.5% (25 mg/g) and prilocaine 2.5% (25 mg/g).

Pharmacology

EMLA cream is a eutectic mixture of amide local anesthetics, lidocaine 2.5% and prilocaine 2.5%, formulated as an oil-in-water emulsion. Both lidocaine and prilocaine stabilize neuronal membranes by inhibiting the ionic fluxes required for the initiation and conduction of impulses, thereby effecting local anesthetic action. At a ratio of 1:1, the melting point of the mixture is 18°C, lower than either compound alone (lidocaine 67°C, prilocaine 37°C). The mixture is an oil at room temperature, and the penetration and subsequent systemic absorption of both prilocaine and lidocaine are enhanced. The amount absorbed is determined by the area over which it is applied and the duration of application under occlusion. The onset, depth, and duration of dermal analgesia depend primarily on the duration of application. Dermal analgesia can be expected to increase for up to 3 hours under occlusive dressing.

Pharmacokinetics

Onset of Action: <20 minutes.
Peak Effect: Satisfactory dermal analgesia: 45 minutes (adults), 60 minutes (children). Maximum dermal analgesia: 2–3 hours.
Duration of Action: 1–5 hours.

Interactions

Methemoglobinemia at high doses and with concomitant administration of methemoglobin-inducing agents (e.g., sulfonamides, acetaminophen, acetanilid, aniline dyes, benzocaine, chloroquine, dapsone, naphthalene, nitrates, nitrites, nitrofurantoin, nitroglycerin, sodium nitroprusside, pamaquine, *para*-aminosalicylic acid, phenacetin, phenobarbital, phenytoin, primaquine, and quinine); additive cardiac effects with other antiarrhythmics (e.g., tocainide, mexiletine).

Toxicity

Toxic Range: Lidocaine, >5µg/mL; prilocaine, >6µg/mL.

Manifestations: Seizures, arrhythmias, circulatory collapse, methemoglobinemia, respiratory depression, cardiac arrest.

Antidote: No specific antidote.

Management: Discontinue or reduce medication. Support ventilation and circulation (patent airway, oxygen, IV fluids, vasopressors). Benzodiazepines (diazepam IV 0.05–0.2mg/kg, midazolam IV/IM 0.025–0.1mg/kg) or barbiturates (thiopental sodium IV 0.5–2.0mg/kg) to control seizures. Prolonged cardiopulmonary resuscitation with cardiac arrest: Sodium bicarbonate IV 1–2mEq/kg to treat cardiac toxicity (sodium channel blockade); bretylium IV 5mg/kg; DC cardioversion/defibrillation for ventricular arrhythmias. Remove ingested drug by induced emesis followed by activated charcoal. Treat methemoglobinemia with oxygen and methylene blue (1–2mg/kg injected over 5 minutes). Hypersensitivity reactions: Remove from further exposure and treat dermatitis.

Guidelines/Precautions

1. EMLA cream is not recommended for use on mucous membranes due to the risk of systemic toxicity. EMLA cream should be used with caution in the external auditory canal. Penetration or

migration beyond the tympanic membrane into the middle ear may result in ototoxicity.

2. The amount of lidocaine and prilocaine systemically absorbed is directly related to the duration of application and the area over which the cream is applied.

3. Toxic plasma levels may occur with application of EMLA cream to broken or inflamed skin or to $2000\,cm^2$ or more of skin.

4. EMLA cream properly applied is a safe and non-invasive method of anesthesia for neonatal circumcision. However, it is less effective than a ring block or dorsal penile nerve block.

5. EMLA cream is contraindicated in patients with congenital or idiopathic methemoglobinemia and in infants younger than 12 months who are receiving treatment with methemoglobin-inducing agents. EMLA cream should be used with caution in patients with glucose-6-phosphate deficiencies, who are more susceptible to methemoglobinemia.

6. Treat methemoglobinemia with methylene blue (IV 1–2 mg/kg injected over 5 minutes).

7. Dermal application of EMLA cream may cause a transient local blanching, followed by redness or erythema.

8. EMLA cream should be used with caution in patients who may be more sensitive to the systemic effects of lidocaine and prilocaine, including acutely ill, debilitated, elderly patients or those with severe hepatic disease.

9. Avoid contact of EMLA cream with the eye. If eye contact occurs, immediately wash out the eye

with water or saline and protect the eye until sensation returns.

10. The patient should avoid inadvertent trauma to the treated area, and avoid exposure to hot or cold temperatures until complete sensation has returned.

Principal Adverse Reactions

Cardiovascular: Hypotension, bradycardia.
Pulmonary: Respiratory depression, bronchospasm.
CNS: Euphoria, confusion, tinnitus, seizures, blurred vision.
Dermatologic: Blanching, pallor, erythema, edema, urticaria, pruritus, anaphylactoid reactions (rare).
Other: Methemoglobinemia.

EPHEDRINE SULFATE

Class: Sympathomimetic

Uses: Treatment of hypotension occurring during regional or general anesthesia, treatment of bronchospasm.

Dosing: *Hypotension*

IV: 5–20 mg [100–200 µg/kg].

IM/SC: 25–50 mg.

If necessary, dose may be repeated in 5–10 minutes. Maximum parenteral dose: 150 mg (3 mg/kg) in 24 hours.

Bronchospasm

IV/IM/SC: 5–20 mg [100–200 µg/kg]; IM: 25–50 mg. Further dosage should be determinted by patient response.

PO: 25–50 mg every 3–4 hours as needed.

Elimination: Hepatic, renal.

Preparations

Ephedrine sulfate **(Ephedrine Sulfate)**
   Injection: 25 mg/mL, 50 mg/mL.
   Capsules: 25 mg, 50 mg.

Pharmacology

Ephedrine is a noncatecholamine sympathomimetic with mixed direct and indirect actions. It is resistant to metabolism by monoamine oxidase (MAO) and catechol-*O*-methyltransferase (COMT), resulting in prolonged duration of action. Ephedrine increases cardiac output, blood pressure, and heart rate by α- and β-adrenergic stimulation. It increases coronary and skeletal blood flow and produces bronchodilatation by stimulation of β$_2$-receptors. Ephedrine has minimal effects on uterine blood flow. However, it restores uterine blood flow when used to treat epidural or spinal hypotension in pregnant patients.

Pharmacokinetics

Onset of Action: IV, almost immediate; IM, few minutes.
Peak Effect: IV, 2–5 minutes; IM, <10 minutes.
Duration of Action: IV/IM, 10–60 minutes.

Interactions

Increased risk of arrhythmias with volatile anesthetic agents; potentiated by tricyclic antidepressants.

Toxicity

Toxic Range: Not routinely monitored.
Manifestations: Hypertension, arrhythmias.

Antidote: α-adrenergic blockers (e.g., phentolamine IV/IM 2.5–5.0 mg).

Management: Discontinue or reduce infusion. Support ventilation and circulation (patent airway, oxygen, IV fluids, vasodilators). Symptomatic treatment.

Guidelines/Precautions

1. Tolerance may develop, but temporary cessation of the drug restores its original effectiveness.
2. Use cautiously in patients with hypertension and ischemic heart disease.
3. Ephedrine has unpredictable effects in patients in whom endogenous catecholamines are depleted.
4. Ephedrine may produce an unacceptable degree of CNS stimulation, resulting in insomnia.

Principal Adverse Reactions

Cardiovascular: Hypertension, tachycardia, arrhythmias.

Pulmonary: Pulmonary edema.

CNS: Anxiety, tremors.

Metabolic: Hyperglycemia, transient hyperkalemia then hypokalemia.

Dermatologic: Necrosis at site of injection.

EPINEPHRINE HYDROCHLORIDE

Class: Sympathomimetic

Uses: Inotrope; bronchodilator; prolongation of duration of local anesthetics; treatment of allergic reactions, postintubation, and infectious croup; resuscitation.

Dosing: *Cardiac arrest*

Standard dose: IV bolus 1 mg or 0.02 mg/kg (10 mL or 0.2 mL/kg of 1:10,000 solution). Administer every 3–5 minutes as necessary. If no response after second dose, administer high dose.

High dose (acceptable, possibly helpful): IV bolus 5–10 mg or 0.1–0.2 mg/kg (5–10 mL of a 1:3000 solution) every 3–5 minutes as necessary.

If intravenous access is not available, dilute 5–10 mg or 0.1–0.2 mg/kg (5–10 mL of a 1:3000 solution) in an equal volume of sterile normal saline and inject via an endotracheal tube.

Inotropic support: Infusion 2–20 μg/min (0.1–1.0 μg/kg/min).

Anaphylaxis or severe asthma

Adults: SC/IM 0.1 to 0.5 mg (0.1–0.5 mL of a 1:3000 solution).

Children: SC/IM 0.01 mg/kg (0.01 mL/kg of a 1:3000 solution), not to exceed 0.5 mg. Subcutaneous doses may be repeated at 10- to 15-minute intervals in patients with anaphylactic shock and at 20-minute to 4-hour intervals in patients with asthma.

Bronchodilator/Croup therapy

Inhalation: Nebulization with oxygen: 2.25% racemic epinephrine or 1% (1:100) epinephrine. Dilute 1 mL in 3 mL normal saline. Give one to three inhalations and repeat after 5 minutes if necessary. Administer treatments every 2–6 hours. No less than 30 minutes between treatments. [Children: 0.5% (1:200) epinephrine or 1.25% racemic epinephrine. Dilute 0.5 mL in 1.5 mL normal saline. Give every 2–6 hours.]

Metered aerosol: 160–250 µg (one inhalation). Repeat once if necessary after at least 1 minute. Subsequent doses should not be administered for at least 4 hours. Rebound effect with increasing obstruction may follow an initial clearing of the airway. Monitor patient closely.

Test dose in regional anesthesia (marker for accidental intravascular injection): 10–15 µg (2–3 mL of 1:200,000 epinephrine solution mixed with local anesthetic). Intravascular injections detected by increase in heart rate (>10 beats per minute) within 30–45 seconds.

Prolongation of infiltration/plexus/epidural/caudal/interpleural anesthesia: 1:200,000 to 1:100,000 solution mixed with local anesthetic (0.1 mg epinephrine diluted in 20 mL local anesthetic gives 1:200,000 solution or 5 µg/mL). Maximum dose 250 µg (3–5 µg/kg).

Prolongation of spinal anesthesia: 0.1–0.4 mg (0.1–0.4 mL of a 1:1000 solution) added to anesthetic spinal fluid mixture. (Children: 5 µg/kg or epinephrine wash.)

Elimination: Enzymatic degradation (hepatic, renal, and GI tract).

Preparations

Epinephrine hydrochloride **(Epinephrine, Adrenaline, Anaguard Epinephrine, Epi-Pen):** Injection: 0.01 mg/mL (1 : 100,000), 0.1 mg/mL (1 : 10,000), 0.5 mg/mL (1 : 2000), 1 mg/mL (1 : 1000).

Epinephrine hydrochloride **(Adrenaline, Adreno-Mist):** Solution for nebulization: 1% (1 : 100) epinephrine.

Racepinephrine hydrochloride **(Vaponefrin, Breath-easy, Asthma-nefrin, Racepinephrine, microNefrin, Nephron, S-2 Inhalant):** Solution for nebulization: 1.25% racemic epinephrine, 2.25% racemic epinephrine.

Epinephrine **(Epinephrine Mist, Primatene Mist, Bronkaid Mist):** Aerosol: 200 µg/metered spray, 220 µg/metered spray, 250 µg/metered spray.

Epinephrine **(Sus-Phrine):** Parenteral suspension: 5 mg/mL.

Epinephrine bitartrate **(AsthmaHaler, Bronitin Mist, Bronkaid Mist, Primatene Mist, Primatene Mist Suspension):** Aerosol: 160 µg/metered spray.

Dilution for Infusion: 3 mg in 250 mL D5W or normal saline (12 µg/mL).

Pharmacology

Epinephrine is an endogenous catecholamine that activates both α- and β-adrenergic receptors. At therapeutic parenteral doses, the prominent effects are on β-adrenergic receptors. There is increased myocardial contractility and heart rate, relaxation of the smooth muscle of the bronchial tree, dilation of skeletal muscle vasculature, and a decrease in total peripheral resistance. At higher doses, α-adrenergic effects predominate and there is an increase in total peripheral resistance. Epinephrine increases uterine activity, produces uterine vasoconstriction, and decreases uterine blood flow. Epinephrine decreases the rate of absorption of local anesthetics. It prolongs the duration of anesthesia and decreases the risk of systemic toxicity. Analgesic effects of epinephrine at the spinal cord level may be due partly to α_2-agonist effects and suppressed activity of wide dynamic range neurons.

Pharmacokinetics

Onset of Action: IV, 30–60 seconds. SC, 6–15 minutes. Intratracheal, 5–15 seconds. Inhalation, 3–5 minutes.
Peak Effect: IV, within 3 minutes.
Duration of Action: IV, 5–10 minutes. Intratracheal, 15–25 minutes. Inhalation/SC, 1–3 hours.

Interactions

Ventricular arrhythmias (increased risk with use of volatile anesthetics, especially halothane); reduction of renal blood flow and urinary outflow; enhanced effect with tricyclic antidepressants and bretylium; decreases onset time and improves quality of epidural and spinal anesthetics (α_2-adrenergic effects).

Toxicity

Toxic Range: Not routinely monitored.
Manifestations: Hypertension, hypotension, ischemic EKG changes, supraventricular tachyarrhythmias, bradycardia, ventricular arrhythmias, myocardial infarction, pulmonary edema, headache, nausea and vomiting, abdominal pain, cyanosis, diaphoresis, precordial chest

tightness or pain, tingling of extremities, hyperglycemia, transient hyperkalemia.

Antidote: No specific antidote.

Management: Discontinue or reduce medication. Monitor vital signs carefully for development of myocardial infarction. Support ventilation and circulation. Treat hypertension cautiously because hypotension may occur, requiring vasopressor therapy.

Guidelines/Precautions

1. Use with digitalis or volatile anesthetics may result in arrhythmias.
2. Use with caution in patients with cardiovascular disease, hypertension, diabetes, or hyperthyroidism.
3. Use with caution for obstetric regional anesthesia, especially in high-risk parturients with uteroplacental insufficiency. The α-adrenergic effects may decrease uterine blood flow, and the β-adrenergic effects may slow labor and increase the need for oxytocic supplementation.
4. Contraindicated for IV regional anesthesia or local anesthesia of end organs (digits, penis, ears).
5. In cardiopulmonary resuscitation, intratracheal administration may be advantageous in bypassing the sluggish blood flow, hemodilution, and significant degradation in the blood stream attending injection of the drug into a peripheral vein. The absorption rate, duration, and pharmacologic effects of intratracheal drug administration compare favorably with the IV route.
6. Avoid intramuscular injections of epinephrine oil suspension into the buttocks. Gas gangrene may occur because epinephrine reduces oxygen tension

of the tissues, encouraging the growth of anaerobic organisms.

Principal Adverse Reactions

Cardiovascular: Hypertension, tachycardia, arrhythmias, angina.
Pulmonary: Pulmonary edema.
CNS: Anxiety, headache, cerebrovascular hemorrhage.
Dermatologic: Necrosis at site of injection.
Metabolic: Hyperglycemia, transient hyperkalemia, hypokalemia.

ERGOTAMINE TARTRATE

Class: Ergot Alkaloid

Uses: Prophylaxis and treatment of vascular headaches, including migraine and cluster headaches.

Dosing: *Treatment*

PO/SL: 2mg initially, then 1–2mg at 30-minute intervals until the attack has abated or a maximum dose of 6mg is given. Maximum daily dose 6mg. Maximum weekly dose 10mg.

Inhalation: 360µg (1 inhalation). May repeat at 5-minute intervals if indicated. Maximum daily dose 2.16mg (6 inhalations). Maximum weekly dose 5.4mg (15 inhalations).

Rectal: 2mg initially. May repeat in 1 hour. Maximum rectal dose 4mg for one attack. Maximum weekly rectal dose 10mg.

> *Prophylaxis (for series of attacks)*
> PO/SL: 1–2 mg at bedtime for 10–14 days.
> Rectal: 2–4 mg at bedtime for 10–14 days.

Elimination: Hepatic.

Preparations

Ergotamine tartrate and caffeine **(Ercaf, Lanatrate, Wigraine):** Tablets: Ergotamine tartrate 1 mg and caffeine 100 mg.

Ergotamine tartrate, levorotatory belladonna alkaloids, and phenobarbital **(Bellergal-S, Bel-Phen-Ergot S, Phenerbel-S):** Tablets: Ergotamine tartrate 0.6 mg, belladonna alkaloids 0.2 mg, and phenobarbital 40 mg.

Pharmacology

A naturally occurring ergot alkaloid, ergotamine constricts peripheral and cranial blood vessels and depresses central vasomotor centers. Ergotamine stimulates α-adrenergic receptors and may inhibit the reuptake of norepinephrine. At high doses and in very hypertonic vessels, ergotamine may manifest α-adrenergic blocking activity and produce vasodilatation. Depending on the site, ergotamine has partial agonist or antagonist activity at serotonin and dopamine receptors. The drug reduces extracranial blood flow, causes a decline in the amplitude of pulsation in the cranial arteries, and decreases hyperperfusion of the basilar artery territory. Ergotamine does not reduce cerebral hemispheric blood flow. It stimulates the chemoreceptor trigger zone and has potent emetic effects. Ergotamine may stimulate uterine contractions, especially in the gravid uterus. The effects on blood pressure are unpredictable but usually minimal at therapeutic doses.

Pharmacokinetics

Onset: PO, variable.
Peak Effect: PO, 30 minutes to 3 hours.
Duration of Action: PO, 3 hours.

Interactions

Increased hypertensive effects with concomitant propranolol; increased serum levels and toxic effects (severe vasospasm) of ergotamine with concomitant troleandomycin, erythromycin; additive toxicity with other ergot alkaloids.

Toxicity

Toxic Range: Not routinely monitored.
Manifestations: Nausea, vomiting, chest pain, delirium, hypertension, peripheral vasospasm, seizures, ischemic bowel disease, renal failure, shock, death.
Antidote: No specific antidote.
Management: Discontinue or reduce medication. Support ventilation and circulation (patent airway, oxygen, IV fluids, vasodilators). Treat peripheral vasospasm by keeping affected extremities warm. For impending ischemia, administer vasodilators such as sodium nitroprusside or tolazoline (IV 10–50 mg four times daily or intra-arterial 25–75 mg one or two times daily). To minimize thrombosis caused by stasis and endothelial damage, administer heparin and/or dextran 40. Symptomatic treatment. Hemodialysis.

Guidelines/Precautions

1. Avoid prolonged administration and excessive dosage due to the danger of ergotism and gangrene.
2. Contraindicated in patients with hypersensitivity to ergot alkaloids, peripheral vascular disease (thromboangiitis obliterans, syphilitic arteritis, severe arteriosclerosis, thrombophlebitis, Raynaud's disease), hepatic or renal disease, severe pruritus, coronary artery disease, hypertension, sepsis, or malnutrition.
3. Do not administer ergotamine in women who are or may become pregnant.

Principal Adverse Reactions

Cardiovascular: Chest pain, hypotension, hypertension, tachycardia, bradycardia, arterial spasm, myocardial infarction.
CNS: Headache, depression.
Gastrointestinal: Nausea, vomiting, abdominal pain, diarrhea.
Genitourinary: Polydipsia, renal artery vasoconstriction.
Dermatologic: Pruritus.
Extremities: Weakness in the legs, paresthesias, pulselessness, gangrene.

ETIDOCAINE HYDROCHLORIDE

Class: Local Anesthetic

Uses: Regional anesthesia.

Dosing: *Infiltration, peripheral nerve block:* 50–400 mg (1% solution).

   Epidural

      Bolus: 100–300 mg (10–20 mL of 1.0–1.5% solution).

      Infusion: 6–12 mL/hr (0.25–0.5% solution with or without epidural narcotics).

   Caudal: 100–300 mg (10–30 mL of 1% solution). Children 0.4–0.7–1.0 mL/kg for L2-T10-T7 level of anesthesia.

   Maximum safe dose: 3 mg/kg without epinephrine; 4 mg/kg with epinephrine. Solutions containing preservatives should not be used for epidural or caudal block. Except where contraindicated, vasoconstrictor drugs may be added to increase effect and prolong local or regional anesthesia. For dosage/route guidelines, see the Dosing section of Epinephrine (p. 204). Do not use vasoconstrictor drugs for local anesthesia of end organs (digits, penis, ears).

Elimination: Hepatic

Preparations

Etidocaine **(Duranest):** Injection: 1% solution with or without epinephrine 1:200,000; 1.5% solution with epinephrine 1:200,000.

Pharmacology

An amino amide and a long-acting local anesthetic, etidocaine stabilizes neuronal membrane by inhibiting the ionic fluxes required for the initiation and conduction of impulses. The drug produces a profound degree of motor blockade and abdominal muscle relaxation when used for peridural analgesia. Toxic blood levels may cause seizures and cardiovascular collapse secondary to a decrease in peripheral vascular resistance and direct myocardial depression. High plasma levels (as occur in paracervical blocks) produce uterine vasoconstriction and decrease in uterine blood flow. Vasoconstrictor agents decrease rate of absorption and prolong duration of action.

Pharmacokinetics

Onset of Action: Infiltration, 3–5 minutes. Epidural, 5–15 minutes.
Peak Effect: Infiltration, 5–15 minutes. Epidural, 15–20 minutes.
Duration of Action: Infiltration, 2–3 hours; with epinephrine, 3–7 hours. Epidural, 3–5 hours.

Interactions

Reduced clearance with concomitant use of β-blocking agents or cimetidine; benzodiazepines, barbiturates, and volatile anesthetics increase seizure threshold; duration of local or regional anesthesia prolonged by vasoconstrictor agents (e.g., epinephrine) or α_2-agonists (e.g., clonidine); alkalinization increases rate of onset and potency of local or regional anesthesia.

Toxicity

Toxic Range: Not routinely monitored.

Manifestations: Seizures, arrhythmias, circulatory collapse, respiratory depression, cardiac arrest.

Antidote: No specific antidote.

Management: Discontinue or reduce medication. Support ventilation and circulation (patent airway, oxygen, IV fluids, vasopressors). Benzodiazepines (diazepam IV 0.05–0.2 mg/kg, midazolam IV/IM 0.025–0.1 mg/kg) or barbiturates (thiopental sodium IV 0.5–2.0 mg/kg) to control seizures. Prolonged cardiopulmonary resuscitation with cardiac arrest: Sodium bicarbonate IV 1–2 mEq/kg to treat cardiac toxicity (sodium channel blockade); bretylium IV 5 mg/kg; DC cardioversion/ defibrillation for ventricular arrhythmias. Remove ingested drug by induced emesis followed by activated charcoal. Hypersensitivity reactions: Remove from further exposure and treat dermatitis. Exchange transfusions in newborns with toxicity.

Guidelines/Precautions

1. Do not use for spinal anesthesia.
2. Due to profound motor blockade, etidocaine is not recommended for epidural anesthesia in normal delivery.
3. Use with caution in patients with hypovolemia, severe congestive heart failure, shock, and all forms of heart block. The increased cardiac toxicity of etidocaine (compared with lidocaine or mepivacaine) results from a greater decrease in myocardial contractility and depression of cardiac conduction.
4. Contraindicated in patients with hypersensitivity to amide-type local anesthetics.

5. Use for paracervical block may be associated with fetal bradycardia.
6. The level of sympathetic blockade (bradycardia with block above T5) determines the degree of hypotension (often heralded by nausea and vomiting) following epidural or intrathecal etidocaine. Fluid hydration (10–20 mL/kg normal saline or lactated Ringer's solution), vasopressor agents (e.g., ephedrine), and left uterine displacement in pregnant patients may be used for prophylaxis and/or treatment. Administer atropine to treat bradycardia.
7. Epidural or caudal injections should be avoided when the patient has hypovolemic shock, septicemia, infection at the injection site, or coagulopathy.

Principal Adverse Reactions

Cardiovascular: Bradycardia, hypotension.
Pulmonary: Respiratory depression.
CNS: Euphoria, tinnitus, seizures.
Allergic: Urticaria, edema, anaphylactoid symptoms.
Epidural/Caudal: High spinal, loss of bladder and bowel control, loss of perineal sensation and sexual function, persistent motor sensory and/or autonomic (sphincter control) deficit.

ETODOLAC

Class: Nonsteroidal Anti-inflammatory Drug

Uses: Symptomatic treatment of mild to moderate inflammatory and degenerative arthritis, posttraumatic pain, chronic pain, cancer pain (especially with bone metastasis).

Dosing: *Pain and inflammatory diseases*

> Etodolac: PO 200–400 mg (4–8 mg/kg) every 6 to 12 hours. Maximum dose 1200 mg daily.
>
> Etodolac XL (extended release): PO 400–1000 mg once daily.
>
> Administer analgesic regularly (not as needed). Addition of opioid analgesics, antidepressant agents, and use of nondrug therapies such as transcutaneous electrical nerve stimulation (TENS) may enhance analgesia (see pages xxvi–xliv for drug combinations). Etodolac is not recommended for treatment of rheumatoid arthritis, as some of the other NSAIDs are more effective. In geriatric patients and patients with decreased renal or hepatic function, decrease doses by one-third to one-half. The incidence of etodolac-induced gastropathy may be decreased by administration with meals, milk, antacids, or sucralfate (PO 1 g four times daily). Misoprostol (PO 100–200 µg four times daily) may be used to prevent gastric ulcers in high-risk patients.

Elimination: Hepatic, renal.

Preparations

Etodolac **(Lodine):** Capsules: 200 mg, 300 mg, 400 mg.
Etodolac extended release **(Lodine XL):** Capsules: 400 mg, 600 mg.

Pharmacology

An indoleacetic acid derivative and nonsteroidal anti-inflammatory drug (NSAID), etodolac has analgesic and anti-inflammatory activities that are about three times that of aspirin and are partly due to the inhibition of prostaglandin synthesis and/or release secondary to the inhibition of cyclooxygenase. Cyclooxygenase enzyme (prostaglandin G/H synthetase) catalyzes the formation of prostaglandin precursors—endoperoxide intermediate prostaglandin G_2 (PGG_2)—from arachidonic acid. PGG_2 is reduced by peroxidase activity to another endoperoxide intermediate, prostaglandin H_2 (PGH_2). These endoperoxide intermediates are the common precursors for the synthesis of prostaglandins, prostacyclins, and thromboxanes. The inhibition of cyclooxygenase, and thus prostanoid synthesis, by etodolac and other NSAIDs is associated with side effects such as irritation and ulcer formation in the upper gastrointestinal tract and impairment of kidney function. However, etodolac is better tolerated than indomethacin, naproxen, or ibuprofen, and equipotent doses are associated with less gastric mucosal abnormalities.

It has been recognized recently that mammalian cells express two forms of cyclooxygenase (COX) activity. COX-1 is expressed in many normal tissues and is the major form present in platelets, kidney, and the gastrointestinal tract. COX-2 is induced in response to proinflammatory cytokines, lipopolysaccharide (LPS), and growth factors and is subjected to repression by glucocorticosteroids. This second form is generally not detected in healthy tissues but is found in elevated levels in inflammatory exudates. This has led to the hypotheses that COX-1 is mainly associated with homeostasis (including cytoprotection in the stomach and regulation of kidney function) and that COX-2 is associated with the edematous, nociceptive, and pyretic effects of inflammation. Most classic NSAIDs, including flurbiprofen and ibuprofen, show little specificity of inhibition toward COX isoforms. Etodolac demonstrates a favorable balance of COX-2 to COX-1 suppression. In contrast, indomethacin, piroxicam, and phenylbutazone are preferential inhibitors of COX-1. Ulcerogenic-sparing selective COX-2 inhibition does not inhibit cytoprotective stomach PGE_2 production.

The antipyretic activity of etodolac may occur secondary to inhibition of pyrogen-induced release of prostaglandins in the central nervous system (including the hypothalamus) and possibly to centrally mediated peripheral vasodilatation. Etodolac (like other NSAIDs) exhibits a ceiling effect for analgesia. Exceeding recommended doses results in increased toxicity without improvement in analgesia. Inhibition of prostaglandin synthesis may result in decreased uterine tone and contractility and prolonged gestation in the parturient and premature closure of the ductus arteriosus in the fetus. Etodolac inhibits platelet aggregation and prolongs bleeding time. The drug has no uricosuric activity.

Pharmacokinetics

Onset of Action: PO, analgesic effect 15–30 minutes.
Peak Effect: PO, analgesic effect 1–2 hours.
Duration of Action: PO, analgesic effect 4–6 hours.

Interactions

Risks of bleeding increased with concomitant NSAIDs, anticoagulant or heparin therapy, alcohol ingestion; decreases antihypertensive effects of β-adrenergic blocking agents; serum levels of etodolac may be decreased by concomitant aspirin; serum levels of etodolac increased by concomitant probenecid; serum levels and toxic effects of digoxin, cyclosporine, methotrexate, and lithium increased by concomitant etodolac; GI absorption of etodolac delayed by food and milk.

Toxicity

Toxic Range: Not routinely monitored.

Manifestations: *Acute:* Drowsiness, nausea, vomiting, lethargy, paresthesia, disorientation, abdominal pain, GI bleeding.

Antidote: None.

Management: Discontinue or reduce medication. Correct fluid, electrolyte, and acid-base disturbances. Support ventilation and circulation (patent airway, oxygen, IV fluids, vasopressors). Airway-protected, ipecac syrup–induced emesis (30 mL or 0.5 mL/kg ipecac syrup followed by 200 mL or 4 mL/kg of water or clear fluid) or gastric lavage (with drug ingestion) followed by administration of activated charcoal (PO 50–100 g or 1–2 g/kg). Symptomatic treatment.

Guidelines/Precautions

1. Use with caution in patients with active GI lesions (e.g., erosive gastritis, peptic ulcer), a history of recurrent GI lesions, hepatic or renal dysfunction, preexisting hypoprothrombinemia, or vitamin K

deficiency. Etodolac may decrease glomerular filtration rate and cause peripheral edema. The drug should be used cautiously in patients with heart failure, hypertension, or conditions associated with fluid retention.

2. Renal prostaglandins may have a supportive role in maintaining renal perfusion in patients with prerenal conditions. Etodolac should be avoided in such patients because it may cause a dose-dependent decrease in prostaglandin formation and thus precipitate renal decompensation.

3. Carefully observe patients with coagulation disorders and those receiving drug therapy that interferes with hemostasis.

4. Avoid the use of etodolac during pregnancy. In the third trimester, the drug may produce adverse fetal effects, including constriction of the ductus arteriosus, neonatal primary pulmonary hypertension, and fetal death.

5. Patient response to NSAIDs is variable. Patients who do not respond to or cannot tolerate etodolac may be successfully treated with another NSAID.

6. Etodolac and salicylates should not be administered concomitantly because there may not be any therapeutic advantage and the incidence of adverse GI side effects may be increased.

7. Contraindicated in patients with previously demonstrated hypersensitivity to etodolac or with the complete or partial syndrome of nasal polyps, angioedema, or bronchospastic reactivity to aspirin or other NSAIDs.

8. Signs and symptoms of infection or other diseases

may be masked by the antipyretic and anti-
inflammatory effects of etodolac.
9. Monitor stool for blood every 14 days, and
monitor BUN, serum creatinine, and urinalysis
every 1–2 months when administering etodolac at
chronic high doses.
10. Use of etodolac and other NSAIDs is not recommended during pregnancy (especially during the
last trimester) or during labor and delivery.
Etodolac and other NSAIDs inhibit prostaglandin
synthesis, which may cause dystocia, interfere
with labor, and delay parturition. Prostaglandin
synthesis inhibitors may also have adverse effects
on the fetal cardiovascular system (e.g., premature
closure of ductus arteriosus).

Principal Adverse Reactions

Cardiovascular: Congestive heart failure, peripheral
edema, fluid retention, hypertension, tachycardia,
arrhythmias.
Pulmonary: Dyspnea, bronchospasm.
CNS: Drowsiness, dizziness, headache, anxiety, confusion.
Gastrointestinal: Ulceration, bleeding, dyspepsia, nausea, vomiting, diarrhea, hepatic dysfunction, jaundice.
Genitourinary: Renal dysfunction, acute renal failure,
azotemia, cystitis, hematuria.
Dermatologic: Pruritus, urticaria.
Hematologic: Prolongation of bleeding time, leukopenia, thrombocytopenia, aplastic anemia, hemolytic
anemia.
Other: Tinnitus, blurred vision.

FAMOTIDINE

Class: H_2 Receptor Antagonist

Uses: Treatment of peptic ulcer disease; pathologic hypersecretory states; prophylaxis against acid pulmonary aspiration, stress ulcers, or allergic reactions.

Dosing: IV: 20 mg every 12 hours (dilute in 10 mL normal saline and inject over 2 minutes).
PO: 20 mg twice daily or 20–40 mg at bedtime.

Elimination: Renal.

Preparations

Famotidine **(Pepcid)**
    Tablets: 20 mg, 40 mg.
    Powder for oral suspension: 40 mg per 5 mL when reconstituted.
    Injection: 10 mg/mL.

Pharmacology

This competitive inhibitor of histamine H_2 receptors suppresses acid concentration and volume of gastric secretion. The degree of inhibition is similar to that observed following equipotent doses of cimetidine or ranitidine. Gastric emptying and exocrine pancreatic functions are not affected. Unlike cimetidine, famotidine does not affect the cytochrome P-450 oxidase system and has minimal effects on the elimination of other drugs. Famotidine does not have any cumulative effect with repeated doses.

Pharmacokinetics

Onset of Action: PO, within 1 hour; IV, <30 minutes.
Peak Effect: PO, 1–4 hours; IV, 30 minutes to 3 hours.
Duration of Action: PO/IV, 10–12 hours.

Interactions

Bioavailability enhanced by food and decreased by antacids.

Toxicity

Toxic Range: Not routinely monitored.
Manifestations: Tachycardia, respiratory failure, headache, delirium, psychosis.
Antidote: No specific antidote.
Management: Discontinue or reduce medication. Support ventilation and circulation (patent airway, oxygen, IV fluids, vasopressors). Treat tachycardia. Remove ingested drug by induced airway-protected emesis. Symptomatic treatment.

Guidelines/Precautions

1. Reduce dosage in patients with renal impairment.

Principal Adverse Reactions

Cardiovascular: Palpitations, hypotension.
Pulmonary: Bronchospasm.
CNS: Tinnitus, fatigue, dizziness, depression, paresthesia, headache.
Gastrointestinal: Nausea, vomiting, diarrhea.
Musculoskeletal: Musculoskeletal pain, arthralgia.
Hematologic: Thrombocytopenia.

FENOPROFEN CALCIUM

Class: Nonsteroidal Anti-inflammatory Drug

Uses: Symptomatic treatment of mild to moderate inflammatory and degenerative arthritis, tension headache, postoperative and posttraumatic pain, chronic pain, cancer pain (especially with bone metastasis).

Dosing: *Pain:* PO 200 mg (4 mg/kg) every 4 to 6 hours. Maximum dose 3.2 g daily.

Inflammatory disease or headache: PO 300–600 mg (6–10 mg/kg) every 4 to 6 hours. Maximum dose 3.2 g daily. Patients with rheumatoid or acute gouty arthritis may require larger doses than those with osteoarthritis.

Administer analgesic regularly (not as needed). Addition of opioid analgesics, antidepressant agents, and use of nondrug therapies such as transcutaneous electrical nerve stimulation (TENS) may enhance analgesia (see pages xxvi–xliv for drug combinations). In rheumatoid arthritis or juvenile rheumatoid arthritis, second-line rheumatoid agents may include leflunomide (Arava), etanercept (Enbrel), antimalarials, or methotrexate. In geriatric patients and patients with decreased renal or hepatic function, decrease doses by one-third to one-half. The incidence of fenoprofen-induced gastropathy may be decreased by administration with meals, milk, antacids, or sucralfate (PO 1 g four times daily). Misoprostol (PO 100–200 µg four times daily) may be used to prevent gastric ulcers in high-risk patients.

Elimination: Hepatic, renal.

Preparations

Fenoprofen **(Nalfon)**: Oral capsules: 200 mg, 300 mg.

Pharmacology

A propionic derivative and nonsteroidal anti-inflammatory drug (NSAID), fenoprofen is structurally and pharmacologically related to ibuprofen and naproxen. Like other NSAIDs, the analgesic and anti-inflammatory activities of fenoprofen are partly due to the inhibition of prostaglandin and leukotriene synthesis and to antibradykinin and lysosomal membrane stabilizing activity. The antipyretic activity of fenoprofen may occur secondary to inhibition of pyrogen-induced release of prostaglandins in the central nervous system (including the hypothalamus) and possibly to centrally mediated peripheral vasodilatation. At the recommended dose, fenoprofen has three times the analgesic potency of aspirin (200 mg fenoprofen is equipotent with 650 mg aspirin or 60 mg of codeine). Fenoprofen (and other NSAIDs) exhibits a ceiling effect for analgesia, and higher doses (e.g., 600 mg) are less potent compared with higher doses of codeine. Fenoprofen may be better tolerated than aspirin, and equipotent doses are associated with less gastric mucosal abnormalities. Inhibition of prostaglandin synthesis may result in decreased uterine tone and contractility and prolonged gestation in the parturient and premature closure of the ductus arteriosus in the fetus. Fenoprofen inhibits platelet aggregation and prolongs bleeding time. The drug has no uricosuric activity.

Pharmacokinetics

Onset of Action: PO, analgesic effect 15–30 minutes; anti-inflammatory effect <2 days.
Peak Effect: PO, analgesic effect 1–2 hours; anti-inflammatory effect 2–3 weeks.
Duration of Action: PO, analgesic effect 4–6 hours.

Interactions

Risks of bleeding increased with concomitant NSAIDs, anticoagulant or heparin therapy, alcohol ingestion; decreases antihypertensive effects of β-adrenergic blocking agents; serum levels of fenoprofen decreased by concomitant aspirin, phenobarbital; GI absorption of fenoprofen delayed by food and milk; prostaglandin-mediated natriuretic effects of loop diuretics antagonized by fenoprofen.

Toxicity

Toxic Range: Not routinely monitored.
Manifestations: *Acute:* Coma, hypotension, metabolic acidosis, respiratory depression, acute renal failure, proteinuria, tachycardia.
Antidote: None.
Management: Discontinue or reduce medication. Correct fluid, electrolyte, and acid-base disturbances. Support ventilation and circulation (patent airway, oxygen, IV fluids, vasopressors). Airway-protected, ipecac syrup–induced emesis (30 mL or 0.5 mL/kg ipecac syrup followed by 200 mL or 4 mL/kg of water or clear fluid) or gastric lavage (with drug ingestion)

followed by administration of activated charcoal (PO 50–100 g or 1–2 g/kg). Forced alkaline diuresis with IV sodium bicarbonate (IV furosemide if necessary) after correction of dehydration. Symptomatic treatment.

Guidelines/Precautions

1. Use with caution in patients with active GI lesions (e.g., erosive gastritis, peptic ulcer), a history of recurrent GI lesions, hepatic or renal dysfunction, preexisting hypoprothrombinemia, or vitamin K deficiency.
2. Carefully observe patients with coagulation disorders and those receiving drug therapy that interferes with hemostasis.
3. Use with caution in pregnancy and only where the perceived benefits outweigh the risks.
4. Patient response to NSAIDs is variable. Patients who do not respond to or cannot tolerate fenoprofen may be successfully treated with another NSAID.
5. Fenoprofen and salicylates should not be administered concomitantly because there may not be any therapeutic advantage and the incidence of adverse GI side effects may be increased.
6. Contraindicated in patients with previously demonstrated hypersensitivity to fenoprofen or with the complete or partial syndrome of nasal polyps, angioedema, or bronchospastic reactivity to aspirin or other NSAIDs.
7. Signs and symptoms of infection or other diseases may be masked by the antipyretic and anti-inflammatory effects of fenoprofen.

8. Monitor stool for blood every 14 days, and monitor BUN, serum creatinine, and urinalysis every 1–2 months when administering fenoprofen at chronic high doses.

Principal Adverse Reactions

Cardiovascular: Peripheral edema, fluid retention, hypertension, palpitation.
Pulmonary: Dyspnea, bronchospasm.
CNS: Drowsiness, dizziness, headache, anxiety, confusion.
Gastrointestinal: Ulceration, bleeding, dyspepsia, nausea, vomiting, diarrhea, hepatic dysfunction.
Genitourinary: Renal dysfunction, acute renal failure, azotemia, cystitis, hematuria.
Dermatologic: Pruritus, urticaria.
Hematologic: Prolongation of bleeding time, leukopenia, thrombocytopenia, aplastic anemia, hemolytic anemia.
Other: Tinnitus, blurred vision.

FENTANYL CITRATE

Class: Narcotic Agonist

Uses: Treatment of acute, chronic, and cancer pain.

Dosing: *Pain*

Oral transmucosal: 200–400 µg (adult 5 µg/kg, children 5–15 µg/kg, elderly 2.5–5 µg/kg) every 4–6 hours. Oralets should be sucked and not chewed. Oralets are contraindicated in doses >5 µg/kg in adults and >15μg/kg in children. Do not exceed a maximum dose of 400μg for adults or children.

Transdermal system

Initial: 25–50μg/hr.

Maintenance: 25–100μg/hr. Base dose on prior 24-hour analgesic requirements. 60mg IM morphine dose = 360mg PO morphine dose = 100–200μg/hr transdermal fentanyl dose. Doses >50μg/hr should be used only in patients who are already receiving and have developed some tolerance to opioids. Each transdermal application provides 72 hours of reliable analgesic delivery. Therapeutic concentrations are not achieved until 12 to 24 hours after initial application. Initial dosage may be increased after 3 days. Further titration should be evaluated after two applications (6 days) on the new dose. To maintain adequate pain control, add short-acting opioids as needed for breakthrough pain.

IV/IM: 25–100μg (0.7–2μg/kg).

Epidural

Bolus: 50–100μg (1–2μg/kg).

Infusion: 10–60μg/hr (0.2–0.7μg/kg/hr).

Spinal: Bolus, 5–20μg (0.1–0.4μg/kg).

Cancer pain: Initial dose is 200μg Actiq transmucosal. Dose may be repeated in 30 minutes. Patients should be prescribed an initial titration supply not exceeding six 200-μg Actiq units. Titrate dose upward every 1–2 days until the patient reaches a dose that provides adequate analgesia using a single Actiq dosage unit per breakthrough cancer pain episode. Once a successful dose has been found, patients should limit consumption to four or fewer units per day. If consumption increases above four units per day, the dose of the long-acting opioid used for persistent cancer pain should be re-evaluated. Actiq oralets are intended for use only in treatment of breakthrough cancer pain in patients who are already receiving and tolerant to opioid therapy for their underlying cancer pain. Do not use Actiq for acute or postoperative pain.

IV regional block: Add 50μg (1μg/kg) fentanyl to local anesthetic. (See Lidocaine, Prilocaine, or Bupivacaine for dosing and volume.)

Brachial plexus block: Add 50–100μg (1–2μg/kg) fentanyl to 40mL (0.5–0.75mL/kg) local anesthetic.

Patient-controlled analgesia
  IV
    Bolus: 15–75μg (0.3–1.5μg/kg).
    Infusion: 15–100μg/hr (0.3–2μg/kg/hr).
    Lockout interval: 3–10 minutes.
  Epidural
    Bolus: 4–8μg (0.08–0.16μg/kg).
    Infusion: 5–10μg/hr (0.1–0.2μg/kg/hr).
    Lockout interval: 10 minutes.

Administer analgesic regularly (not as needed). Due to impaired elimination, accumulation and excess sedation may occur in patients with hepatic dysfunction. Analgesia may be enhanced by addition of adjuvant drugs such as nonsteroidal anti-inflammatory drugs (NSAIDs) and anti-depressant agents (see pages xxvi–xliv for drug combinations) and use of nondrug therapies such as transcutaneous electrical nerve stimulation (TENS).

Elimination: Hepatic.

Preparations

Fentanyl citrate **(Duragesic):** Transdermal: 25 μg/hr, 50 μg/hr, 75 μg/hr, 100 μg/hr.

Fentanyl citrate **(Fentanyl Oralet):** Transmucosal oralets: 100 μg, 200 μg, 300 μg, 400 μg.

Fentanyl citrate **(Actiq):** Transmucosal oralets: 200 μg, 400 μg, 600 μg, 800 μg, 1200 μg, 1600 μg.

Fentanyl citrate **(Sublimaze):** Injection: 50 μg/mL.

Dilution for Infusion

IV: 500 μg in 100 mL normal saline (5 μg/mL).

Epidural

Bolus: 50–100 μg in 15–20 mL local anesthetic or preservative-free normal saline.

Infusion: 100–500 μg in 100 mL local anesthetic or preservative-free normal saline (1–5 μg/mL).

Pharmacology

This phenylpiperidine derivative is a potent opioid agonist. As an analgesic, fentanyl is 75 to 125 times more potent than morphine. The rapid onset and short duration of action reflect the greater lipid solubility of fentanyl compared with morphine. Depression of ventilation is dose dependent and may last longer than the analgesia. Fentanyl (and other opioids) enhances the action of local anesthetics on peripheral nerve block. This is partly due to weak local anesthetic properties (high doses suppress nerve conduction) and effects on opiate receptors in peripheral nerve terminals. The combination of intrathecal/epidural fentanyl (and other opioids) with local anesthetic (e.g., bupivacaine) is effective in decreasing pain, including visceral discomfort with abdominal malignancies. Fentanyl (and sufentanil) is more lipophilic than morphine, and segmentation of epidural analgesia reflects rapid vascular uptake as well as incorporation in the lipid structures of the spinal space (epidural fat and white matter). The segmental limitation of analgesia requires placement of the epidural catheter at sites adjacent to the dermatomes to be covered. Large volumes of diluent may enable more dermatomes to be included. Lower doses of fentanyl (and other opioids or local anesthetics) are required to prevent pain (by blocking initial nociceptive input and processing at the spinal cord) than to suppress these responses when they occur. Intravenous fentanyl is combined with droperidol to produce neuroleptanalgesia. Fentanyl crosses the placental barrier and may produce depression in the neonate. The drug may appear in breast milk and should be used with caution in nursing mothers.

Pharmacokinetics

Onset of Action: IV, within 30 seconds. IM, <8 minutes. Epidural/Spinal, 4–10 minutes. Transdermal, 12–18 hours. Oral transmucosal, 5–15 minutes.

Peak Effect: IV, 5–15 minutes. IM, <15 minutes. Epidural/Spinal, <30 minutes. Oral transmucosal, 20–30 minutes.

Duration of Action: IV, 30–60 minutes. IM, 1–2 hours. Epidural/Spinal, 1–2 hours. Transdermal, 3 days. Oral transmucosal, 1–2 hours.

Interactions

Circulatory and ventilatory depressant effects potentiated by narcotics, sedatives, volatile anesthetics, nitrous oxide; ventilatory depressant effects potentiated by amphetamines, monoamine oxidase (MAO) inhibitors, phenothiazines, and tricyclic antidepressants; analgesia enhanced and prolonged by α_2-agonists (e.g., epinephrine, clonidine); with high doses, muscle rigidity that may be sufficient to interfere with ventilation; addition of epinephrine to intrathecal/epidural fentanyl results in increased side effects (e.g., nausea).

Toxicity

Toxic Range: Not routinely monitored.

Manifestations: Somnolence, coma, respiratory arrest, apnea, cardiac arrhythmias, combined respiratory and metabolic acidosis, circulatory collapse, cardiac arrest, death.

Antidote: Naloxone IV/IM/SC 0.4–2.0 mg. Repeat dose every 2 to 3 minutes to a maximum of 10–20 mg.

Management: Discontinue or reduce medication. Support ventilation and circulation (patent airway, oxygen, IV fluids, vasopressors). Administer antidote. Monitor blood gases, pH, and electrolytes. Correct acidosis and electrolyte disturbance (lactic acidosis may require sodium bicarbonate IV 1–2mEq/kg). Symptomatic treatment. Airway-protected, ipecac syrup–induced emesis (30mL or 0.5mL/kg ipecac syrup followed by 200mL or 4mL/kg of water or clear fluid) or gastric lavage (with drug ingestion) followed by administration of activated charcoal (PO 50–100g or 1–2g/kg).

Guidelines/Precautions

1. Reduce doses in elderly patients and with concomitant use of sedatives and other narcotics. Incremental doses should be determined from effect of initial dose.
2. Narcotic effects reversed by naloxone (IV 0.2–0.4mg or higher). Duration of reversal may be shorter than duration of narcotic action.
3. High doses may produce increased muscle tone and rigidity, which is reversible by naloxone.
4. Fentanyl crosses the placental barrier, and usage in labor may produce depression of respiration in the neonate. Resuscitation may be required; have naloxone available.
5. Undesirable side effects of epidural, caudal, or intrathecal fentanyl include delayed respiratory depression (up to 8 hours after single dose), pruritus, nausea and vomiting, and urinary retention. Naloxone (IV 0.2–0.4mg as needed or infusion 5–10µg/kg/hr) is effective for prophylaxis and/or treatment of these side effects. Ventilatory support for respiratory depression must be readily available. Antihistamines (e.g., diphenhydramine IV/IM 12.5–25.0mg every 6 hours as needed) may be

used in treating pruritus. Metoclopramide (IV 10 mg every 6 hours) may be used in treating nausea and vomiting. Urinary retention that does not respond to naloxone may require straight bladder catheterization. Bethanechol (Urecholine) PO 15–30 mg three times daily or SC 2.5–5.0 mg three or four times daily as required may be used as an alternative to naloxone. (Bethanechol increases the tone of the detrusor urinae muscle. It should not be given IV or IM, which may result in cholinergic overstimulation. Have atropine available [IV/SC 0.5 mg].)

6. Epidural, caudal, or intrathecal injections should be avoided when the patient has septicemia, infection at the injection site, or coagulopathy.

7. The transmucosal oralets should be removed after consumption or if the patient has shown an adequate sedative/analgesic level or shown signs of respiratory depression. Remove the drug matrix from the handle with tissue paper, and flush down a sink.

8. Accidental dermal exposure to transmucosal oralets should be treated by rinsing the affected area with cool water.

9. Transmucosal oralets are contraindicated in children who weigh less than 15 kg, at home or in any other setting outside a hospital (i.e., outside access to life support equipment), and in patients with known intolerance or hypersensitivity to any of the components (sucrose, liquid glucose, raspberry flavor, carmine, FD&C Blue No. 2 lake dispersion) or the drug fentanyl.

10. Actiq oralets are further contraindicated in the management of acute or postoperative pain and in opioid-intolerant patients. Patients considered opioid tolerant are those taking at least 60 mg morphine per day, 50 µg transdermal fentanyl per hour, or an equally analgesic dose of another opioid for a week or longer.
11. Actiq is not recommended for use in patients who have received MAO inhibitors within 14 days, because severe and unpredictable potentiation by MAO inhibitors has been reported with opioid analgesics.
12. Fentanyl transdermal system is contraindicated in the management of acute or postoperative pain, including use in outpatient surgeries. Deaths have been reported with misuse.
13. Patients should be warned that fentanyl may impair their ability to perform hazardous tasks requiring mental alertness or physical coordination (e.g., driving a motor vehicle, operating heavy machinery).
14. Fentanyl is subject to control under the Federal Controlled Substances Act of 1970 as a Schedule II (C-II) drug.

Principal Adverse Reactions

Cardiovascular: Hypotension, bradycardia.
Pulmonary: Respiratory depression, apnea.
CNS: Dizziness, blurred vision, seizures.
Gastrointestinal: Nausea, emesis, delayed gastric emptying, biliary tract spasm.
Ocular: Miosis.
Musculoskeletal: Muscle rigidity.

FLUOXETINE HYDROCHLORIDE

Class: Selective Serotonin Reuptake Inhibitor— Antidepressant

Uses: Treatment of neurotic and endogenous depression; adjunct treatment of neuropathic pain syndromes, including diabetic neuropathy, postherpetic neuralgia, tic douloureux, and cancer pain; anxiety disorders; phobias; panic disorders; alcohol dependency; enuresis; eating disorders; obesity.

Dosing: *Pain syndromes*
Initial: PO 5–20 mg (0.1–0.4 mg/kg) daily in the morning. Titrate dose upward every 3 to 4 weeks by increments of 5–10 mg as necessary.
Maintenance: PO 5–60 mg (0.1–1 mg/kg) daily in one or two divided doses. Second dose may be given at bedtime if sedation occurs. Doses greater than 20 mg daily may be associated with increased adverse effects. Doses should be decreased if unacceptable side effects occur. Serum levels should be determined if there are signs of toxicity. The higher end of the dose range may be required in the management of painful diabetic neuropathy.
Depression
Initial: PO 5–20 mg daily in the morning.
Maintenance: PO 5–80 mg daily in one or two divided doses. With two divided

doses, administer in the morning and at noon. Second dose may be given at bedtime if sedation occurs. Doses greater than 20 mg daily may be associated with increased adverse effects.

Doses for pain are generally smaller than those used for treatment of affective disorders. Medication should be administered on a fixed schedule and not as needed. After symptoms are controlled, dosage should be gradually reduced to the lowest level that will maintain relief of symptoms. Analgesia may be enhanced by addition of opioid analgesics (see pages xxvi–xliv for drug combinations), non-steroidal anti-inflammatory drugs (NSAIDs), and use of nondrug therapies such as transcutaneous electrical nerve stimulation (TENS). In geriatric patients and patients with decreased renal or hepatic function, decrease doses by one-third to one-half. The possibility for suicide is inherent in depression and may persist until significant remission occurs. The quantity of drug dispensed should reflect this consideration.

Elimination: Hepatic, renal.

Preparations

Fluoxetine hydrochloride **(Prozac)**
   Pulvules: 10 mg, 20 mg.
   Oral solution: 20 mg/5 mL.

Pharmacology

A phenylpropylamine derivative antidepressant agent, fluoxetine differs structurally and pharmacologically from the tricyclic antidepressant agents. The drug is a highly selective serotonin reuptake inhibitor at the presynaptic neuronal membrane. Synaptic concentrations of serotonin are increased, with enhanced serotonergic neurotransmission and numerous CNS effects (e.g., appetite suppression). Fluoxetine has little or no effect on other neurotransmitters. Antidepressant activity is comparable or superior to doxepin or trazodone, with fewer adverse effects, and may be partly due to the highly selective reuptake inhibition of serotonin. Fluoxetine undergoes hepatic demethylation to an active metabolite, norfluoxetine. Fluoxetine may be associated with some anxiety and activation of mania/hypomania. Unlike the tricyclics, sedating and cardiovascular effects are minimal due to the lack of substantial antihistaminic, anticholinergic, α_1-adrenergic-blocking, catecholamine-potentiating, and quinidine-like cardiotoxic effects. Fluoxetine does not appear to affect cardiac conduction and is not arrhythmogenic. Fluoxetine does not inhibit the reuptake of tyramine and has no effect on the pressor response to tyramine. Fluoxetine does not inhibit the monoamine oxidase (MAO) system. Onset of action is comparable to that of the tricyclic antidepressants. Although blockade of neurotransmitter uptake may occur immediately, antidepressant response may take days to weeks.

The analgesic effects of fluoxetine may occur partly through the alleviation of depression, which may be responsible for increased pain suffering, but also by mechanisms that are independent of mood effects. Fluoxetine may potentiate the analgesic effect of opiate agonists possibly by enhancing serotonergic transmission. The drug may produce abnormal EEG patterns and lower the seizure threshold. Therapeutic doses do not affect respiration, but the effects of higher doses remain to be established. Fluoxetine does not appear to have addiction liability. Fluoxetine crosses the placenta and is excreted in breast milk. It should be used with caution in pregnant and nursing mothers.

Pharmacokinetics

Onset of Action: Analgesic effect: PO, <5 days. Antidepressant effect: PO, 1–3 weeks.
Peak Effect: Antidepressant effect: PO, 4 weeks.
Duration of Action: Antidepressant effect: PO, variable.

Interactions

Increased risk of serotonin syndrome (myoclonus, rigidity, hyperreflexia, seizures, hyperthermia, hypertension, restlessness, diaphoresis, shivering, diarrhea, and tremor) with concomitant administration of serotonergics (e.g., clomipramine, tryptophan, pseudoephedrine, tricyclic antidepressant agents, cocaine, lithium, and MAO inhibitors); serum levels and toxic effects of fluoxetine increased by cimetidine; serum levels of fluoxetine decreased by enzyme inducers (e.g., phenytoin, phenobarbital, rifampin); extrapyramidal effects of antipsychotic drugs may be potentiated by fluoxetine; fluoxetine may potentially alter blood glucose concentrations in patients with diabetes mellitus.

Toxicity

Toxic Range: Not routinely monitored.

Manifestations: Serotonin syndrome (myoclonus, rigidity, hyperreflexia, seizures, hyperthermia, hypertension, restlessness, diaphoresis, shivering, diarrhea, and tremor), nausea and vomiting, drowsiness, sinus tachycardia, dilated pupils.

Antidote: Serotonin antagonists: Cyproheptadine (Periactin) PO 4–12 mg stat *or* methysergide PO 2 mg twice daily (three doses may be sufficient).

Management: Discontinue medication. Administer antidote. Correct fluid, electrolyte, and acid-base disturbances. Airway-protected, ipecac syrup–induced emesis (30 mL or 0.5 mL/kg ipecac syrup) or gastric lavage (with drug ingestion) followed by administration of activated charcoal (PO 50–100 g or 1–2 g/kg). Activated charcoal may be administered every 4 to 6 hours during the first 24–48 hours after ingestion. Control seizures: Intravenous benzodiazepines are the first choice; intravenous barbiturates or phenytoin may be useful in refractory seizures. Support ventilation and circulation (patent airway, oxygen, IV fluids, vasoactive drugs). Control hyperpyrexia with ice packs and cooling sponge baths. Hemodialysis or peritoneal dialysis is ineffective because the drug is highly protein bound. Symptomatic treatment. Consider the possibility of multiple drug involvement. Counseling prior to and after discharge for patients who attempted suicide.

Guidelines/Precautions

1. To avoid withdrawal symptoms, the medication should be tapered down over a couple of weeks and not discontinued abruptly.

2. Use with caution in patients with cardiovascular disease, diabetes mellitus, anorexia nervosa, thyroid disease, or seizure disorders.

3. Contraindicated in patients receiving MAO inhibitors (concurrently or within the past 2 weeks), patients in the acute recovery phase following myocardial infarction, and those with demonstrated hypersensitivity to fluoxetine. The combination of fluoxetine and MAO inhibitors may result in the serotonin syndrome, which is characterized by changes in mental status, myoclonus, hyperreflexia, restlessness, diaphoresis, shivering, and tremor. Discontinue the offending medications and treat symptomatically and with a serotonin antagonist (e.g., cyproheptadine).

4. Patients should be warned of the possibility of drowsiness that may impair performance of potentially hazardous tasks such as driving an automobile or operating machinery. Persisting daytime drowsiness may be decreased by administering a lower dose, administering the dose earlier in the evening, or substituting a less sedating alternative.

Principal Adverse Reactions

Cardiovascular: Bradycardia, hypertension.
Pulmonary: Respiratory depression.
CNS: Headache, insomnia, agitation, nervousness, drowsiness, extrapyramidal symptoms, fatigue.
Gastrointestinal: Hepatic dysfunction, jaundice, nausea, vomiting, diarrhea.
Genitourinary: Hyponatremia, urinary frequency, urinary tract infection.

Ocular: Blurred vision, mydriasis, increased intraocular pressure.
Dermatologic: Pruritus, urticaria, petechiae, photosensitivity.
Hematologic: Anemia, thrombocytopenia, eosinophilia, agranulocytosis.
Endocrinologic: Increased or decreased libido, impotence, gynecomastia, SIADH.
Other: Hyperthermia, sexual dysfunction, sexual arousal.

FLUPHENAZINE HYDROCHLORIDE

Class: Phenothiazine

Uses: Antipsychotic, adjunct treatment of neuropathic pain syndromes (e.g., diabetic neuropathy, postherpetic neuralgia).

Dosing: *Pain*

Initial: PO 0.5–1.0 mg (0.01–0.02 mg/kg) every 6 to 8 hours. Titrate dose upward in 0.5-mg increments every few days. Monitor for orthostatic hypotension and extrapyramidal symptoms (e.g., akathisia, cogwheel rigidity).

Maintenance: PO 0.5–2.0 mg (0.01–0.04 mg/kg) every 6 to 8 hours.

Medication should be administered on a fixed schedule (not as needed). After symptoms are controlled, dosage should be gradually reduced to the lowest level that will maintain relief of symptoms. Due to the risk of serious adverse effects (e.g., permanent tardive dyskinesia), fluphenazine is not a drug of first choice for neuropathic pain. It should be used after initial therapy with antidepressants, narcotics, and/or nonsteroidal anti-inflammatory drugs (NSAIDs). It is advisable to obtain informed consent before instituting fluphenazine therapy for chronic pain management.

Psychosis

PO: 0.5–10.0 mg per day (0.01–0.1 mg/kg/day) in divided doses every 6 to 8 hours. Oral doses >20 mg daily should be used with caution. Oral concentrate may be diluted with water or orange, tomato, or grapefruit juice.

IM: 1.25–10.0 mg (0.025–0.2 mg/kg) in divided doses every 6 to 8 hours. IM doses are approximately one-third to one-half the oral dose. IM doses >10 mg daily should be used with caution.

Conversion: 20 mg fluphenazine hydrochloride daily is approximately equal to 25 mg fluphenazine decanoate every 3 weeks.

Observe for hypotension.

Elimination: Hepatic.

Preparations

Fluphenazine decanoate **(Fluphenazine Decanoate, Prolixin Decanoate):** Injection: 25 mg/mL.

Fluphenazine enanthate **(Prolixin Enanthate):** Injection: 25 mg/mL.

Fluphenazine hydrochloride **(Prolixin, Permitil)**
   Oral solution: 2.5mg/5mL.
   Solution concentrate: 5mg/mL.
   Tablets: 1mg, 2.5mg, 5mg, 10mg.
   Injection (IM use only): 2.5mg/mL.

Pharmacology

Fluphenazine is a phenothiazine tranquilizer with pharmacologic effects similar to those of chlorpromazine. Fluphenazine is more potent on a weight basis than chlorpromazine. The decanoate ester is longer acting than the hydrochloride salt or enanthate ester. Fluphenazine has weak anticholinergic, antiemetic, and sedative effects. The neuroleptic actions are most likely due to antagonism of dopamine as a synaptic neurotransmitter in the basal ganglia and limbic portions of the forebrain. Significant incidents of extrapyramidal side effects are evidence of interference with the normal actions of dopamine. Weak antiemetic effects are mediated by dopamine receptor blockade in the medullary chemoreceptor trigger zone. At high doses, the antiarrhythmic effects may be evident and due to the direct quinidine-like property or a local anesthetic effect.

Fluphenazine may lower the seizure threshold and cause EEG changes. Therapeutic doses have little effect on respiration, but the drug may enhance respiratory depression produced by other CNS depressants. Fluphenazine may be useful in chronic pain syndromes by altering the perception of pain and, where applicable, relieving psychosis and/or anxiety. Fluphenazine is occasionally useful in postherpetic neuralgia and other neuropathies in which burning dyesthetic pain and lancinating sensations are prominent features. Unlike the anticonvulsant drugs, fluphenazine appears to be helpful in the management of both qualities of pain.

Pharmacokinetics

Onset: Antipsychotic effects: Fluphenazine hydrochloride, PO/IM, within 1 hour; fluphenazine decanoate, within 24–72 hours.

Peak Effect: Antipsychotic effects: Fluphenazine hydrochloride, PO, variable; fluphenazine decanoate, IM, variable.

Duration of Action: Antipsychotic effects: Fluphenazine hydrochloride, PO/IM, 6–8 hours; fluphenazine decanoate, IM, 1–6 weeks.

Interactions

Potentiates depressant effects of barbiturates, narcotics, anesthetics; additive anticholinergic effects with atropine, glycopyrrolate, and other anticholinergics; decreases hepatic metabolism and increases serum levels and pharmacologic/toxic effects of tricyclic antidepressants; neuronal uptake and antihypertensive effects of guanethidine inhibited; paradoxical hypotension with epinephrine; may potentiate neuromuscular blockade in conjunction with polypeptide antibiotics; interferes with metabolism of phenytoin and may precipitate toxicity; lithium reduces bioavailability; mephentermine, epinephrine, thiazide diuretics potentiate fluphenazine-induced hypotension; concomitant administration of propranolol increases plasma levels of both drugs.

Toxicity

Toxic Range: Not routinely monitored.
Manifestations: Hypotension, tardive dyskinesia (rhythmic involuntary movement of the tongue, face,

mouth, or jaw), extrapyramidal symptoms (akathisia, cogwheel rigidity, oculogyric crisis), neuroleptic malignant syndrome (hyperpyrexia, muscle rigidity, altered mental status, autonomic instability).

Antidote: No specific antidote.

Management: Discontinue or reduce medication. Support ventilation and circulation (patent airway, oxygen, IV fluids, vasopressors). Phenylephrine or norepinephrine should be used to treat hypotension; epinephrine should not be used because it may paradoxically further lower the blood pressure. Treat extrapyramidal symptoms with anticholinergic antiparkinsonian agents (e.g., benztropine IV/PO 1–2 mg two or three times daily, or trihexyphenidyl PO 5–15 mg daily) or with H_1 receptor antagonists such as diphenhydramine (IV/PO 25 mg). Treat neuroleptic malignant syndrome symptomatically and with dantrolene (IV 1.0–2.5 mg/kg every 6 hours for up to two days) or bromocriptine (PO 2.5–10.0 mg three times daily). Symptomatic treatment.

Guidelines/Precautions

1. Fluphenazine may suppress laryngeal reflex with possible aspiration of vomitus.
2. The drug may lower seizure threshold.
3. Use cautiously in geriatric patients, patients with glaucoma, prostatic hypertrophy, or seizure disorders, and children with acute illnesses (e.g., chickenpox, measles).
4. Neuroleptic malignant syndrome, a rare but potentially fatal side effect, may manifest with hyperpyrexia, muscle rigidity, altered mental status, and evidence of autonomic instability (irregular pulse

or blood pressure, tachycardia, diaphoresis, arrhythmias). Discontinue fluphenazine; treat symptomatically and with dantrolene or bromocriptine.

5. Extrapyramidal reactions may consist of dystonic reactions, feelings of motor restlessness (akathisia), and parkinsonian signs and symptoms. Dystonic reactions occur more frequently in children, especially those with acute infections, whereas parkinsonian symptoms predominate in geriatric patients.

6. Do not use epinephrine to treat fluphenazine-associated hypotension. Phenothiazines cause a reversal of epinephrine's vasopressor effects (α-adrenergic effects of epinephrine are blocked, leaving unopposed β activity) and a further lowering of blood pressure. Treat the drug-induced hypotension with norepinephrine or phenylephrine.

Principal Adverse Reactions

Cardiovascular: Hypotension, tachycardia, bradycardia.

CNS: Extrapyramidal reactions, seizures, syncope, drowsiness, exacerbation of psychosis.

Allergic: Urticaria, photosensitivity.

Hematologic: Agranulocytosis, hemolytic anemia.

Other: Neuroleptic malignant syndrome.

GABAPENTIN

Class: Anticonvulsant

Use(s): Adjunct treatment of partial seizures with or without secondary generalization, treatment of neuropathic pain syndromes including sympathetic mediated pain, trigeminal neuralgia, postherpetic neuralgia, post-thoracotamy neuralgia, diabetic neuropathy, and phantom pain.

Dosing: *Anticonvulsant, sympathetic mediated pain, and neuropathic pain*

Initial: PO, day 1, 300 mg once a day; day 2, 300 mg twice a day; day 3, 300 mg three times a day.

Maintenance: PO 900–1800 mg per day in one to three divided doses. Dose may be titrated upward in increments of 300 mg daily every 5–7 days. Doses of up to 2400 mg daily may be required. For treatment of neuropathic pain, drowsiness and sedation may be minimized by administering the majority of the dose at bedtime. It is not necessary to monitor serum levels to optimize therapy.

Dosage should be decreased (by 50% to 75%) in patients with compromised renal function or undergoing hemodialysis. Discontinuation of gabapentin or addition of another anticonvulsant should be done gradually over a minimum of one week.

Elimination: Renal.

Preparations

Gabapentin **(Neurontin):** Capsules: 100 mg, 300 mg, 400 mg.

Pharmacology

A structural analogue of the neurotransmitter γ-aminobutyric acid (GABA), gabapentin has an unknown mechanism for its anticonvulsant activity. Binding of the drug occurs in the outer layers of the isocortex and the hippocampus. The drug does not bind to GABA, benzodiazepine, glutamate, glycine, opiate, or *N*-methyl D-aspartate receptors and may have an uncommon binding site in the CNS. Gabapentin has a unique pharmacokinetic profile for an anticonvulsant drug, including no binding to plasma proteins, primary elimination by the kidney, and dose-dependent oral absorption at high dosages. No drug interactions occur with other anticonvulsants. Gabapentin alleviates burning, aching, and dysthetic components, as well as lancinating, shooting paroxysmal pain in peripheral and central neuropathic pain syndromes. It has an exclusively central site of action, whereas lidocaine acts primarily in the periphery (by reducing the rate of continuing discharge of injured afferent fibers) and amitriptyline has both peripheral and central components. The beneficial effects of gabapentin in alleviating the peripheral manifestations of sympathetic mediated pain (hyperpathia, allodynia, edema, stiffness, discoloration, and vasomotor and sudomotor changes) may be due to inhibitory action at its receptor sites and an increase in the bioavailability of serotonin, with consequent decrease in catecholamine outflow and production of antidepressant effects. Gabapentin crosses the blood-brain barrier and may produce CNS side effects (e.g., somnolence, memory impairment).

Pharmacokinetics

Onset of Action: Neuropathicsympathetic mediated pain: 30–60 min.
Peak Effect: Anticonvulsant effect: PO, <12 weeks.

Duration of Action: Anticonvulsant effect/Sympathetic mediated pain: PO, variable.

Interactions

Decreased oral bioavailability with concomitant administration of antacids; does not interfere with the metabolism of carbamazepine, phenytoin, phenobarbital, or valproic acid.

Toxicity

Toxic Range: Not routinely monitored.
Manifestations: Postural hypotension, drowsiness, dizziness, tremors, ataxia, amnesia, diplopia, nausea, vomiting.
Antidote: No specific antidote.
Management: Discontinue or reduce medication. Support ventilation and circulation (patent airway, oxygen, IV fluids). Symptomatic treatment. Hemodialysis.

Guidelines/Precautions

1. Patients should be advised that gabapentin may cause dizziness, somnolence, and other symptoms and signs of CNS depression. They should be advised not to drive a car or operate other complex machinery until they have gained sufficient experience on gabapentin to gauge whether or not it affects their mental and/or motor performance adversely.
2. Gabapentin may be used in combination with other antiepileptic drugs without concern for alteration of the blood concentrations of gabapentin or the antiepileptic drugs.
3. Gabapentin is contraindicated in patients who have demonstrated hypersensitivity to the drug or its ingredients.

Principal Adverse Reactions

Cardiovascular: Hypotension, angina pectoris, arrhythmia, palpitation.

Pulmonary: Rhinitis, pharyngitis, coughing, bronchospasm.

CNS: Somnolence, amnesia, dizziness, ataxia, fatigue, depression, nystagmus, hyperkinesia, dyskinesia, dysarthria, paresthesia.

Gastrointestinal: Dyspepsia, dry mouth, constipation, increased appetite, gingivitis.

Genitourinary: Impotence.

Dermatologic: Abrasions, pruritus.

Other: Decreased white blood count, myalgia.

GUANETHIDINE MONOSULFATE

Class: α-Adrenergic Blocker

Use(s): Treatment of hypertension, sympathetic mediated pain, and Raynaud's disease; reversal of arterial spasm.

Dosing: *Hypertension*

Initial: PO 10 mg/day.

Maintenance: PO 10–50 mg/day. Dose may be titrated upward in increments of 12.5–25.0 mg daily every 5–7 days.

Sympathetic mediated pain: IV regional sympathetic block: 10–30 mg (0.2–0.4 mg/kg) diluted in 20–30 mL of normal saline or 0.5% lidocaine (upper extremity) *or* 40 mg (0.5 mg/kg) diluted in 40–50 mL of normal saline or 0.5% lidocaine (lower extremity). Initial series of blocks may be repeated every 4 days and then every 2 to 3 weeks as indicated. Methylprednisolone (80 mg) may be added to the solution to decrease the postmanipulation edema. Administer 500 mL of fluid immediately after tourniquet release to prevent orthostasis.

Raynaud's disease: IV regional sympathetic block: 15–30 mg (0.25 mg/kg) diluted in 20–30 mL of normal saline or 0.5% lidocaine. Heparin 500 IU may be added if desired.

Reversal of arterial spasm: Intra-arterial injection: 5 mg in 5 mL normal saline with or without intravenous regional blockade.

Elimination: Renal.

Preparations

Guanethidine monosulfate **(Ismelin):** Tablets: 10 mg, 25 mg.

Guanethidine monosulfate and hydrochlorothiazide **(Esimil):** Tablets: Guanethidine monosulfate 10 mg and hydrochlorothiazide 25 mg.

The parenteral formulation is designated an orphan drug and is not available commercially. If you wish to acquire the product, you may contact the manufacturer, Ciba-Geigy, at 556 Morris Avenue, Summit, NJ 07901 (908-277-5691).

Dilution for Infusion: 2 g in 500 mL D5W or normal saline (4 mg/mL).

Pharmacology

A postganglionic adrenergic blocking agent, guanethidine produces a selective block of efferent peripheral sympathetic pathways. Guanethidine reaches its site of action by active transport into the neuron. The drug decreases norepinephrine stores from adrenergic nerve endings (but not from the adrenal medulla) and prevents release of norepinephrine from adrenergic nerve endings in response to sympathetic stimulation. Chronic administration of guanethidine results in increased sensitivity of adrenergic receptors to catecholamines. Unlike ganglionic blocking agents, guanethidine does not produce central or parasympathetic blockade. Following oral administration of therapeutic doses, depletion of catecholamine stores from adrenergic nerve endings occurs at a very slow rate, producing a gradual prolonged fall in blood pressure (mainly systolic) that is usually associated with bradycardia and decreased pulse pressure. Guanethidine reduces or eliminates cardiovascular reflexes, and thus orthostatic hypotension may be common. Intravenous regional sympathetic blockade with guanethidine is more effective than reserpine or bretylium in alleviating the peripheral manifestations of sympathetic mediated pain (reflex sympathetic dystrophy and causalgia). Unlike reserpine, guanethidine does not cross the blood-brain barrier and does not produce CNS side effects. Compared with local anesthetic sympathetic blocks (e.g., stellate ganglion), the incidence of toxicity is lower and duration of pain relief is longer.

Pharmacokinetics

Onset of Action: Antihypertensive effect: PO, <2 days.
Peak Effect: Antihypertensive effect: PO, 14 days.
Duration of Action: Antihypertensive effect: PO, 1–3 weeks. IV regional (pain relief in reflexive sympathetic dystrophy): 3–6 weeks.

Interactions

Hypotensive effects potentiated with diuretics, alcohol, methotrimeprazine, or other hypotensive agents; hypotensive effects antagonized by monoamine oxidase (MAO) inhibitors; pressor effects of norepinephrine, phenylephrine, and metaraminol may be potentiated by guanethidine; resistance to antiadrenergic (hypotensive) effects in patients receiving tricyclic antidepressants (which block the uptake of guanethidine), haloperidol, mephentermine, ephedrine, methylphenidate, amphetamines, oral contraceptives; risks of bradycardia increased with concomitant digoxin.

Toxicity

Toxic Range: Not routinely monitored.
Manifestations: Postural hypotension, dizziness, blurred vision, syncope, bradycardia, diarrhea.
Antidote: No specific antidote.
Management: Discontinue or reduce medication. Support ventilation and circulation (patent airway, oxygen, IV fluids; vasopressors should be used with caution). Airway-protected, ipecac syrup–induced emesis (30 mL or 0.5 mL/kg ipecac syrup followed by 200 mL or 4 mL/kg of water or clear fluid) or gastric lavage (with drug ingestion) followed by administration of activated charcoal (PO 50–100 g or 1–2 g/kg). Correct fluid, electrolytes, and acid-base balance. Symptomatic treatment.

Guidelines/Precautions

1. Guanethidine should be discontinued 2 to 3 weeks prior to elective surgery to reduce the possibility of cardiovascular collapse and cardiac arrest during

anesthesia. If emergency procedures are necessary, preanesthetic and anesthetic agents should be administered cautiously in reduced dosages. Vasopressors should be used with caution since the response to these drugs may be increased.

2. MAO inhibitors should be discontinued for at least 1 week prior to administration of guanethidine.

3. Use with caution in patients with impaired renal function, incipient cardiac decompensation, or severe heart failure.

4. Contraindicated in patients with known or suspected pheochromocytoma or frank congestive heart failure not caused by hypertension.

5. Severe hypotension should be treated with appropriate fluid therapy and vasopressor agents such as dopamine or norepinephrine.

6. In intravenous regional blocks, when normal saline is used as the diluent, the cuff may be deflated cautiously after 10 minutes. If a local anesthetic is used as the diluent (e.g., lidocaine 0.5%), the cuff should be deflated after 40 minutes and after no less than 20 minutes. Between 20 and 40 minutes, the cuff may be deflated, reinflated immediately, and finally deflated after a minute to reduce the sudden absorption of local anesthetic into the systemic circulation.

Principal Adverse Reactions

Cardiovascular: Hypotension, bradycardia.
Pulmonary: Dyspnea.
CNS: Dizziness, syncope, weakness.
Gastrointestinal: Increased frequency of bowel movements, explosive diarrhea, nausea, vomiting.

Genitourinary: Urinary retention, inhibition of ejaculation.

Other: Hypoglycemia in patients with diabetes mellitus, edema, nasal congestion.

HALOPERIDOL

Class: Butyrophenone

Use(s): Antipsychotic, adjunct treatment of neuropathic pain (e.g., diabetic neuropathy, postherpetic neuralgia).

Dosing: *Pain:* PO 0.5–10.0 mg (0.01–0.2 mg/kg) in divided doses. Medication should be administered on a fixed schedule (not as needed). After symptoms are controlled, dosage should be gradually reduced to the lowest level that will maintain relief of symptoms. Due to the risk of serious adverse effects (e.g., permanent tardive dyskinesia), haloperidol is not a drug of first choice for neuropathic pain. It should be used after initial therapy with antidepressants, narcotics, and/or nonsteroidal anti-inflammatory drugs (NSAIDs). It is advisable to obtain informed consent before instituting haloperidol therapy for chronic pain management.

    Antipsychotic

        IM: Haloperidol lactate 2–5 mg. (Do not administer intravenously.)

        IM: Haloperidol decanoate (for chronic

psychotic patients). Give 10 to 15 times the daily oral dose. Interval between doses is 4 weeks. (Do not administer intravenously.)

PO: 0.5–5.0 mg two or three times daily. Children, 0.05–0.15 mg/kg/day.

Elimination: Hepatic.

Preparations

Haloperidol **(Haldol):** Tablets: 0.5 mg, 1 mg, 2 mg, 5 mg, 10 mg, 20 mg.

Haloperidol lactate **(Haldol, Haloperidol)**
  Oral concentrate: 2 mg/mL.
  Injection (for IM use only): 5 mg/mL.

Haloperidol decanoate **(Haldol Decanoate):** Injection (for IM use only): 50 mg/mL, 100 mg/mL.

Pharmacology

A butyrophenone derivative, haloperidol has pharmacologic effects similar to those of the piperazine-derived phenothiazines. The drug reduces dopaminergic neurotransmission in the CNS and may antagonize the effect of glutamic acid in the extrapyramidal system. Haloperidol has weak anticholinergic, α-adrenergic, and ganglionic blocking effects. The strong antiemetic effects may be mediated by dopamine receptor blockade in the medullary chemoreceptor trigger zone. Haloperidol produces less sedation, hypotension, and hypothermia than chlorpromazine. The drug may lower the seizure threshold and cause EEG changes. Therapeutic doses have little effect on respiration, but respiratory depression produced by other CNS depressants may be enhanced. Haloperidol reduces the anxiety accompanying psychosis but is less effective against acute situational anxiety. Haloperidol may be useful in chronic pain syndromes by altering the perception of pain and, where applicable, relieving psychosis and/or anxiety. Haloperidol may be useful in postherpetic neuralgia and other neuropathies in which burning dyesthetic pain and lancinating sensations are prominent features. Unlike the anticonvulsant drugs, haloperidol may be helpful in the management of both qualities of pain.

Pharmacokinetics

Onset of Action: Antiemetic effects: IM, 10–30 minutes; PO, 1–2 hours.
Peak Effect: Antiemetic effects: IM, 30–45 minutes; PO, 2–4 hours.
Duration of Action: Antiemetic effects: 12–38 hours (half-life).

Interactions

Potentiates depressant effects of barbiturates, narcotics, anesthetics; additive anticholinergic effects with atropine, glycopyrrolate, and other anticholinergics; decreases hepatic metabolism and increases serum levels and pharmacologic/toxic effects of tricyclic antidepressants; inhibits neuronal uptake and antihypertensive effects of guanethidine; paradoxical hypotension with epinephrine; may potentiate neuromuscular blockade in conjunction with polypeptide antibiotics; interferes with metabolism of phenytoin and may precipitate toxicity; encephalopathic syndrome with coadministration of lithium; mephentermine, epinephrine, and thiazide diuretics potentiate haloperidol-induced hypotension; concomitant administration of propranolol increases plasma levels of both drugs.

Toxicity

Toxic Range: Not routinely monitored.

Manifestations: Hypotension, QT interval prolongation, respiratory depression, tardive dyskinesia (rhythmic involuntary movement of the tongue, face, mouth, or jaw), extrapyramidal symptoms (akathisia, cogwheel rigidity, oculogyric crisis), neuroleptic malignant syndrome (hyperpyrexia, muscle rigidity, altered mental status, autonomic instability).

Antidote: No specific antidote.

Management: Discontinue or reduce medication. Support ventilation and circulation (patent airway, oxygen, IV fluids, vasopressors). Phenylephrine or norepinephrine should be used to treat hypotension. Epinephrine should not be used because it may paradoxically further lower the blood pressure (the α-adrenergic effects of epinephrine are blocked, leaving unopposed β activity). Treat extrapyramidal symptoms with anticholinergic antiparkinsonian agents (e.g., benztropine IV/PO 1–2 mg two or three times daily, or trihexyphenidyl PO 5–15 mg daily) or with H_1 receptor antagonists such as diphenhydramine (IV/PO 25 mg). Treat neuroleptic malignant syndrome symptomatically and with dantrolene (IV 1.0–2.5 mg/kg every 6 hours for up to 2 days) or bromocriptine (PO 2.5–10.0 mg three times daily). Symptomatic treatment.

Guidelines/Precautions

1. Extrapyramidal reactions may consist of dystonic reactions, feelings of motor restlessness (akathisia), and parkinsonian signs and symptoms. Dystonic reactions occur more frequently in children, whereas parkinsonian symptoms predominate in geriatric patients.

2. Use cautiously in geriatric patients; patients with glaucoma, prostatic hypertrophy, or seizure disorders; and children with acute illnesses (e.g., chickenpox, measles).

3. Neuroleptic malignant syndrome, a rare but potentially fatal side effect, may manifest with hyperpyrexia, muscle rigidity, altered mental status, and evidence of autonomic instability (irregular pulse or blood pressure, tachycardia, diaphoresis, arrhythmias).

4. Contraindicated in Parkinson's disease.

Principal Adverse Reactions

Cardiovascular: Tachycardia, hypotension, hypertension.

Pulmonary: Laryngospasm, bronchospasm.

CNS: Extrapyramidal reaction, tardive dyskinesia.

Gastrointestinal: Hypersalivation, diarrhea, nausea and vomiting.

Metabolic: Hyperglycemia, hypoglycemia, hyponatremia.

Ocular: Retinopathy, visual disturbance.

HYDROCODONE BITARTRATE

Class: Narcotic Agonist and Antitussive

Use(s): Acute pain, chronic pain, cancer pain, coughing induced by chemical or mechanical irritation of the respiratory system.

Dosing: *Analgesia:* PO 5–10 mg (0.1–0.2 mg/kg) every 4 to 6 hours.

Antitussive: PO 5 mg (0.1 mg/kg) every 4–6 hours. Titrate dose to effect. Use the smallest effective dose. Maximum daily dose 90 mg.

Maximum daily dose of nonopioid ingredient in fixed-combination preparations (e.g., Vicodin): Acetaminophen 4 g, aspirin 6 g, ibuprofen 1 g.

Warning: Chronic ingestion of acetaminophen doses as low as 3 g have caused liver damage. Acetaminophen-free hydrocodone capsules may be prepared by compounding pharmacists.

Administer analgesic regularly (not as needed). Due to impaired elimination, accumulation and excess sedation may occur in patients with renal or hepatic dysfunction. Analgesia may be enhanced by addition of adjuvant drugs such as nonsteroidal anti-inflammatory drugs (NSAIDs) and antidepressant agents (see pages xxvi–xliv for drug combinations) and use of nondrug therapies such as transcutaneous electrical nerve stimulation (TENS).

Elimination: Hepatic, renal.

Preparations

Hydrocodone bitartrate and acetaminophen **(Lortab 2.5/500):** Tablets: Hydrocodone bitartrate 2.5 mg and acetaminophen 500 mg.

Hydrocodone bitartrate and acetaminophen **(Dolacet, Hydrocet, Lorcet, Zydone):** Capsules: Hydrocodone bitartrate 5 mg and acetaminophen 500 mg.

Hydrocodone bitartrate and acetaminophen **(Anexsia, Anodynos-DHC, Co-Gesic, DuoCet, Duradyne DHC, Hy-Phen, Lorcet, Lortab, Norcet, Vicodin):** Tablets: Hydrocodone bitartrate 5 mg and acetaminophen 500 mg.

Hydrocodone bitartrate and acetaminophen **(Lortab 5/500):** Tablets: Hydrocodone bitartrate 5 mg and acetaminophen 500 mg.

Hydrocodone bitartrate and acetaminophen **(Lortab 7.5/500):** Tablets: Hydrocodone bitartrate 7.5 mg and acetaminophen 500 mg.

Hydrocodone bitartrate and acetaminophen **(Anexsia 7.5/650, Lorcet Plus, Norcet 7.5 mg):** Tablets: Hydrocodone bitartrate 7.5 mg and acetaminophen 650 mg.

Hydrocodone bitartrate and acetaminophen **(Vicodin ES):** Tablets: Hydrocodone bitartrate 7.5 mg and acetaminophen 750 mg.

Hydrocodone bitartrate and acetaminophen **(Vicodin HP, Anexsia 10/650, Lorcet 10/650):** Tablets: Hydrocodone bitartrate 10 mg and acetaminophen 650 mg.

Hydrocodone bitartrate and acetaminophen **(Norco 10/325):** Tablets: Hydrocodone bitartrate 10 mg and acetaminophen 325 mg.

Hydrocodone bitartrate and aspirin **(Azdone, Damason-P, Lortab ASA):** Tablets: Hydrocodone bitartrate 5 mg and aspirin 500 mg.

Hydrocodone bitartrate and acetaminophen **(Lortab Liquid):** Suspension: Hydrocodone bitartrate 2.5 mg/ 5 mL and acetaminophen 120 mg/5 mL.

Hydrocodone bitartrate and ibuprofen **(Vicoprofen):**

Tablets: Hydrocodone bitartrate 7.5 mg and ibuprofen 200 mg.

Pharmacology

A synthetic phenanthrene-derivative opiate agonist and antitussive, hydrocodone is the hydrogenated ketone derivative of codeine. The analgesic activity is mild and comparable to that of codeine. Hydrocodone is often used in combination with non-narcotic analgesics (e.g., aspirin, acetaminophen) for the treatment of mild to moderate pain. The drug is an effective antitussive and is used as a cough suppressant. Abuse liability is less than that of morphine and occurs rarely after oral analgesic use. Hydrocodone produces minimal sedation, nausea, vomiting, and constipation. Hydrocodone crosses the placental barrier and may produce depression in the neonate. The drug may appear in breast milk, but at usual doses the effects on the infant may not be clinically significant.

Pharmacokinetics

Onset of Action: PO, 15–30 minutes.
Peak Effect: PO, 30–60 minutes.
Duration of Action: PO, 4–8 hours.

Interactions

Potentiates CNS and circulatory depressant effects of other narcotic analgesics, volatile anesthetics, phenothiazines, sedative-hypnotics, alcohol, and tricyclic antidepressants; analgesia enhanced and prolonged by narcotic and non-narcotic analgesics (e.g., aspirin, acetaminophen) and α_2-agonists (e.g., clonidine).

Toxicity

Toxic Range: Not routinely monitored.

Manifestations: Somnolence, coma, respiratory arrest, apnea, cardiac arrhythmias, combined respiratory and metabolic acidosis, circulatory collapse, cardiac arrest, death.

Antidote: Naloxone IV/IM/SC 0.4–2.0 mg. Repeat dose every 2 to 3 minutes to a maximum of 10–20 mg.

Management: Discontinue or reduce medication. Support ventilation and circulation (patent airway, oxygen, IV fluids, vasopressors). Administer antidote. Monitor blood gases, pH, and electrolytes. Correct acidosis and electrolyte disturbance (lactic acidosis may require sodium bicarbonate IV 1–2 mEq/kg). Symptomatic treatment. Airway-protected, ipecac syrup–induced emesis (30 mL or 0.5 mL/kg ipecac syrup followed by 200 mL or 4 mL/kg of water or clear fluid) or gastric lavage (with drug ingestion) followed by administration of activated charcoal (PO 50–100 g or 1–2 g/kg).

Guidelines/Precautions

1. Reduce dosage in elderly patients and with concomitant use of narcotics and sedative-hypnotics.
2. Prescribe or supply an antiemetic (e.g., metoclopramide) for use in the event of nausea and/or vomiting.
3. Constipation may be more difficult to control than pain. Prevent and/or treat by daily administration of laxatives and stool softeners, for example, Colace (docusate sodium) 100–300 mg/day. Do not administer bulk-forming agents that contain methylcellu-

lose, psyllium, or polycarbophil. Temporary arrest in the passage through the gastrointestinal tract may lead to fecal impaction or bowel obstruction.

4. Tolerance may develop in all patients taking narcotic analgesics for more than a couple of weeks. It may be a function of dose, frequency, and route of administration, since IV and spinal infusions of narcotics are associated with rapid development of tolerance. The first sign is a decrease in duration of effective analgesia. To delay the development of tolerance, add adjuvant drugs (e.g., NSAIDs, antidepressant agents, dextromethorphan) or switch to alternative opioids (starting at one-half the equianalgesic dose) or supplement with nondrug therapies (e.g., TENS).

5. Physical dependence may be revealed with abrupt discontinuation of chronically administered opioids (>2 weeks). Withdrawal symptoms may manifest by anxiety, nervousness, irritability, chills alternating with hot flashes, diaphoresis, insomnia, abdominal cramps, nausea, vomiting, and myoclonus. To avoid withdrawal, doses should be reduced slowly (e.g., dose reduction of 75% every 2 days). Withdrawal should be treated symptomatically.

6. Addiction (psychological dependence) is characterized by a continued craving for a narcotic and the need to use the narcotic for effects other than for pain relief. The patient exhibits drug-seeking behavior. Most patients with psychological dependence are also physically dependent, but the reverse is rare in patients using narcotics for the management of pain.

7. Drug combinations with adjuvant drugs enhance analgesia (see pages xxvi–xliv).
8. Adjuvant drug therapies also include regional blockade, trigger-point injections (with local anesthetics and steroids), and intravenous regional anesthesia.
9. Adjuvant nondrug therapies include TENS and modalities such as ice or heat application, ultrasound, and soft tissue mobilization.
10. Patients should be warned that hydrocodone may impair their ability to perform hazardous tasks requiring mental alertness or physical coordination (e.g., driving a motor vehicle, operating heavy machinery).
11. The drug preparation may contain sulfites, which may cause allergic reactions or anaphylaxis in susceptible individuals.
12. Hydrocodone is subject to control under the Federal Controlled Substances Act as a Schedule III (C-III) drug.

Principal Adverse Reactions

Cardiovascular: Hypotension, circulatory depression, bradycardia, syncope.
Pulmonary: Respiratory depression.
CNS: Sedation, somnolence, euphoria, dysphoria, disorientation.
Genitourinary: Urinary retention.
Gastrointestinal: Nausea, vomiting, abdominal pain, biliary tract spasm, constipation, anorexia, hepatic dysfunction.
Ocular: Miosis.
Allergic: Rash, pruritus, urticaria.

HYDROMORPHONE HYDROCHLORIDE

Class: Narcotic Agonist

Use(s): Treatment of acute, chronic, and cancer pain; control of persistent nonproductive cough.

Dosing: *Pain*

> PO: 2–4 mg every 4–6 hours.
> IM/SC: 2–4 mg (0.04–0.08 mg/kg) every 4–6 hours.
> Rectal: 3 mg every 6–8 hours.
> Slow IV: 0.5–2.0 mg (0.01–0.04 mg/kg).
> Spinal: 0.1–0.2 mg (2–4 µg/kg).
> Epidural
>> Bolus: 1–2 mg (20–40 µg/kg). Dilute in 10 mL preservative-free normal saline or local anesthetic.
>> Infusion: 0.15–0.3 mg/hr (2.0–3.5 µg/kg/hr).
>
> *Patient-controlled analgesia IV*
>> Bolus: 0.1–0.5 mg (2–10 µg/kg).
>> Infusion: 0.1–0.5 mg/hr (2–10 µg/kg/hr).
>> Lockout interval: 5–15 minutes.
>
> *Patient-controlled analgesia epidural*
>> Bolus: 0.15–0.3 mg (3–6 µg/kg).
>> Infusion: 0.15–0.3 mg/hr (3–6 µg/kg/hr).
>> Lockout interval: 15–30 minutes.

Antitussive: PO 0.5–1.0 mg every 3–4 hours.

Administer analgesic regularly (not as needed). Due to impaired elimination, accumulation and excess sedation may occur in patients with renal hepatic dysfunction. Analgesia may be enhanced by addition of adjuvant drugs such as non-steroidal anti-inflammatory drugs (NSAIDs) and antidepressant agents (see pages xxvi–xliv for drug combinations) and use of nondrug therapies such as transcutaneous electrical nerve stimulation (TENS).

Elimination: Hepatic.

Preparations

Hydromorphone hydrochloride **(Dilaudid)**
    Injection: 1 mg/mL, 2 mg/mL, 3 mg/mL, 4 mg/mL.
    Tablets: 1 mg, 2 mg, 3 mg, 4 mg.
    Rectal suppositories: 3 mg.
Hydromorphone hydrochloride **(Dilaudid HP):** Injection: 10 mg/mL.

Dilution for Infusion

IV: 5 mg in 100 mL normal saline (50 μg/mL).
Epidural
    Bolus: 1–2 mg in 10 mL local anesthetic or preservative-free normal saline.
    Infusion: 5 mg in 100 mL local anesthetic or preservative-free normal saline (50 μg/mL).

Pharmacology

An opiate agonist that is a hydrogenated ketone of morphine, hydromorphone is seven times more potent than morphine as an analgesic. Primary effects are on the central nervous system and organs containing smooth muscle. Excitatory synaptic pain transmission is decreased by hydromorphone-induced inhibition of neurotransmitter release (e.g., bradykinin at site of tissue injury, substance P in the dorsal horn, and dopamine in the basal ganglia). In addition, hydromorphone (and other opioids) may alter cognitive and emotional processing of painful input by acting on limbic and cortical opioid receptors. Hydromorphone produces analgesia, drowsiness, euphoria, and dose-related depression of respiration. The drug releases histamine, which can cause pruritus. It may induce nausea and vomiting by activating the chemoreceptor trigger zone. It depresses the cough reflex by a direct effect on the cough centers in the medulla. Hydromorphone crosses the placental barrier and may produce depression in the neonate. The drug may appear in breast milk and should be used with caution in nursing mothers.

Pharmacokinetics

Onset of Action: IV, almost immediate. IM/PO/SC, 15–30 minutes. Rectal, 10–15 minutes. Epidural, 5 minutes.

Peak Effect: IV, 5–20 minutes. IM/PO/SC/Rectal, 30–60 minutes. Epidural, 30 minutes.

Duration of Action: IV, 2–4 hours. IM/PO/SC, 4–6 hours. Rectal, 6–8 hours. Epidural, 6–16 hours.

Interactions

CNS and circulatory depressant effects potentiated by alcohol, sedatives, narcotics, antihistamines, phenothiazines, butyrophenones, monoamine oxidase (MAO) inhibitors, and tricyclic antidepressants; analgesia enhanced and prolonged by α_2-agonists (e.g., clonidine); addition of epinephrine to intrathecal/epidural hydromorphone results in increased side effects (e.g., nausea); hydromorphone may decrease the effect of diuretics in patients with congestive heart failure.

Toxicity

Toxic Range: Not routinely monitored.

Manifestations: Somnolence, coma, respiratory arrest, apnea, cardiac arrhythmias, combined respiratory and metabolic acidosis, circulatory collapse, cardiac arrest, death.

Antidote: Naloxone IV/IM/SC 0.4–2.0 mg. Repeat dose every 2 to 3 minutes to a maximum of 10–20 mg.

Management: Discontinue or reduce medication. Support ventilation and circulation (patent airway, oxygen, IV fluids, vasopressors). Administer antidote. Monitor blood gases, pH, and electrolytes. Correct acidosis and electrolyte disturbance (lactic acidosis may require sodium bicarbonate IV 1–2 mEq/kg). Symptomatic treatment. Airway-protected, ipecac syrup–induced emesis (30 mL or 0.5 mL/kg ipecac syrup followed by 200 mL or 4 mL/kg of water or clear fluid) or gastric lavage (with drug ingestion) followed by administration of activated charcoal (PO 50–100 g or 1–2 g/kg).

Guidelines/Precautions

1. Reduce dose in elderly patients and with concomitant use of sedatives and other narcotics.
2. The narcotic antagonist naloxone is a specific antidote (IV/IM/SC 0.2–0.4 mg or higher). Reversal of narcotic effect may lead to onset of pain and release of catecholamines.
3. Crosses the placental barrier, and usage in labor may produce depression of respiration in the neonate. Resuscitation may be required; have naloxone available.
4. Do not confuse the highly concentrated Dilaudid

HP (10 mg/mL) with other standard parenteral formulations. It is intended for use in narcotic-tolerant patients.

5. Undesirable side effects of epidural, caudal, or intrathecal hydromorphone include delayed respiratory depression, pruritus, nausea and vomiting, and urinary retention. Naloxone (IV 0.2–0.4 mg as needed or infusion 5–10 μg/kg/hr) is effective for prophylaxis and/or treatment of these side effects. Ventilatory support for respiratory depression must be readily available. Antihistamines such as diphenhydramine (IV/IM 12.5–25.0 mg every 6 hours as needed) may be used in treating pruritus. Metoclopramide (IV 10 mg every 6 hours as needed) may be used in treating nausea and vomiting. Urinary retention that does not respond to naloxone may require an "in and out" bladder catheter. Bethanechol (Urecholine) PO 15–30 mg three times daily or SC 2.5–5.0 mg three or four times daily as required may be used as an alternative to naloxone. (Bethanechol increases the tone of the detrusor urinae muscle. It should not be given IV or IM, which may result in cholinergic overstimulation. Have atropine available [IV/SC 0.5 mg].)

6. Epidural, caudal, or intrathecal injections should be avoided when the patient has septicemia, infection at the injection site, or coagulopathy.

7. Patients should be warned that hydromorphone may impair their ability to perform hazardous tasks requiring mental alertness or physical coordination (e.g., driving a motor vehicle, operating heavy machinery).

8. Hydromorphone is subject to control under the Controlled Substances Act of 1970 as a Schedule II (C-II) drug.

Principal Adverse Reactions

Cardiovascular: Hypotension, hypertension, bradycardia, arrhythmias.
Pulmonary: Bronchospasm, laryngospasm.
CNS: Blurred vision, syncope, euphoria, dysphoria.
Genitourinary: Urinary retention, antidiuretic effect, ureteral spasm.
Gastrointestinal: Biliary tract spasm, constipation, anorexia, nausea, vomiting.
Ocular: Miosis.
Allergic: Pruritus, urticaria.
Musculoskeletal: Chest wall rigidity.

HYDROXYZINE HYDROCHLORIDE

Class: Antihistamine

Use(s): Antiemetic; sedative; adjunct treatment of acute, chronic, and cancer pain; adjunct treatment of migraine and tension headache; treatment of pruritus due to allergic conditions (e.g., chronic urticaria and histamine-mediated pruritus).

Dosing: *Pain:* PO/IM 25–100 mg (0.5–2.0 mg/kg) four times daily or every 6 to 8 hours. Medication should be administered on a fixed schedule (not as needed). Dose should be adjusted according to symptom response. After symptoms are controlled, dosage should be gradually reduced to the lowest level that will maintain relief of symptoms. Analgesia may be enhanced by addition of opioid analgesics (see pages xxvi–xliv for drug combinations), nonsteroidal anti-inflammatory drugs (NSAIDs), antidepressant agents, and use of nondrug therapies such as transcutaneous electrical nerve stimulation (TENS).

Sedation/Nausea/Emesis: PO/IM 25–100 mg (0.5–2.0 mg/kg) every 6 hours as indicated.

Elimination: Hepatic.

Preparations

Hydroxyzine hydrochloride **(Atarax)**
 Oral solution: 2 mg/mL.
 Tablets: 10 mg, 25 mg, 50 mg, 100 mg.
Hydroxyzine hydrochloride **(Vistaril, Hyzine, Vistaject, Vistacon, Vistazine, Neucalm, Quiess):** Injection: 25 mg/mL, 50 mg/mL.
Hydroxyzine pamoate **(Hy-Pam, Vistaril)**
 Oral solution: 5 mg/mL (equivalent to hydroxyzine hydrochloride).
 Capsules: 25 mg, 50 mg, 100 mg (equivalent to hydroxyzine hydrochloride).

Pharmacology

This piperazine-derivative antihistamine has anticholinergic, antiemetic, antispasmodic, and local anesthetic activity. The sedative and tranquilizing effects may result principally from suppression of activity at subcortical levels of the central nervous system (CNS). The antiemetic and anti-motion sickness effects may result from central anticholinergic and CNS depressant properties. Hydroxyzine has intrinsic analgesic activity with a ceiling effect at doses beyond 150 mg. Hydroxyzine potentiates the sedative and analgesic effects of opioids and enables a decrease in opioid dose and reduction of side effects such as nausea and vomiting. The nonaddicting anxiolytic effects are useful in the management of chronic pain syndromes. Hydroxyzine is effective alone or in combination with acetaminophen or NSAIDs in the relief of migraine or tension headache. Hydroxyzine may cross the placenta. It is not known if the drug is distributed in breast milk. Hydroxyzine should not be used in early pregnancy or in nursing mothers.

Pharmacokinetics

Onset: Antiemetic/Sedative effects: PO, 15–30 minutes.
Peak Effect: Antiemetic/Sedative effects: PO, 2–3 hours.
Duration of Action: Antiemetic/Sedative effects: PO, 4–6 hours. Analgesic effects: IM, 6 hours.

Interactions

Potentiates depressant effects of alcohol, sedatives, barbiturates, narcotics, volatile anesthetics; additive anticholinergic effects with atropine, glycopyrrolate, and other anticholinergics; α-adrenergic effects of epinephrine blocked, leaving unopposed β activity.

Toxicity

Toxic Range: Not routinely monitored.
Manifestations: Excessive sedation, hypotension.
Antidote: No specific antidote.
Management: Discontinue or reduce medication. Airway-protected, ipecac syrup–induced emesis (30 mL or 0.5 mL/kg ipecac syrup followed by 200 mL or 4 mL/kg of water or clear fluid) or gastric lavage (with drug

ingestion) followed by administration of activated charcoal (PO 50–100 g or 1–2 g/kg). Support ventilation and circulation (patent airway, oxygen, IV fluids, vasopressors). Phenylephrine, norepinephrine, or metaraminol should be used to treat hypotension; epinephrine should not be used because it may paradoxically further lower the blood pressure. Symptomatic treatment.

Guidelines/Precautions

1. Local discomfort, sterile abscesses, erythema, and tissue necrosis may occur at the site of IM injection. Subcutaneous tissue induration may result from extravasation of the drug. Intra-arterial injection may result in thrombosis and gangrene. IM administration should be performed with caution to avoid extravasation and inadvertent subcutaneous or intra-arterial injection.
2. Patients should be warned that hydroxyzine may impair their ability to perform activities requiring mental alertness or physical coordination (e.g., operating heavy machinery, driving a motor vehicle).
3. Do not use epinephrine to treat hydroxyzine-associated hypotension. Hydroxyzine may cause a reversal of epinephrine's vasopressor effects and a further lowering of blood pressure. Treat the drug-induced hypotension with norepinephrine or phenylephrine.
4. Contraindicated during early pregnancy.

Principal Adverse Reactions

Cardiovascular: Hypotension, tachycardia, bradycardia.

Pulmonary: Wheezing, tightness of the chest.
CNS: Excessive sedation, dizziness, slurred speech, headache, ataxia, disinhibition, tremor, seizures.
Gastrointestinal: Nausea, increased GI peristalsis.
Other: Tissue necrosis, tissue slough, abscess, petechial hemorrhage.

IBUPROFEN

Class: Nonsteroidal Anti-Inflammatory Drug

Use(s): Symptomatic treatment of mild to moderate inflammatory and degenerative arthritis, primary dysmenorrhea, tension headache, postoperative and posttraumatic pain, chronic pain, cancer pain (especially with bone metastasis), symptomatic relief of fever and symptoms associated with the common cold (in combination with pseudoephedrine).

Dosing: *Pain, inflammatory disease, or headache:* Ibuprofen PO 200–800 mg (8–16 mg/kg) every 6 hours. Maximum dose 4.2 g daily.

Acute pain: Ibuprofen 200 mg/hydrocodone 7.5 mg: PO one tablet every 4 to 6 hours. Maximum dose five tablets daily. Indicated for short-term (<10 days) treatment of acute pain. Not indicated for long-term treatment of osteoarthritis or rheumatoid arthritis.

Administer analgesic regularly (not as needed). Addition of opioid analgesics, antidepressant agents, and use of nondrug therapies such as TENS may enhance analgesia (see pages xxvi–xliv for drug combinations). In rheumatoid arthritis or juvenile rheumatoid arthritis, second-line rheumatoid agents may include leflunomide (Arava), etanercept (Enbrel), antimalarials, or methotrexate. In geriatric patients and patients with decreased renal or hepatic function, decrease doses by one-third to one-half. The incidence of ibuprofen-induced gastropathy may be decreased by administration with meals, milk, antacids, or sucralfate (PO 1 g four times daily). Misoprostol (PO 100–200 µg four times daily) may be used to prevent gastric ulcers in high-risk patients.

Relief of cold symptoms: PO ibuprofen 200 mg/pseudoephedrine 30 mg. One or two tablets every 4 to 6 hours. Maximum dose six tablets daily.

Elimination: Hepatic, renal.

Preparations

Ibuprofen **(Advil):** Oral suspension: 100 mg/5 mL.

Ibuprofen **(Motrin):** Tablets: 200 mg, 300 mg, 400 mg, 600 mg, 800 mg.

Ibuprofen **(Advil, Motrin, Genpril, Nuprin, Ibuprin, Medipren, Menadol):** Tablets, film coated: 200 mg, 300 mg, 400 mg, 600 mg, 800 mg.

Ibuprofen and pseudoephedrine hydrochloride **(Co-Advil, Advil Cold & Sinus):** Tablets, film coated: Ibuprofen 200 mg and pseudoephedrine hydrochloride 30 mg.

Ibuprofen and hydrocodone bitartrate **(Vicoprofen):** Tablets: Ibuprofen 200 mg and hydrocodone bitartrate 7.5 mg.

Pharmacology

Ibuprofen is a propionic derivative and nonsteroidal anti-inflammatory drug (NSAID). As with aspirin, the analgesic and anti-inflammatory activities of ibuprofen are partly due to the inhibition of prostaglandin and leukotriene synthesis and to antibradykinin and lysosomal membrane stabilizing activity. The antipyretic activity of ibuprofen may occur secondary to inhibition of pyrogen-induced release of prostaglandins in the central nervous system (including the hypothalamus) and possibly to centrally mediated peripheral vasodilatation. The analgesic and anti-inflammatory potency of ibuprofen is about equal to that of salicylates and less than that of indomethacin or phenylbutazone. Ibuprofen (like other NSAIDs) exhibits a ceiling effect for analgesia. Exceeding recommended doses results in increased toxicity without improvement in analgesia. The drug is better tolerated than aspirin or naproxen, and equipotent doses are associated with less gastric mucosal abnormalities. Inhibition of prostaglandin synthesis may result in decreased uterine tone and contractility and prolonged gestation in the parturient and premature closure of the ductus arteriosus in the fetus. Ibuprofen inhibits platelet aggregation and prolongs bleeding time, but it does not affect prothrombin time or clotting time. The drug has no uricosuric activity.

Pharmacokinetics

Onset of Action: PO, analgesic effect <30 minutes; antipyretic effect <1 hour; anti-inflammatory effect <7 days.

Peak Effect: PO, antipyretic effect 2–4 hours; anti-inflammatory effect 1–2 weeks.

Duration of Action: PO, antipyretic effect 6–8 hours; analgesic effect 4–6 hours.

Interactions

Risks of bleeding increased with concomitant NSAIDs, anticoagulant or heparin therapy, alcohol ingestion; decreases antihypertensive effects of β-adrenergic blocking agents; serum levels of ibuprofen increased by concomitant aspirin; GI absorption of ibuprofen delayed by food and milk; prostaglandin-mediated natriuretic effects of loop diuretics antagonized by ibuprofen.

Toxicity

Toxic Range: Not routinely monitored.
Manifestations: *Acute:* Apnea, cyanosis, drowsiness, dizziness, nystagmus.
Antidote: None.
Management: Discontinue or reduce medication. Correct fluid, electrolyte, and acid-base disturbances. Support ventilation and circulation (patent airway, oxygen, IV fluids, vasopressors). Airway-protected, ipecac syrup–induced emesis (30 mL or 0.5 mL/kg ipecac syrup followed by 200 mL or 4 mL/kg of water or clear fluid) or gastric lavage (with drug ingestion) followed by administration of activated charcoal (PO 50–100 g or 1–2 g/kg). Forced alkaline diuresis with IV sodium bicarbonate (IV furosemide if necessary) after correction of dehydration. Symptomatic treatment.

Guidelines/Precautions

1. Use with caution in patients with active GI lesions (e.g., erosive gastritis, peptic ulcer), a history of

recurrent GI lesions, hepatic or renal dysfunction, preexisting hypoprothrombinemia, or vitamin K deficiency. Ibuprofen may cause sodium retention and peripheral edema by suppression of renal prostaglandin synthesis. The drug should be used cautiously in patients with heart failure, hypertension, or other conditions associated with fluid retention.

2. Carefully observe patients with coagulation disorders and those receiving drug therapy that interferes with hemostasis.

3. Renal prostaglandins may have a supportive role in maintaining renal perfusion in patients with prerenal conditions. Ibuprofen should be avoided in such patients because it may cause a dose-dependent decrease in the production of vasodilatory prostaglandins and thus precipitate renal decompensation.

4. Patient response to NSAIDs is variable. Patients who do not respond to or cannot tolerate ibuprofen may be successfully treated with another NSAID.

5. Ibuprofen and salicylates should not be administered concomitantly because there may not be any therapeutic advantage and the incidence of adverse GI side effects may be increased.

6. Contraindicated in patients with previously demonstrated hypersensitivity to ibuprofen or with the complete or partial syndrome of nasal polyps, angioedema, or bronchospastic reactivity to aspirin or other NSAIDs.

7. Signs and symptoms of infection or other diseases may be masked by the antipyretic and anti-inflammatory effects of ibuprofen.

8. Monitor stool for blood every 14 days, and monitor BUN, serum creatinine, and urinalysis every 1 to 2 months when administering ibuprofen at chronic high doses.
9. Do not administer a fixed-combination preparation of ibuprofen and pseudoephedrine to patients on monoamine oxidase (MAO) inhibitor drugs or less than 2 weeks after stopping the MAO inhibitors.
10. Use of ibuprofen and other NSAIDs is not recommended during pregnancy (especially during the last trimester) or during labor and delivery. Ibuprofen and other NSAIDs inhibit prostaglandin synthesis, which may cause dystocia, interfere with labor, and delay parturition. Prostaglandin synthesis inhibitors may also have adverse effects on the fetal cardiovascular system (e.g., premature closure of ductus arteriosus).

Principal Adverse Reactions

Cardiovascular: Peripheral edema, fluid retention, hypertension, palpitation.
Pulmonary: Dyspnea, bronchospasm.
CNS: Drowsiness, dizziness, headache, anxiety, confusion.
Gastrointestinal: Ulceration, bleeding, dyspepsia, nausea, vomiting, diarrhea, hepatic dysfunction.
Genitourinary: Renal dysfunction, acute renal failure, azotemia, cystitis, hematuria.
Dermatologic: Pruritus, urticaria.
Hematologic: Prolongation of bleeding time, leukopenia, thrombocytopenia, aplastic anemia, hemolytic anemia.
Other: Tinnitus, blurred vision.

IMIPRAMINE HYDROCHLORIDE

Class: Tricyclic Antidepressant

Use(s): Treatment of neurotic and endogenous depression; migraine prophylaxis; adjunct treatment of neuropathic pain syndromes, including diabetic neuropathy, postherpetic neuralgia, tic douloureux, and cancer pain; anxiety disorders; phobias; panic disorders; enuresis; eating disorders.

Dosing: *Pain syndromes*

Initial: PO 25–100 mg (0.5–2.0 mg/kg) daily at bedtime. Titrate dose upward every 3 to 4 weeks by increments of 25–50 mg as necessary.

Maintenance: PO 25–200 mg (0.5–4.0 mg/kg) daily at bedtime. Doses should be decreased if unacceptable side effects occur. Serum levels should be determined if there are signs of toxicity. The higher end of the dose range may be required in the management of painful diabetic neuropathy.

Depression

Initial PO: 75–100 mg daily in one to four divided doses.

Maintenance PO: 50–300 mg daily in one to four divided doses. Doses greater than 200 mg daily are not recommended for outpatients.

IM: 100 mg daily in divided doses. Replace with oral medication as soon as possible. Do not administer intravenously.

Doses for pain are generally smaller than those used for treatment of affective disorders. Medication should be administered on a fixed schedule and not as needed. Administration of the entire daily dose at bedtime may reduce daytime sedation. After symptoms are controlled, dosage should be gradually reduced to the lowest level that will maintain relief of symptoms. Analgesia may be enhanced by addition of opioid analgesics (see pages xxvi–xliv for drug combinations), nonsteroidal anti-inflammatory drugs (NSAIDs), and use of nondrug therapies such as transcutaneous electrical nerve stimulation (TENS). In geriatric patients and patients with decreased renal or hepatic function, decrease doses by one-third to one-half. The possibility for suicide is inherent in depression and may persist until significant remission occurs. The quantity of drug dispensed should reflect this consideration.

Elimination: Hepatic, renal.

Preparations

Imipramine hydrochloride **(Tofranil)**
   Tablets: 10 mg, 25 mg, 50 mg.
   Injection: 12.5 mg/mL.
Imipramine hydrochloride **(Janimine):** Tablets, film coated: 10 mg, 25 mg, 50 mg.
Imipramine pamoate **(Tofranil-PM):** Capsules: 75 mg, 100 mg, 125 mg, 150 mg. Dosages expressed as imipramine hydrochloride equivalents.

Pharmacology

A dibenzazepine derivative and a tertiary amine tricyclic antidepressant, imipramine is structurally related to the phenothiazine antipsychotic agents. Antidepressant activity may be partly due to inhibition of the amine-pump uptake of neurotransmitters (e.g., norepinephrine and serotonin) at the presynaptic neuron and down-regulation of β-receptor sensitivity. Anticholinergic effects of imipramine are similar to doxepin. Compared with doxepin or amitriptyline, imipramine produces less sedation or hypotension. Although blockade of neurotransmitter uptake may occur immediately, anti-depressant response may take days to weeks. Patients with low norepinephrine levels may respond better to imipramine compared with serotonin-deficient patients. Imipramine does not inhibit the monoamine oxidase (MAO) system. Imipramine is demethylated in the liver to the active metabolite, desipramine.

The analgesic effects of imipramine may occur partly through the alleviation of depression, which may be responsible for increased pain suffering, but also by mechanisms that are independent of mood effects. Serotonin and norepinephrine activity may be increased in descending pain inhibitory pathways. Activation of these pathways decreases the transmission of nociceptive impulses from primary afferent neurons to first-order cells in laminae I and V of the spinal cord dorsal horn. Imipramine may also potentiate the analgesic effect of opioids by increasing their binding efficacy to opioid receptors. Imipramine has varying degrees of efficacy in different pain syndromes and may be better at relieving the burning, aching, and dyesthetic component of neuropathic pain. The drug is seldom useful in the management of lancinating, shooting paroxysmal pain. At full antidepressant dosages, imipramine (and other tricyclic antidepressants) is especially effective in chronic low back pain with associated major depression. Patients with uncomplicated low back pain (i.e., without major depression) do not respond as well. The antimigraine activity of imipramine is relatively independent of its antidepressant effects. Low doses of imipramine are more effective for chronic tension headache compared with barbiturates and benzodiazepines. Imipramine produces varying degrees of sedation and blocks α_1-adrenergic, H_1, and H_2 receptors. Imipramine may be as effective as cimetidine in enhancing ulcer healing.

The drug may produce abnormal EEG patterns and lower the seizure threshold. Therapeutic doses do not affect respiration, but toxic doses may lead to respiratory depression. The direct quinidine-like effects may manifest at toxic doses and produce cardiovascular disturbances (e.g., conduction blockade). Imipramine does not have addiction liability and its use is not associated with drug-seeking behavior. Withdrawal symptoms, including sleep disruption with vivid dreams, may be precipitated by acute withdrawal. Tolerance develops to the sedative and anticholinergic effects, but there are no reports of tolerance to the analgesic effects. Imipramine crosses the placenta and use in pregnancy may be associated with fetal malformations. The drug is excreted in breast milk and has a potential for serious adverse effects in nursing infants.

Pharmacokinetics

Onset of Action: Analgesic effect: PO, <5 days. Antidepressant effect: PO, 1–2 weeks.
Peak Effect: Antidepressant effect: PO, 2–4 weeks.
Duration of Action: Antidepressant effect: PO, variable.

Interactions

Increased risk of hyperthermia with concomitant administration of anticholinergics (e.g., atropine), phenothiazines, thyroid medications; serum levels and toxic effects of imipramine increased by concomitant methylphenidate, fluoxetine, cimetidine, phenothiazines, and haloperidol; ventilatory and circulatory depressant effects of CNS depressant drugs and alcohol potentiated by imipramine; increases the pressor and cardiac effects of sympathomimetics (e.g., isoproterenol, phenylephrine, norepinephrine, epinephrine, amphetamine); decreases serum levels and pharmacologic effects of levodopa and phenylbutazone; increases serum levels and toxic effects of dicumarol; onset of therapeutic effects shortened and adverse cardiac effects of imipramine increased with concomitant administration of levothyroxine and liothyronine; fatal hyperpyretic crisis or seizures with concomitant use of MAO inhibitors; uptake-dependent efficacy of IV regional bretylium decreased by imipramine.

Toxicity

Toxic Range: Not routinely monitored. Blood and urine levels may not correlate with the degree of intoxication and are not reliable guides for clinical management.

Manifestations: *Chronic:* Dream and sleep disturbances, akathisia, anxiety, chills, coryza, malaise, myalgia, headache, dizziness, nausea and vomiting. *Acute:* In addition to the previously listed symptoms, CNS stimulation with excitement, delirium, hallucinations, hyperreflexia, myoclonus, choreiform movements, parkinsonian symptoms, seizures, hyperpyrexia, then CNS depression with drowsiness, areflexia, hypothermia, respiratory depression, cyanosis, hypotension, coma; peripheral anticholinergic symptoms, including urinary retention, dry mucous membranes, mydriasis, constipation, adynamic ileus; cardiac irregularities, including tachycardia, QRS prolongation; metabolic and/or respiratory acidosis; polyradiculoneuropathy; renal failure; vomiting; ataxia; dysarthria; bullous cutaneous lesions; pulmonary consolidation.

Antidote: None.

Management: Discontinue or reduce medication. Correct fluid, electrolyte, and acid-base disturbances. Airway-protected, ipecac syrup–induced emesis (30 mL or 0.5 mL/kg ipecac syrup) or gastric lavage (with drug ingestion) followed by administration of activated charcoal (PO 50–100 g or 1–2 g/kg). These purging actions should be performed even if several hours have elapsed after ingestion because the anticholinergic effects may delay gastric emptying, and the drug may also be secreted into the stomach. Control seizures: Intravenous benzodiazepines are the first choice because IV barbiturates may enhance respiratory depression; however, IV barbiturates or phenytoin may be useful in refractory seizures. Support ventilation and circulation (patent airway, oxygen, IV fluids, vasopressors). Continuous EKG monitoring. Treat cardiac arrhythmias with IV lidocaine or propranolol. Digoxin, quinidine, procainamide, and diisopyramide should be avoided because they may further depress myocardial conduction and/or contractility. Temporary pacemakers may be necessary in patients with advanced atrioventricular block, severe bradycardia, and/or life-threatening ventricular arrhythmias unresponsive to drug therapy. Control hyperpyrexia with ice packs and cooling sponge baths. Physostigmine (slow IV 1–3 mg) may be used in the treatment of life-threatening anticholinergic toxicity. Routine use of physostigmine is not advisable due to its serious adverse effects (e.g., seizures, bronchospasm, and severe bradyarrhythmias). Hemodialysis or peritoneal dialysis is ineffective because the drug is highly protein bound. Symptomatic treatment. Consider the possibility of multiple drug involvement. Counseling prior to and after discharge for patients who attempted suicide.

Guidelines/Precautions

1. To avoid withdrawal symptoms, the medication should be tapered down over a couple of weeks and not discontinued abruptly.
2. Use with caution in patients with cardiovascular disease, thyroid disease, or seizure disorders and in those in whom excessive anticholinergic activity may be harmful (e.g., patients with benign prostatic hypertrophy, a history of urinary retention, or increased intraocular pressure). The drug should be used in close-angle glaucoma only when the glaucoma is adequately controlled by drugs and closely monitored.
3. Contraindicated in patients receiving MAO

inhibitors (concurrently or within the past 2 weeks), patients in the acute recovery phase following myocardial infarction, and those with demonstrated hypersensitivity to imipramine. Cross-sensitivity with other tricyclic antidepressants may occur.

4. Certain formulations of imipramine may contain sulfites and/or tartrazine dye, which may cause allergic reactions in susceptible individuals.

5. Patients should be warned of the possibility of drowsiness that may impair performance of potentially hazardous tasks such as driving an automobile or operating machinery. Persisting daytime drowsiness may be decreased by administering a lower dose, administering the dose earlier in the evening, or substituting a less sedating alternative.

Principal Adverse Reactions

Cardiovascular: Postural hypotension, arrhythmias, conduction disturbances, hypertension, sudden death.

Pulmonary: Respiratory depression.

CNS: Confusion, disorientation, extrapyramidal symptoms.

Gastrointestinal: Hepatic dysfunction, jaundice, nausea, vomiting, constipation, decrease in lower esophageal sphincter tone.

Genitourinary: Urinary retention, paradoxical nocturia, urinary frequency.

Ocular: Blurred vision, mydriasis, increased intraocular pressure.

Dermatologic: Pruritus, urticaria, petechiae, photosensitivity.

Hematologic: Leukopenia, thrombocytopenia, eosinophilia, agranulocytosis, purpura.
Endocrinologic: Increased or decreased libido, impotence, gynecomastia, SIADH.
Other: Hyperthermia.

INDOMETHACIN

Class: High-Potency Anti-inflammatory Agent

Use(s): Symptomatic treatment of moderate to severe inflammatory and degenerative arthritis, primary dysmenorrhea, tension headache, ankylosing spondylitis, gouty arthritis, Reiter's syndrome, posttraumatic pain, chronic pain, cancer pain (especially with bone metastasis or hypercalcemia secondary to prostaglandin-mediated osteolytic activity); closure of patent ductus arteriosus in premature infants.

Dosing: *Pain, inflammatory diseases, and headache*
Indomethacin: PO 25–50 mg (0.5–1.0 mg/kg) two to four times daily. Maximum dose 200 mg daily.
Indomethacin (extended release): PO 75 mg (1.5 mg/kg) once or twice daily.
Parenteral indomethacin is available in the United States only for treatment of patent ductus arteriosus.
Administer analgesic regularly (not as needed). Indomethacin may cause serious adverse effects. It is not a drug of first choice, and should not be used as a simple analgesic or antipyretic. Extended-release

preparations are not recommended for use in acute gouty arthritis. Analgesia may be enhanced by addition of opioid analgesics (see pages xxvi–xliv for drug combinations), antidepressant agents, and use of nondrug therapies such as transcutaneous electrical nerve stimulation (TENS). In rheumatoid arthritis or juvenile rheumatoid arthritis, second-line rheumatoid agents may include leflunomide (Arava), etanercept (Enbrel), antimalarials, or methotrexate. In geriatric patients and patients with decreased renal or hepatic function, decrease doses by one-third to one-half. The incidence of indomethacin-induced gastropathy may be decreased by administration with meals, milk, antacids, or sucralfate (PO 1 g four times daily). Misoprostol (PO 100–200 µg four times daily) may be used to prevent gastric ulcers in high-risk patients.

Elimination: Hepatic, renal.

Preparations

Indomethacin **(Indocin)**
   Capsules: 25 mg, 50 mg, 75 mg.
   Oral suspension: 25 mg/5 mL.
   Rectal suppositories: 50 mg.
Indomethacin **(Indocin SR):** Capsules, extended release 75 mg.

Pharmacology

An indoleacetic acid derivative and nonsteroidal anti-inflammatory drug (NSAID), indomethacin is structurally and pharmacologically related to sulindac. As with other NSAIDs, the analgesic and anti-inflammatory activities of indomethacin are partly due to the inhibition of prostaglandin synthesis and/or release secondary to the inhibition of cyclooxygenase. Indomethacin is one of the most potent inhibitors of the cyclooxygenase enzyme that catalyzes the formation of prostaglandin precursors (endoperoxides) from arachidonic acid. Indomethacin (and some other NSAIDs) may interfere with prostaglandin-mediated formation of autoantibodies that are involved in the inflammatory process. Indomethacin permits closure of prostaglandin-induced patent ductus arteriosus in premature infants. The anti-inflammatory effects of indomethacin are comparable with colchicine in the treatment of gouty arthritis. The drug has no uricosuric activity and is not useful in the management of chronic gout. The antipyretic activity of indomethacin may occur secondary to inhibition of pyrogen-induced release of prostaglandins in the central nervous system (including the hypothalamus) and possibly to centrally mediated peripheral vasodilatation. Indomethacin is more effective than aspirin in relieving the pain of primary dysmenorrhea. On a weight basis, the analgesic potency of indomethacin is about 20 times that of aspirin.

Indomethacin (like other NSAIDs) exhibits a ceiling effect for analgesia. Exceeding recommended doses results in increased toxicity without improvement in analgesia. Indomethacin may cause gastric mucosal damage that may result in ulceration or bleeding. Inhibition of prostaglandin synthesis may result in decreased uterine tone and contractility and prolonged gestation in the parturient and premature closure of the ductus arteriosus in the fetus. Indomethacin inhibits platelet aggregation and prolongs bleeding time. However, unlike the irreversible effects of aspirin, these effects are transient, and platelet function and aggregation return to normal within 24 hours.

Pharmacokinetics

Onset of Action: PO, analgesic effect 15–30 minutes; anti-inflammatory effect <7 days.
Peak Effect: PO, analgesic effect 1–2 hours; anti-inflammatory effect 1–2 weeks.
Duration of Action: PO, analgesic effect 4–6 hours.

Interactions

Risks of bleeding increased with concomitant NSAIDs, anticoagulant or heparin therapy, alcohol ingestion; decreases antihypertensive effects of β-adrenergic blocking agents; serum levels of indomethacin decreased slightly by concomitant aspirin; serum levels of indomethacin increased by concomitant probenecid; renal elimination decreased and serum levels and toxic effects of methotrexate and lithium increased by concomitant indomethacin; GI absorption of indomethacin delayed by food and milk; antihypertensive effects of thiazide diuretics, β-adrenergic blocking agents antagonized by indomethacin; prostaglandin-mediated natriuretic effects of loop diuretics antagonized by indomethacin.

Toxicity

Toxic Range: Not routinely monitored.
Manifestations: *Acute:* Drowsiness, nausea, vomiting, lethargy, paresthesia, disorientation, seizures, abdominal pain, GI bleeding.
Antidote: None.

Management: Discontinue or reduce medication. Correct fluid, electrolyte, and acid-base disturbances. Support ventilation and circulation (patent airway, oxygen, IV fluids, vasopressors). Airway-protected, ipecac syrup–induced emesis (30 mL or 0.5 mL/kg ipecac syrup followed by 200 mL or 4 mL/kg of water or clear fluid) or gastric lavage (with drug ingestion) followed by administration of activated charcoal (PO 50–100 g or 1–2 g/kg). Symptomatic treatment. Monitor for several days due to the risk of delayed GI ulceration.

Guidelines/Precautions

1. Use with caution in patients with active GI lesions (e.g., erosive gastritis, peptic ulcer), a history of recurrent GI lesions, hepatic or renal dysfunction, preexisting hypoprothrombinemia, or vitamin K deficiency. Indomethacin may cause sodium retention and peripheral edema by suppression of renal prostaglandin synthesis. The drug should be used cautiously in patients with heart failure, hypertension, or other conditions associated with fluid retention.
2. Renal prostaglandins may have a supportive role in maintaining renal perfusion in patients with prerenal conditions. Indomethacin should be avoided in such patients because it may cause a dose-dependent decrease in the production of vasodilatory prostaglandins and thus precipitate renal decompensation.
3. Carefully observe patients with coagulation disorders and those receiving drug therapy that interferes with hemostasis.

4. Avoid the use of indomethacin during pregnancy. In the third trimester, the drug may produce adverse fetal effects, including constriction of the ductus arteriosus, neonatal primary pulmonary hypertension, and fetal death.

5. Indomethacin and salicylates should not be administered concomitantly because there may not be any therapeutic advantage and the incidence of adverse GI side effects may be increased.

6. Patient response to NSAIDs is variable. Patients who do not respond to or cannot tolerate indomethacin may be successfully treated with another NSAID.

7. Contraindicated in patients with previously demonstrated hypersensitivity to indomethacin or with the complete or partial syndrome of nasal polyps, angioedema, or bronchospastic reactivity to aspirin or other NSAIDs.

8. Signs and symptoms of infection or other diseases may be masked by the antipyretic and anti-inflammatory effects of indomethacin.

9. Monitor stool for blood every 14 days, and monitor BUN, serum creatinine, and urinalysis every 1 to 2 months when administering indomethacin at chronic high doses.

Principal Adverse Reactions

Cardiovascular: Congestive heart failure, peripheral edema, fluid retention, hypertension, tachycardia, arrhythmias.

Pulmonary: Dyspnea, bronchospasm.

CNS: Drowsiness, dizziness, headache, anxiety, confusion.

Gastrointestinal: Ulceration, bleeding, dyspepsia, nausea, vomiting, diarrhea, hepatic dysfunction, jaundice.

Genitourinary: Renal dysfunction, acute renal failure, azotemia, cystitis, hematuria.

Dermatologic: Pruritus, urticaria.

Hematologic: Prolongation of bleeding time, leukopenia, thrombocytopenia, aplastic anemia, hemolytic anemia.

Other: Tinnitus, blurred vision.

KETAMINE HYDROCHLORIDE

Class: NMDA Receptor Antagonist

Use(s): Dissociative anesthetic, sedation, systemic and topical analgesia.

Dosing: *Sedation/Analgesia*
> IV: 0.5–1.0 mg/kg.
> IM/Rectal: 2.5–5.0 mg/kg.
> PO: 5–6 mg/kg. Dilute injectate solution in 5–10 mL (0.2 mL/kg) cola-flavored drink.
> Epidural/Caudal: 0.5 mg/kg. Dilute in preservative-free normal saline or local anesthetic (1 mL/kg).
> Topical (not available commercially): 1–15% ketamine in PLO gel placed in calibrated applicators. 10–700 mg (0.1–9.0 mg/kg) per single application. Apply one to three times daily until pain relief is obtained, then apply as needed.

Elimination: Hepatic.

Preparations

Ketamine hydrochloride **(Ketalar):** Injection: 10 mg/mL, 50 mg/mL, 100 mg/mL. Store at room temperature (15–30°C). Protect from light and heat.

Dilution for Infusion: 250 mg in 250 mL D5W or normal saline (1 mg/mL).

Pharmacology

This phencyclidine derivative produces rapid-acting dissociative anesthesia characterized by normal or slightly enhanced pharyngeal-laryngeal reflexes and skeletal muscle tone, respiratory stimulation, and occasionally a transient and minimal respiratory depression. Anesthetic effects of ketamine may be partly due to an antagonist effect on *N*-methyl D-aspartate (NMDA) receptors, a subgroup of opioid receptors. The activation of small-diameter primary afferents is capable of producing a prolonged alteration in the excitability of neurons in the spinal cord, modifying the way these neurons respond to subsequent inputs and thereby generating a state of central sensitization. NMDA antagonists such as ketamine block the development of central sensitization and abolish the hypersensitivity if established. By returning an abnormally excitable spinal cord to its normal level of excitability, NMDA antagonists will return a pathologic situation in which low-intensity or innocuous stimuli begin to produce pain (allodynia) to the normal physiologic state in which pain is produced by noxious stimuli. The same dose of the NMDA antagonist that is required to prevent the establishment of central sensitization also abolishes it once it has been induced. This differs from preemptive analgesia with opioids, wherein higher doses are required to abolish than to prevent central sensitization.

Analgesic doses of ketamine administered parenterally or topically may relieve symptoms of neuropathic pain and chronic regional pain syndrome. Ketamine may act on norepinephrine, serotonin, and muscarinic cholinergic receptors in the CNS. The central sympathetic stimulation, neuronal release of catecholamines, and inhibition of neuronal uptake of catecholamines usually override the direct myocardial depressant effects of ketamine. Hemodynamic effects (that depend on intact sympathetic responses) include increases in systemic and pulmonary arterial pressure, heart rate, and cardiac output. Ketamine is a useful anesthetic agent in patients with hemodynamic compromise based on either hypovolemia or intrinsic cardiac (but not coronary artery) disease (e.g., cardiac tamponade, cyanotic heart disease). It is a bronchial smooth muscle relaxant and is as effective as the inhalational anesthetics in preventing experimentally induced bronchospasm. Salivary and tracheobronchial secretions are increased. Ketamine does not release histamine.

Pharmacokinetics

Onset of Action: IV, <30 seconds. IM/Rectal, 3–4 minutes.
Peak Effect: IV, 1 minute. IM/Rectal, 5–20 minutes. PO, 30 minutes.
Duration of Action: IV, 5–15 minutes. IM/Rectal, 12–25 minutes. Epidural, 4 hours.

Interactions

Emergence delirium, hypertension, arrhythmias, myocardial ischemia with concomitant use of sympathomimetics (e.g., epinephrine); hemodynamic depression may occur in presence of α-blockers, β-blockers, calcium channel blockers, benzodiazepines, opioids, volatile-anesthetics, ganglionic blockade, cervical epidural anesthesia, and spinal cord transection; concomitant use with benzodiazepines, barbiturates, volatile anesthetics may prolong recovery; reduction of seizure threshold when administered with aminophylline.

Toxicity

Toxic Range: Not routinely monitored.

Manifestations: Emergence reactions (dreaming, hallucinations, confusion), nystagmus, hypertension, hypotension, laryngospasm, respiratory depression, tonic-clonic movements.

Antidote: None. Premedication with a benzodiazepine may decrease the incidence of emergence reactions.

Management: Discontinue or reduce medication. Correction of fluid, electrolyte, and acid-base disturbances. Support ventilation and circulation (patent airway, oxygen, IV fluids, vasopressors). Symptomatic treatment.

Guidelines/Precautions

1. Critically ill patients with catecholamine depletion may respond to ketamine with unexpected reductions in blood pressure and cardiac output.
2. Emergence reactions (dreaming, hallucinations, confusion) are more common with adults (15–65 years), high doses, and rapid administration and are reduced by premedication with benzodiazepines and droperidol.
3. Do not mix with barbiturates in same syringe—precipitate formation occurs.

4. Use with caution in patients with severe hypertension, ischemic heart disease, aneurysms, or increased intracranial pressure and in chronic alcoholics and the acutely alcohol-intoxicated patient.
5. Increased salivary secretions may cause upper airway obstruction and laryngospasm, especially in children. Administer an antisialagogue (e.g., glycopyrrolate) preoperatively.

Principal Adverse Reactions

Cardiovascular: Hypertension, tachycardia, hypotension, arrhythmias, bradycardia.
Pulmonary: Respiratory depression, apnea, laryngospasm.
CNS: Tonic-clonic movements, emergence delirium.
Gastrointestinal: Hypersalivation, nausea, vomiting.
Ocular: Diplopia, nystagmus, slight elevation in intraocular tension.

KETOPROFEN

Class: Nonsteroidal Anti-inflammatory Drug

Use(s): Symptomatic treatment of mild to moderate inflammatory and degenerative arthritis, primary dysmenorrhea, tension headache, postoperative and posttraumatic pain, chronic pain, cancer pain (especially with bone metastasis).

Dosing: *Pain*

Ketoprofen: PO 25–50 mg (0.5–1.0 mg/kg) every 6 to 8 hours. Maximum dose 300 mg daily.

Ketoprofen (extended release): PO 200 mg once daily at bedtime.

Inflammatory disease

Ketoprofen: PO 50–75 mg (1.0–1.5 mg/kg) every 6 to 8 hours. Maximum dose 300 mg daily.

Ketoprofen (extended release): PO 200 mg once daily at bedtime.

Patients with rheumatoid or acute gouty arthritis may require larger doses than those with osteoarthritis.

Administer analgesic regularly (not as needed). Addition of opioid analgesics, antidepressant agents, and use of nondrug therapies such as transcutaneous electrical nerve stimulation (TENS) may enhance analgesia (see pages xxvi–xliv for drug combinations). In rheumatoid arthritis or juvenile rheumatoid arthritis, second-line rheumatoid agents may include leflunomide (Arava), etanercept (Enbrel), antimalarials, or methotrexate. In geriatric patients and patients with decreased renal or hepatic function, decrease doses by one-third to one-half. The incidence of ketoprofen-induced gastropathy may be decreased by administration with meals, milk, antacids, or sucralfate (PO 1 g four times daily). Misoprostol (PO 100–200 µg four times daily) may be used to prevent gastric ulcers in high-risk patients.

Elimination: Hepatic, renal.

Preparations

Ketoprofen **(Orudis):** Oral capsules: 25 mg, 50 mg, 75 mg.

Ketoprofen—nonprescription **(Orudis KT, Actron)**
  Oral caplets: 12.5 mg
  Oral tablets: 12.5 mg

Ketoprofen **(Oruvail):** Oral capsules, extended release: 200 mg.

Pharmacology

A propionic acid derivative and nonsteroidal anti-inflammatory drug (NSAID), ketoprofen is structurally and pharmacologically related to ibuprofen and naproxen. As with other NSAIDs, the analgesic and anti-inflammatory activities of ketoprofen are partly due to the inhibition of prostaglandin and leukotriene synthesis and to antibradykinin and lysosomal membrane stabilizing activity. The antipyretic activity of ketoprofen may occur secondary to inhibition of pyrogen-induced release of prostaglandins in the central nervous system (including the hypothalamus) and possibly to centrally mediated peripheral vasodilatation.

The analgesic potency of ketoprofen is similar to that of indomethacin and about 20 times that of ibuprofen or aspirin. Ketoprofen (like other NSAIDs) exhibits a ceiling effect for analgesia. Exceeding recommended doses results in increased toxicity without improvement in analgesia. Ketoprofen may cause gastric mucosal damage that may result in ulceration or bleeding. Inhibition of prostaglandin synthesis may result in decreased uterine tone and contractility and prolonged gestation in the parturient and premature closure of the ductus arteriosus in the fetus. Ketoprofen inhibits platelet aggregation and prolongs bleeding time (to a greater extent than indomethacin). However, unlike the irreversible effects of aspirin, these effects are transient and platelet function and aggregation return to normal within 24 hours. The drug has no uricosuric activity.

Pharmacokinetics

Onset of Action: PO, analgesic effect 15–30 minutes.
Peak Effect: PO, analgesic effect 1–2 hours.
Duration of Action: PO, analgesic effect 3–4 hours.

Interactions

Risks of bleeding increased with concomitant NSAIDs, anticoagulant or heparin therapy, alcohol ingestion; decreases antihypertensive effects of β-adrenergic blocking agents; serum levels of ketoprofen decreased or increased by concomitant aspirin; serum levels of ketoprofen increased by concomitant probenecid; serum levels and toxic effects of methotrexate, lithium increased by concomitant ketoprofen; GI absorption of ketoprofen delayed by food and milk; prostaglandin-mediated natriuretic effects of loop diuretics antagonized by ketoprofen.

Toxicity

Toxic Range: Not routinely monitored.
Manifestations: *Acute:* Drowsiness, vomiting, abdominal pain, metabolic acidosis.
Antidote: None.
Management: Discontinue or reduce medication. Correct fluid, electrolyte, and acid-base disturbances. Support ventilation and circulation (patent airway,

oxygen, IV fluids, vasopressors). Airway-protected, ipecac syrup–induced emesis (30 mL or 0.5 mL/kg ipecac syrup followed by 200 mL or 4 mL/kg of water or clear fluid) or gastric lavage (with drug ingestion) followed by administration of activated charcoal (PO 50–100 g or 1–2 g/kg). Forced alkaline diuresis with IV sodium bicarbonate (IV furosemide if necessary) after correction of dehydration. Hemodialysis. Symptomatic treatment.

Guidelines/Precautions

1. Use with caution in patients with active GI lesions (e.g., erosive gastritis, peptic ulcer), a history of recurrent GI lesions, hepatic or renal dysfunction, preexisting hypoprothrombinemia, or vitamin K deficiency. Ketoprofen may cause peripheral edema and should also be used cautiously in patients with heart failure, hypertension, or other conditions associated with fluid retention.

2. Renal prostaglandins may have a supportive role in maintaining renal perfusion in patients with prerenal conditions. Ketoprofen should be avoided in such patients because it may cause a dose-dependent decrease in prostaglandin formation and thus precipitate renal decompensation.

3. Carefully observe patients with coagulation disorders and those receiving drug therapy that interferes with hemostasis.

4. Use with caution in pregnancy and only when the perceived benefits outweigh the risks.

5. Patient response to NSAIDs is variable. Patients who do not respond to or cannot tolerate ketoprofen may be successfully treated with another NSAID.

6. Ketoprofen and salicylates should not be administered concomitantly because there may not be any therapeutic advantage and the incidence of adverse GI side effects may be increased.
7. Contraindicated in patients with previously demonstrated hypersensitivity to ketoprofen or with the complete or partial syndrome of nasal polyps, angioedema, or bronchospastic reactivity to aspirin or other NSAIDs.
8. Signs and symptoms of infection or other diseases may be masked by the antipyretic and anti-inflammatory effects of ketoprofen.
9. Monitor stool for blood every 14 days, and monitor BUN, serum creatinine, and urinalysis every 1 to 2 months when administering ketoprofen at chronic high doses.

Principal Adverse Reactions

Cardiovascular: Peripheral edema, fluid retention, hypertension, palpitation.
Pulmonary: Dyspnea, bronchospasm.
CNS: Drowsiness, dizziness, headache, anxiety, confusion.
Gastrointestinal: Ulceration, bleeding, dyspepsia, nausea, vomiting, diarrhea, hepatic dysfunction.
Genitourinary: Renal dysfunction, acute renal failure, azotemia, cystitis, hematuria.
Dermatologic: Pruritus, urticaria.
Hematologic: Prolongation of bleeding time, leukopenia, thrombocytopenia, aplastic anemia, hemolytic anemia.
Other: Tinnitus, blurred vision.

KETOROLAC TROMETHAMINE

Class: Nonsteroidal Anti-inflammatory Drug

Use(s): Symptomatic treatment of acute pain, primary dysmenorrhea, sympathetic mediated pain, postoperative and posttraumatic pain.

Dosing: *Pain—Adults*

Single-dose regimen

IV: 30 mg (0.5 mg/kg).

IM: 60 mg (1 mg/kg).

Multiple-dose regimen

IV/IM: 30 mg (0.5 mg/kg) every 6 hours as needed.

PO: 10–20 mg stat then 10 mg every 4–6 hours.

Maximum total parenteral dose (IV/IM): 120 mg daily. Maximum PO dose: 40 mg daily. IV doses should be infused slowly (>15 seconds) to reduce risk of phlebitis. Combined duration of use for parenteral and oral ketorolac in all patients should not exceed 5 days.

Pain—Elderly (>65 years), children (or patients under 50 kg), and patients with decreased renal function

Single-dose regimen

IV: 15 mg (0.25 mg/kg).

IM: 30 mg (0.5 mg/kg).

Multiple-dose regimen

IV/IM: 15 mg (0.25 mg/kg) every 6 hours as needed.

PO: 10 mg every 4–6 hours.

> Maximum total parenteral dose (IV/IM): 60 mg daily. Maximum PO dose: 40 mg daily.
>
> *Sympathetic mediated pain:* IV regional sympathetic block: 60–120 mg (1–2 mg/kg) diluted in 20–30 mL of normal saline or 0.5% lidocaine (upper extremity), or 120 mg (2 mg/kg) diluted in 40–50 mL of normal saline or 0.5% lidocaine (lower extremity).

Elimination: Hepatic, renal.

Preparations

Ketorolac tromethamine **(Toradol IV/IM)**
   Injection (vial): 15 mg/mL, 30 mg/mL.
   Injection (tubex cartridge–needle unit): 15 mg/mL, 30 mg/mL.
Ketorolac tromethamine **(Toradol ORAL):** Tablets: 10 mg.

Dilution for Infusion: Intravenous piggyback (IVPB): 15–30 mg in 25–50 mL normal saline or D5W. Solution is stable for 24 hours.

Pharmacology

This nonsteroidal anti-inflammatory drug (NSAID) exhibits analgesic, anti-inflammatory, and antipyretic activity. It inhibits synthesis of prostaglandins and may be considered a peripherally acting analgesic. The analgesic potency of ketorolac IM 30 mg is equivalent to morphine 9 mg, with less drowsiness, nausea, and vomiting and no significant change in ventilatory function. The analgesic potency of ketorolac PO 10 or 20 mg is equivalent to aspirin 650 mg or acetaminophen 600 mg with codeine 60 mg. Ketorolac may cause gastric mucosal damage with ulceration and/or bleeding. This may be due to inhibition of synthesis of prostaglandins (e.g., prosta-cyclin, prostaglandins of the E series) that have cytopro-tective effects on GI mucosa. Compared with aspirin, ketorolac causes adverse GI side effects that occur earlier and are more frequent. Due to this potential for serious adverse effects, therapy with ketorolac should be limited to 5 days. Ketorolac inhibits platelet aggregation and pro-longs bleeding time. In patients receiving oral doses up to 200 mg, inhibition of platelet function disappears within 24 to 48 hours after the drug is discontinued. Ketorolac does not affect platelet count, prothrombin time (PT), or partial thromboplastin time (PTT).

Pharmacokinetics

Onset of Action: Analgesic effect: IV, <1 minute; IM, <10 minutes; PO, <1 hour.
Peak Effect: Analgesic effect: IV/IM/PO, 1–3 hours.
Duration of Action: Analgesic effect: IV/IM/PO, 3–7 hours.

Interactions

Effects potentiated by concomitant use of salicylates; enhances toxicity of lithium, methotrexate; increased risk of bleeding with concomitant NSAIDs, anticoagu-lant or low-dose heparin therapy; GI absorption of ketorolac delayed by food and milk; prostaglandin-mediated natriuretic effects of loop diuretics antago-nized by ketorolac.

Toxicity

Toxic Range: Not routinely monitored.
Manifestations: Drowsiness, headache, dyspepsia, nausea, GI ulceration, metabolic acidosis, hematoma, edema, palpitation.
Antidote: None.

Management: Discontinue or reduce medication. Support ventilation and circulation (patent airway, oxygen, IV fluids, vasopressors). Symptomatic treatment. Dialysis does not significantly clear ketorolac from the bloodstream.

Guidelines/Precautions

1. Use with caution in patients with active GI lesions (e.g., erosive gastritis, peptic ulcer), a history of recurrent GI lesions, hepatic or renal dysfunction, preexisting hypoprothrombinemia, or vitamin K deficiency. Ketorolac may cause fluid retention and edema in patients with cardiac decompensation or hypertension. The drug may precipitate renal failure in patients with impaired renal function, heart failure, or liver dysfunction, in patients on diuretic therapy, and in the elderly.

2. Carefully observe patients with coagulation disorders and those receiving drug therapy that interferes with hemostasis.

3. Patient response to NSAIDs is variable. Patients who do not respond to or cannot tolerate ketorolac may be successfully treated with another NSAID.

4. Ketorolac is contraindicated in patients receiving aspirin or other NSAIDs and in patients receiving probenecid. The drug is contraindicated in patients with a history of peptic ulcer disease or gastrointestinal bleeding, or with advanced renal impairment; patients at risk of volume depletion; patients with suspected or confirmed cerebrovascular bleeding, hemorrhagic diasthesis, or incomplete hemostasis; patients with high risk of bleeding; and patients with previously demonstrated hyper-

sensitivity to ketorolac or with the complete or partial syndrome of nasal polyps, angioedema, or bronchospastic reactivity to aspirin or other NSAIDs. Use as a prophylactic analgesic prior to major surgery is contraindicated as well as use intraoperatively when hemostasis is critical.

5. Epidural and intrathecal administration of ketorolac is contraindicated due to the alcohol content of the drug formulation.

6. Ketorolac is contraindicated during labor and delivery because it may adversely affect fetal circulation and inhibit uterine contractions. Ketorolac is excreted in breast milk and is contraindicated in nursing mothers.

7. Ketorolac is not recommended for premedication because it prolongs bleeding time.

8. Ketorolac is incompatible and should not be mixed with solutions of morphine sulfate, meperidine, promethazine, or hydroxyzine.

9. Signs and symptoms of infection or other diseases may be masked by the antipyretic and anti-inflammatory effects of ketorolac.

10. Monitor stool for blood every 14 days, and monitor BUN, serum creatinine, and urinalysis every 1 to 2 months when administering ketorolac at chronic high doses (which are not recommended).

Principal Adverse Reactions

Cardiovascular: Vasodilatation, pallor, angina.
Pulmonary: Dyspnea, asthma.
CNS: Drowsiness, dizziness, headache, sweating, depression, euphoria.

Gastrointestinal: Ulceration, bleeding, dyspepsia, nausea, vomiting, diarrhea, gastrointestinal pain.

Genitourinary: Hematuria, proteinuria, interstitial nephritis, renal papillary necrosis.

Dermatologic: Pruritus, urticaria.

LEFLUNOMIDE

Class: Disease-Modifying Antirheumatic Drug

Use(s): Treatment of rheumatoid arthritis.

Dosing: *Rheumatoid arthritis*

Initial Loading: PO 100 mg once daily for 3 days.

Maintenance: PO 20 mg once daily. If not well tolerated, dose may be decreased to 10 mg once daily. Maintenance doses higher than 20 mg once daily are not recommended due to greater incidence of side effects.

Dosage recommendations are not available for children at this time. The use of leflunomide in patients less than 18 years of age is not recommended. Exclude pregnancy prior to administration to women of childbearing potential. Liver enzymes should be monitored prior to the initiation of treatment and monthly thereafter.

Patients with hepatic impairment: Leflunomide is not recommended in patients with preexisting hepatic impairment. If ALT elevations greater than twice the upper limits of normal (ULN) occur while on leflunomide treatment, a dose reduction to PO 10 mg once daily may allow continued administration of the drug. Patients should continue to be monitored clinically and with frequent serum liver function test (LFT) measurements. Patients who have persistent elevations greater than twice but less than or equal to three times the ULN despite dose reduction should have a liver biopsy before the physician decides to continue treatment. Dose reduction or discontinuation of treatment is recommended for patients with ALT elevations greater than three times the ULN. Treatment may require the use of the drug elimination protocol with cholestyramine (see below). If elevations of hepatic enzymes persist, leflunomide should be discontinued, cholestyramine should be readministered, and close clinical monitoring should continue. Retreatment with cholestyramine may be needed to lower leflunomide M1 levels to less than 0.02 mg/L.

Patients with renal impairment: There are no specific dosing guidelines. Leflunomide M1 serum levels may be doubled in dialysis patients. Use with caution.

Dose adjustments may be necessary during treatment with leflunomide. Due to the prolonged half-life of the active metabolite of leflunomide, patients should be carefully observed after dose reduction, as it may take several weeks for the metabolite level to decline. After stopping treatment with leflunomide, if it is desirable to rapidly obtain plasma levels less than 0.02 mg/L, a drug elimination procedure with cholestyramine is recommended (see below). The procedure can lower serum leflunomide (M1) concentrations by 40% within 24 hours. Without the procedure, it may take 2 years for concentrations to decrease to this level.

Drug elimination procedure: Cases of pregnancy, significant overdose or toxicity, or other circumstances that require rapid lowering of leflunomide M1 plasma levels.

1. Stop leflunomide.
2. Administer cholestyramine PO 8 g three times daily for 11 days.
3. Verify plasma levels of the leflunomide M1 metabolite are less than 0.02 mg/L by two separate tests at least 14 days apart. If plasma M1 levels are higher than 0.02 mg/L, additional cholestyramine treatment should be considered.
4. Alternatively, administer activated charcoal suspensions orally or via a nasogastric tube: 50 g every 6 hours for 24 hours. Plasma concentrations of M1 have been reduced by 48% within 48 hours by this method. Repeat administration may be necessary.

Elimination: Hepatic, renal.

Preparations

Leflunomide **(Arava):** Tablets: 10 mg, 20 mg, 100 mg.

Pharmacology

An isoxazole derivative and pyrimidine synthesis inhibitor, leflunomide is the first agent for rheumatoid arthritis that is indicated for both symptomatic improvement and retardation of structural joint damage based on radiographic evidence of its disease-modifying activity. Leflunomide exhibits essentially all of its pharmacologic activity via its active primary metabolite M1. M1 inhibits dihydroorotate dehydrogenase (DHODH), an enzyme involved in de novo pyrimidine synthesis. Suppression of pyrimidine synthesis in T and B lymphocytes interferes with RNA and protein synthesis within the cells. T and B cell collaborative actions are interrupted and immunoglobulin production is suppressed. The effect appears to be cytostatic and not cytotoxic. Leflunomide M1 may also have anti-inflammatory properties secondary to reduction of histamine release and inhibition of cyclooxygenase-2 (COX-2) enzyme induction. Leflunomide may decrease proliferation, aggregation, and adhesion of peripheral and synovial fluid mononuclear cells. Decrease in the activity of lymphocytes leads to reduced cytokine- and antibody-mediated destruction of the synovial joints and attenuation of the inflammatory process. After 52 weeks of treatment in clinical trials, leflunomide showed similar improvements in tender and swollen joint counts, pain, and other symptoms when compared to methotrexate and sulfasalazine. Leflunomide was significantly superior to placebo in time to progression of structural disease as evidenced by Sharp x-ray scores. Sharp scores were not consistently different between leflunomide and methotrexate. Leflunomide has a fast onset of action (4 weeks) relative to other disease-modifying agents. The drug has a uricosuric effect and may produce hypophosphaturia in some individuals.

Pharmacokinetics

Onset of Action: Within 4 weeks.
Peak Effect: Variable.
Duration of Action: Variable.

Interactions

Clearance increased by GI binding with cholestyramine; may inhibit the metabolism of some NSAIDs; additive hepatotoxicity with other hepatotoxic drugs (e.g., methotrexate, azathioprine, sulfasalazine, cyclosporine, isoniazid, INH, ketoconazole, tacrine, troglitazone) and with heavy ethanol use; serum levels of leflunomide M1 increased by rifampin; increases serum levels of tolbutamide.

Toxicity

Toxic Range: <0.02 mg/L or 0.02 µg/mL.
Manifestations: Nausea, vomiting, diarrhea, abdominal pain, anorexia, oral ulceration, headache, immune suppression, elevated liver enzymes, rash, back pain, weight loss.
Antidote: Drug elimination with cholestyramine or activated charcoal.
Management: Discontinue or reduce medication. Administer cholestyramine PO 8 g three times daily for 11 days; *or* administer activated charcoal (powder made into a suspension) PO or via a nasogastric tube: 50 g every 6 hours for 24 hours. Repeat administration may be necessary. Symptomatic treatment. Forced diuresis,

alkalinization of urine, peritoneal dialysis, hemodialysis or hemoperfusion may not be useful due to high protein binding of leflunomide M1.

Guidelines/Precautions

1. Loading doses are necessary at the initiation of leflunomide treatment because of the long half-life of M1. Without a loading dose it may take almost 2 months of dosing to attain steady state plasma concentrations of M1.
2. Aspirin, NSAIDs, or low-dose corticosteroids may be continued during treatment with leflunomide. Concomitant use with other disease-modifying agents has not been adequately studied.
3. Leflunomide is contraindicated in patients with known hypersensitivity to the drug or any of the components of the drug formulation.
4. The drug is contraindicated in breast feeding, as there is a potential for serious adverse reactions in nursing infants. Breast feeding should be discontinued upon initiation of leflunomide. Alternative methods of feeding should be pursued.
5. Leflunomide is pregnancy Category X and can cause fetal harm when administered to a pregnant woman. The drug is absolutely contraindicated in pregnancy or in women who may become pregnant. Women of child-bearing potential must not be started on leflunomide until pregnancy is excluded and it has been confirmed that they are using reliable contraception. Before starting treatment, fully counsel patients on the potential for serious risk to the fetus. If the drug is used during

pregnancy, or if the patient becomes pregnant while taking the drug, apprise the patient of the potential hazard. A woman who wishes to become pregnant after starting leflunomide treatment should not pursue pregnancy until the medication has been discontinued and the proper drug elimination procedure for leflunomide has been completed (see above). Men who wish to father a child should consider discontinuing leflunomide and completing the appropriate drug elimination procedure.

6. Leflunomide is not recommended in patients with significant hepatic impairment or positive hepatitis B or C serologies. Leflunomide should be used with caution in patients with renal impairment.

7. Due to the potential for immune suppression, leflunomide is not recommended for patients with severe immunodeficiency, bone marrow dysplasia, or uncontrolled infections. Administration of live virus vaccines (i.e., smallpox) is not recommended. Consider the long half-life of leflunomide when contemplating administration of a live vaccine after stopping the medication if the drug elimination procedure has not been performed.

Principal Adverse Reactions

Cardiovascular: Hypertension, chest pain.

Pulmonary: Bronchitis, increased cough, rhinitis, sinusitis.

CNS: Dizziness, headache, anxiety, depression.

Gastrointestinal: Abdominal pain, anorexia, diarrhea, dyspepsia, gastroenteritis, hepatic dysfunction, elevated liver enzymes, cholelithiasis, oral ulceration, weight loss.

Genitourinary: Urinary tract infection.

Immunologic: Alopecia.

Dermatologic: Pruritus, dermatitis, acne, rash.

Hematologic: Anemia (including iron deficiency anemia), ecchymosis.

Endocrine: Diabetes mellitus, hyperthyroidism.

Other: Allergic reaction, asthenia, flu syndrome, hypokalemia, weight loss.

LEVORPHANOL TARTRATE

Class: Narcotic Agonist

Use(s): Treatment of acute, chronic, and cancer pain.

Dosing: *Analgesia*

> PO/SC: 2–4 mg every 4–6 hours.
> Slow IV: 1 mg (0.02 mg/kg).

> Administer analgesic regularly (not as needed). Due to impaired elimination, accumulation and excess sedation may occur in patients with renal or hepatic dysfunction. Analgesia may be enhanced by addition of adjuvant drugs such as nonsteroidal anti-inflammatory drugs (NSAIDs) and antidepressant agents (see pages xxvi–xliv for drug combinations) and use of nondrug therapies such as transcutaneous electrical nerve stimulation (TENS).

Elimination: Hepatic, renal.

Preparations

Levorphanol **(Levo-Dromoran)**
    Tablets: 2 mg.
    Injection: 2 mg/mL.

Pharmacology

A synthetic morphinan derivative that is structurally related to the phenanthrene-derivative opiate agonists, levorphanol exerts its potent analgesic actions on the central nervous system. In analgesic efficacy, 1 mg of parenteral levorphanol is equivalent to 5 mg of parenteral morphine sulfate. Levorphanol produces less nausea, vomiting, and constipation and more sedation and smooth muscle stimulation than equianalgesic doses of morphine sulfate. Levorphanol crosses the placental barrier and may produce depression in the neonate. The drug may appear in breast milk and should be used with caution in nursing mothers.

Pharmacokinetics

Onset of Action: IV, 10–15 minutes.
Peak Effect: IV, <20 minutes; SC, 60–90 minutes.
Duration of Action: IV/SC, 6–8 hours.

Interactions

Potentiates CNS and circulatory depressant effects of other narcotic analgesics, volatile anesthetics, phenothiazines, sedative-hypnotics, alcohol, tricyclic antidepressants; analgesia enhanced and prolonged by narcotic and non-narcotic analgesics (e.g., aspirin, acetaminophen), α_2-agonists (e.g., clonidine).

Toxicity

Toxic Range: Not routinely monitored.

Manifestations: Somnolence, coma, respiratory arrest, apnea, cardiac arrhythmias, combined respiratory and metabolic acidosis, circulatory collapse, cardiac arrest, death.

Antidote: Naloxone IV/IM/SC 0.4–2.0 mg. Repeat dose every 2 to 3 minutes to a maximum of 10–20 mg.

Management: Discontinue or reduce medication. Support ventilation and circulation (patent airway, oxygen, IV fluids, vasopressors). Administer antidote. Monitor blood gases, pH, and electrolytes. Correct acidosis and electrolyte disturbance (lactic acidosis may require sodium bicarbonate IV 1–2 mEq/kg). Symptomatic treatment. Airway-protected, ipecac syrup–induced emesis (30 mL or 0.5 mL/kg ipecac syrup followed by 200 mL or 4 mL/kg of water or clear fluid) or gastric lavage (with drug ingestion) followed by administration of activated charcoal (PO 50–100 g or 1–2 g/kg).

Guidelines/Precautions

1. Reduce dosage in elderly patients and with concomitant use of narcotics and sedative-hypnotics.
2. The drug formulation may contain sodium metabisulfite, which may cause allergic reactions or anaphylaxis in susceptible individuals.
3. Prescribe or supply an antiemetic (e.g., metoclopramide) for use in the event of nausea and/or vomiting.
4. Constipation may be more difficult to control than

pain. Prevent and/or treat by daily administration of laxatives and stool softeners, for example, Colace (docusate sodium) 100–300 mg/day. Do not administer bulk-forming agents that contain methylcellulose, psyllium, or polycarbophil. Temporary arrest in the passage through the gastro-intestinal tract may lead to fecal impaction or bowel obstruction.

5. Tolerance is manifested by decreased duration of effect and increasing need for the drug. In these cases, add adjuvant drugs (e.g., NSAIDs, antidepressant agents) or switch to alternative opioids (starting at one-half the equianalgesic dose) or supplement with nondrug therapies (e.g., TENS).

6. Abrupt discontinuation of opioids in patients with physical dependence may manifest with withdrawal symptoms. To avoid withdrawal, doses should be reduced slowly (e.g., dose reduction of 75% every 2 days). Withdrawal should be treated symptomatically.

7. Addiction occurs rarely (frequency of less than 1:3000) and should not be considered in deciding the proper dose and schedule of levorphanol.

8. Drug combinations with adjuvant drugs enhance analgesia (see pages xxvi–xliv).

9. Adjuvant drug therapies also include regional blockade, trigger-point injections (with local anesthetics and steroids), and intravenous regional anesthesia.

10. Adjuvant nondrug therapies include TENS and modalities such as ice or heat application, ultrasound, and soft tissue mobilization.

11. Patients should be warned that levorphanol may impair their ability to perform hazardous tasks requiring mental alertness or physical coordination (e.g., driving a motor vehicle, operating heavy machinery).
12. Levorphanol is subject to control under the Controlled Substances Act of 1970 as a Schedule II (C-II) drug.

Principal Adverse Reactions

Cardiovascular: Hypotension, circulatory depression, bradycardia, syncope.
Pulmonary: Respiratory depression.
CNS: Sedation, somnolence, euphoria, dysphoria, disorientation.
Genitourinary: Urinary retention.
Gastrointestinal: Nausea, vomiting, abdominal pain, biliary tract spasm, constipation, anorexia, hepatic dysfunction.
Ocular: Miosis.
Allergic: Rash, pruritus, urticaria.

LIDOCAINE HYDROCHLORIDE

Class: Local Anesthetic, Antiarrhythmic

Use(s): Regional anesthesia; treatment of ventricular arrhythmias, especially when associated with acute myocardial infarction or cardiac surgery; systemic analgesia for treatment of migraine, neuropathic pain (e.g., diabetic neuropathy), reflex sympathetic dystrophy (chronic regional pain syndrome).

Dosing: *Antiarrhythmic*

>Slow IV bolus: 1–1.5 mg/kg (1–2% solution) followed by 0.5 mg/kg every 2–5 minutes (to maximum of 200–300 mg in 1 hour). Patients with congestive heart failure or cardiogenic shock may require smaller bolus doses.
>
>Slow IV infusion: (0.1–0.4% solution) 1–4 mg/min (20–50 μg/kg/min).
>
>When arrhythmias appear during constant infusion, a small bolus dose (e.g., 0.5 mg/kg may be administered to rapidly increase plasma concentrations and the infusion rate may be maintained or increased. The infusion should be terminated as soon as the patient's basic cardiac rhythm appears to be stable or at the earliest sign of toxicity.
>
>IM: 200–400 mg (4–6 mg/kg). May be repeated 60–90 minutes later.
>
>Reduce doses in the elderly, patients with heart failure or liver disease, or patients who are receiving β-blockers or cimetidine.

Local anesthesia

>Topical: 0.6–3.0 mg/kg (2–4% solution).
>
>Infiltration/Peripheral nerve block: 0.5–5.0 mg/kg (0.5–2.0% solution).
>
>Transtracheal: 80–120 mg (2–3 mL of 4% solution).
>
>Superior laryngeal nerve: 40–60 mg (2–3 mL of 2% solution on each side).

Intravenous regional block
Upper extremities: 200–250 mg (40–50 mL of 0.5% solution).

Lower extremities: 250–300 mg (100–120 mL of 0.25% solution).

Do not add epinephrine for intravenous regional block. If desired, add fentanyl 50 μg to enhance the block and/or muscle relaxant (pretreatment doses only), for example, pancuronium 0.5 mg. This combination may enable the use of lower concentrations of the local anesthetic (e.g., lidocaine 50 mL of 0.25% for upper extremity block).

Brachial plexus block: 300–750 mg (30–50 mL of 1.0–1.5% solution); children 0.5–0.75 mL/kg. With high doses (>4 mg/kg), add epinephrine 1 : 200,000 to decrease systemic toxicity (in the absence of any contraindications). Regional blockade may be potentiated by addition of tetracaine 0.5–1.0 mg/kg or fentanyl 1–2 μg/kg or morphine (0.05–0.1 mg/kg).

Stellate ganglion block: 10–20 mL of 1% solution (100–200 mg) with or without epinephrine 1 : 200,000.

Lumbar sympathetic block: 10–15 mL of 1% solution (100–150 mg) with or without epinephrine 1 : 200,000.

Posterior tibial nerve sympathetic block: 2.0–2.5 mL of 1% solution (20–25 mg) with or without epinephrine 1 : 200,000 and with or without steroids (e.g., triamcinolone ace-tonide). Note: The posterior tibial sympathetics control 85% of the sympathetics to the foot, including all four muscle layers and the vital structures of the sole of the foot. Such selective sympathectomy may be preferable to a lumbar paravertebral block for reflexive sympathetic dystrophy (RSD) of the foot.

Celiac plexus block: 20–25 mL of 1% solution (200–250 mg) with or without epinephrine 1:200,000.

Caudal: 150–300 mg (15–20 mL of 1% or 1.5% solution). Children 0.4–0.7–1.0 mL/kg (L2-T10-T7 level of anesthesia). At higher volumes (>0.6 mL/kg), utilize lower concentrations of lidocaine.

Epidural

    Bolus: 200–400 mg (1–2% solution); children 7–9 mg/kg.

    Infusion: 6–12 mL/hr (0.5% solution with or without epidural narcotics); children 0.2–0.35 mL/kg/hr.

    Rate of onset and potency of local anesthetic action may be enhanced by carbonation. (Add 1 mL of 7.5% or 8.4% sodium bicarbonate with 10 mL of 0.5–2.0% lidocaine. Do not use if there is precipitation.)

Spinal bolus/infusion: 50–100 mg (0.5–5.0% solution with or without glucose 7.5%). 1.5% solution provides a shorter time to ambulation, full motor recovery, and discharge compared with 5% solution for spinal anesthesia. Intrathecal doses that exceed 75 mg may be associated with increased incidences of neurologic deficit. The addition of epinephrine or 7.5% glucose to lidocaine may contribute to persistent neurologic injury.

Acute migraine: Sphenopalatine ganglion block

Intranasal: 1.5 mL of 4% lidocaine three times daily.

Slow IV: 100 mg or 2 mg/kg (0.1% solution) with or without droperidol 2.5 mg (50 μg/kg) or promethazine 25 mg (0.5 mg/kg). Administer over 20–30 minutes (rate of 5 mg/min). May combine with oxygen inhalation (10 L/min). Observe for symptoms of toxicity (e.g., hypotension, slurred speech, drowsiness) and adjust rate accordingly.

Neuropathic pain/RSD

IM: 200–400 mg once weekly (4–6 mg/kg). Use 2% solution for infiltration and nerve block. Maximum 10 mL at any site. Use contralateral thigh/deltoid if more than one site is required.

Slow IV: 50–300 mg (1–5 mg/kg of 0.1% solution). Administer over 10–60 minutes (rate of 5 mg/min). Observe for symptoms of toxicity (e.g., slurred speech) and adjust rate accordingly. If there is long-lasting pain relief with parenteral lidocaine, patient may benefit from oral mexiletine (100–150 mg one to three times daily).

Subcutaneous bolus: 2 mg/kg. Administer over 1 hour.

Subcutaneous infusion: 2 mg/kg/hr (adult range of 100–160 mg/hr). Use 10% solution. Monitor serum levels regularly and adjust dose to keep levels within 2–5 μg/mL. Discontinue infusion with relief of symptoms or signs of toxicity. Patients have been maintained on continuous subcutaneous lidocaine infusions in combination with other pharmacologic therapies (including intrathecal opioids) for up to 6 months. Avoid IM injection of concentrated lidocaine (10%). It may cause muscle inflammation and necrosis.

Therapeutic level: 1.5–6.0 μg/mL. Maximum safe dose: 4 mg/kg without epinephrine, 7 mg/kg with epinephrine 1:200,000.

IV: Use only lidocaine injection without preservatives and clearly labeled for IV use. Doses for epidural or spinal anesthesia should be reduced in pregnant patients. Solutions containing preservatives should not be used for spinal, epidural, or caudal block. Except where contraindicated, vasoconstrictor drugs may be added to increase effect and prolong local or regional anesthesia. For dosage and route guidelines, see Epinephrine. Do not use vasoconstrictor drugs for IV regional anesthesia or local anesthesia of end organs (digits, penis, ears).

Elimination: Hepatic, pulmonary.

Preparations

Lidocaine hydrochloride **(Xylocaine, Lidocaine, Dilo-
caine, Lidoject, Nervocaine, Lignocaine)**
Parenteral administration
IM injection: 10%.
Injection for direct IV: 1%, 2%.
Injection for IV admixture: 4%, 10%, 20%.
Injection for IV infusion: 0.2%, 0.4%, 0.8%.
Infiltration/Peripheral nerve block: 0.5%, 1%, 1.5%,
2% with or without epinephrine 1:50,000,
1:100,000, 1:200,000.
Epidural: 1%, 1.5%, 2% preservative free.
Spinal (hyperbaric solution): 1.5%, 5% solution with
7.5% dextrose/glucose.
Laryngotracheal (with laryngotracheal cannula): 4%
sterile solution.

Dilution for Infusion

IV: 500mg to 2g in 500mL D5W (1–4mg/mL or
0.1–0.4% solution).
Epidural: 20mL 1% in 20mL preservative-free normal
saline (0.5% solution).

Pharmacology

This amide-derivative local anesthetic has a rapid
onset of action. It stabilizes neuronal membrane by
inhibiting the sodium flux required for the initiation
and conduction of impulses. The drug is also a class 1B
antiarrhythmic agent that suppresses automaticity and
shortens the effective refractory period and action
potential duration of the His/Purkinje system. The
action potential duration and effective refractory period
of ventricular muscle are also decreased. When admin-

istered parenterally, lidocaine may produce central analgesia. This may be due to local anesthetic effects, inhibition of release of neurotransmitters (e.g., substance P,
ATP from nociceptive afferent C fibers), modulation of
information transfer along primary afferents, and central
sympathetic blockade with decrease in pain-induced
reflex vasoconstriction. Only minimal amounts of lidocaine enter the circulation following subcutaneous
injection, but lidocaine blood levels increase with repeat
or continuous dosing due to gradual accumulation of
the drug or its active metabolite monoethylglycinexyli-
dide (MEGX). Subcutaneous infusion of lidocaine may
stop sympathetic activation of wide dynamic range
neurons mediated by peripheral mechanoreceptors.
High plasma levels (as occur in paracervical blocks)
produce uterine vasoconstriction and decrease in
uterine blood flow. Therapeutic doses of lidocaine do
not significantly decrease systemic arterial blood pressure, myocardial contractility, or cardiac output.
Repeated doses cause significant increases in blood
level due to slow accumulation.

Pharmacokinetics

Onset: IV (antiarrhythmic effects), 45–90 seconds. Intratracheal (antiarrhythmic effects), 10–15 seconds. Infiltration, 0.5–1.0 minutes. Epidural, 5–15 minutes.
Peak Effect: IV (antiarrhythmic effects), 1–2 minutes.
IM (antiarrhythmic effects), 10–15 minutes. IV (analgesic effects), 15–20 minutes. Infiltration/Epidural, <30
minutes.
Duration of Action: IV (antiarrhythmic effects), 10–20
minutes. Intratracheal (antiarrhythmic effects), 30–50
minutes. Infiltration, 0.5–1.0 hour; with epinephrine,
2–6 hours. Epidural, 1–3 hours.

Interactions

Cardiac effects with other antiarrhythmics, such as phenytoin, procainamide, propranolol, or quinidine, may be additive or antagonistic; may potentiate the neuromuscular blocking effect of succinylcholine, tubocurarine; reduced clearance with concomitant use of β-blocking agents, cimetidine; seizures, respiratory and circulatory depression at high plasma levels; benzodiazepines, barbiturates, and volatile anesthetics increase seizure threshold; duration of regional anesthesia prolonged by vasoconstrictor agents (e.g., epinephrine), α_2-agonists (e.g., clonidine), and narcotics (e.g., fentanyl); alkalinization increases rate of onset and potency of local or regional anesthesia.

Toxicity

Toxic Range: 6–10 µg/mL.

Manifestations: Initial: CNS stimulation such as anxiety, apprehension, headache, tremors, restlessness, nervousness, disorientation, confusion, dizziness, perioral numbness, tinnitus, blurred vision, tremors, nausea/vomiting, shivering, seizures. Subsequent: CNS depression including drowsiness, slurred speech, unconsciousness, respiratory depression and arrest. Cardiovascular toxicity including myocardial depression, sinus bradycardia, arrhythmias, hypotension, circulatory collapse, and cardiac arrest.

Antidote: No specific antidote.

Management: Discontinue or reduce medication. Support ventilation and circulation (patent airway, oxygen, IV fluids, vasopressors). Control seizures with benzodiazepines (diazepam IV 0.05–0.2 mg/kg, midazolam IV/IM 0.025–0.1 mg/kg) or barbiturates (thiopental sodium IV 0.5–2.0 mg/kg). Prolonged cardiopulmonary resuscitation with cardiac arrest: Sodium bicarbonate IV 1–2 mEq/kg to treat cardiac toxicity (sodium channel blockade); bretylium IV 5 mg/kg; DC cardioversion/defibrillation for ventricular arrhythmias. Remove ingested drug by induced emesis followed by activated charcoal. Hypersensitivity reactions: Remove from further exposure and treat dermatitis.

Guidelines/Precautions

1. Use with caution in patients with hypovolemia, G6PD deficiency, severe congestive heart failure, shock, all forms of heart block, and methemoglobinemia. Lidocaine may induce or exacerbate preexisting methemoglobinemia.
2. Lidocaine is contraindicated in patients with hypersensitivity to amide-type local anesthetics.
3. Benzodiazepines increase seizure threshold for lidocaine and other local anesthetics.
4. Use of lidocaine for paracervical block is associated with fetal bradycardia and acidosis.
5. If intravenous access is not available, the drug may be diluted 1:1 in sterile normal saline and injected via an endotracheal tube. The absorption rate, duration, and pharmacologic effects of intratracheal drug administration compare favorably with the IV route.
6. In intravenous regional blocks, deflate the cuff after 40 minutes and not less than 20 minutes. Between 20 and 40 minutes, the cuff can be deflated, reinflated immediately, and finally deflated after a minute to reduce the sudden

absorption of anesthetic into the systemic circulation.

7. Cauda equina syndrome with permanent neurologic deficit has occurred in patients receiving greater than 100 mg of a 5% lidocaine solution with a continuous spinal technique. Transient neurologic deficits have occurred with bolus injections of hyperbaric 5% lidocaine (in 7.5% dextrose) or isobaric 2% lidocaine. There is a sevenfold increase of postspinal radiculopathy with the patient in lithotomy flexion, wherein perfusion of the cauda equina may be compromised and the nerves may be more vulnerable to chemical injury. Consistent neurologic damage is significantly more common with lidocaine (at any concentration) than with bupivacaine or tetracaine. Positioning in lithotomy flexion has no adverse impact on spinal anesthesia when bupivacaine or tetracaine is used.

8. The recommended volumes for brachial plexus block are consistent with available data on plasma levels (subtoxic) after brachial plexus block. The risks of systemic toxicity may be decreased by adding epinephrine to the local anesthetic and avoiding IV injection, which may result in an immediate toxic reaction.

9. The level of sympathetic blockade (bradycardia with block above T5) determines the degree of hypotension (often heralded by nausea and vomiting) following epidural or intrathecal lidocaine. Fluid hydration (10–20 mL/kg normal saline or lactated Ringer's solution), vasopressor agents (e.g., ephedrine), and left uterine displacement in pregnant patients may be used for prophylaxis

and/or treatment. Administer atropine to treat bradycardia.

10. Epidural motor blockade may be reversed by the epidural injection of 20 mL of 0.9% saline.

11. Epidural, caudal, or intrathecal injections should be avoided when the patient has hypovolemic shock, septicemia, infection at the injection site, or coagulopathy.

Principal Adverse Reactions

Cardiovascular: Hypotension, bradycardia, arrhythmias, heart block.

Pulmonary: Respiratory depression, arrest.

CNS: Tinnitus, seizures, loss of hearing, euphoria, anxiety, diplopia, postspinal headache, arachnoiditis, palsies.

Allergic: Urticaria, pruritus, angioneurotic edema.

Epidural/Caudal/Spinal: High spinal; loss of bladder and bowel control; permanent motor, sensory, and autonomic (sphincter control) deficit of lower segments.

LORAZEPAM

Class: Benzodiazepine

Use(s): Sedative, treatment of chemotherapy-induced or postoperative nausea and vomiting.

Dosing: *Sedation*

   PO: 2–3 mg twice or three times daily. Elderly, 1–2 mg/day in divided doses.

   IV/IM: 1–4 mg (0.02–0.08 mg/kg). Dilute with equal volume of D5W or normal saline.

  Antiemetic

   PO: 1–2 mg two or three times daily.

   IV: 0.5–1.0 mg (0.01–0.02 mg/kg).

Elimination: Hepatic, renal.

Preparations

Lorazepam **(Ativan)**
  Tablets: 0.5 mg, 1 mg, 2 mg.
  Injection: 2 mg/mL, 4 mg/mL.
Lorazepam **(Lorazepam Intensol):** Oral solution concentrate: 2 mg/mL.

Pharmacology

This benzodiazepine produces a dose-related sedation and relief of anxiety. Like other benzodiazepines, the drug is thought to influence the effect of γ-aminobutyric acid (GABA), an inhibitory neurotransmitter, in the brain. In chronic pain syndromes, relief of anxiety and agitation may increase the pain threshold. Lorazepam does not have intrinsic analgesic activity and should be used in combination with analgesics (e.g., opioids, NSAIDs, antidepressant agents). It produces minimal depressant effects on ventilation and circulation in the absence of other CNS depressant drugs. The drug is intermediate in speed of onset compared with other benzodiazepines.

Pharmacokinetics

Onset of Action: IV, 1–5 minutes. IM, 15–30 minutes. PO, 20–30 minutes.
Peak Effect: IV, 15–20 minutes. PO, 2 hours.
Duration of Action: IV/IM/PO, 6–10 hours.

Interactions

CNS and circulatory depressant effects potentiated by alcohol, narcotics, sedatives, barbiturates, phenothiazines, monoamine oxidase (MAO) inhibitors, and volatile anesthetics; decreases requirements for volatile anesthetics; effects antagonized by flumazenil.

Toxicity

Toxic Range: Not routinely monitored.
Manifestations: Respiratory depression, apnea, hypotension, confusion, coma, seizures.
Antidote: Flumazenil IV 0.2–2.0 mg.
Management: Discontinue or reduce medication. Administer antidote. Support ventilation and circulation (patent airway, oxygen, IV fluids, vasopressors). Symptomatic treatment. Airway-protected, ipecac syrup–induced emesis (30 mL or 0.5 mL/kg ipecac syrup followed by 200 mL or 4 mL/kg of water or clear fluid) or gastric lavage (with drug ingestion) followed by administration of activated charcoal (PO 50–100 g or 0.5–1.0 g/kg). Hemodialysis is not useful. Treat withdrawal hyperactivity with low-dose barbiturate.

Guidelines/Precautions

1. Intra-arterial injection may produce arteriospasm resulting in gangrene. Treat with local infiltration of phentolamine (5–10 mg in 10 mL normal saline) and, if necessary, sympathetic block.
2. Unexpected hypotension and respiratory depression may occur when combined with opioids.
3. Use with caution in elderly patients since excessive sedation and hypoventilation may occur.
4. The drug is not for use in children younger than 12 years.
5. Patients should be warned that lorazepam may impair their ability to perform activities requiring mental alertness or physical coordination (e.g.,

operating heavy machinery, driving a motor
vehicle).
6. Contraindicated in patients with known hypersensitivity to benzodiazepines or any ingredients in the
parenteral formulation (i.e., polyethylene glycol,
propylene glycol, or benzyl alcohol) and in
patients with acute close-angle glaucoma.
7. Lorazepam is subject to control under the Federal
Controlled Substances Act of 1970 as a Schedule IV
(C-IV) drug.

Principal Adverse Reactions

Cardiovascular: Hypotension, hypertension, bradycar-
dia, tachycardia.
Pulmonary: Respiratory depression.
CNS: Sedation, dizziness, weakness, depression, agita-
tion, amnesia.
Psychological: Hysteria, psychosis.
Gastrointestinal: Change in appetite.
Other: Visual disturbances, urticaria, pruritus.

MECLOFENAMATE SODIUM

Class: Nonsteroidal Anti-inflammatory Drug

Use(s): Symptomatic treatment of moderate to severe
inflammatory and degenerative arthritis, primary dysmenorrhea, postoperative and posttraumatic pain,
chronic pain, and cancer pain (especially with bone
metastasis).

Dosing: *Pain or inflammatory disease:* PO 200–300 mg
(4–6 mg/kg) daily, in three or four divided
doses. Maximum dose 400 mg daily.

Administer analgesic regularly (not as needed). Meclofenamate may cause serious adverse effects. It is not a drug of first choice, and should not be used as a simple analgesic or antipyretic. Analgesia may be enhanced by addition of opioid analgesics (see pages xxvi–xliv for drug combinations), antidepressant agents, and use of nondrug therapies such as transcutaneous electrical nerve stimulation (TENS). In rheumatoid arthritis or juvenile rheumatoid arthritis, second-line rheumatoid agents may include leflunomide (Arava), etanercept (Enbrel), antimalarials, or methotrexate. In geriatric patients and patients with decreased renal or hepatic function, decrease doses by one-third to one-half. The incidence of meclofenamate-induced gastropathy may be decreased by administration with meals, milk, antacids, or sucralfate (PO 1 g four times daily). Misoprostol (PO 100–200 µg four times daily) may be used to prevent gastric ulcers in high-risk patients.

Elimination: Hepatic, renal.

Preparations

Meclofenamate sodium **(Varions):** Capsules: 50 mg, 100 mg.

Pharmacology

Meclofenamic acid, an anthranilic acid derivative and nonsteroidal anti-inflammatory drug (NSAID), is commercially available as the sodium salt (meclofenamate sodium). Meclofenamate is structurally and pharmacologically related to mefenamic acid. However, the severe hematologic abnormalities commonly associated with mefenamic acid are less prevalent. As with other NSAIDs, the analgesic and anti-inflammatory activities of meclofenamate are partly due to the inhibition of prostaglandin and leukotriene synthesis and to anti-bradykinin and lysosomal membrane stabilizing activity. Unlike other NSAIDs, meclofenamate (and other fenamates) may in addition compete with prostaglandins for binding at the prostaglandin receptor site, thus potentially affecting prostaglandins that have already been formed. The antipyretic activity of meclofenamate may occur secondary to inhibition of pyrogen-induced release of prostaglandins in the central nervous system (including the hypothalamus) and possibly to centrally mediated peripheral vasodilatation.

The analgesic and anti-inflammatory potency of meclofenamate is similar to that of piroxicam and about three times that of ibuprofen or aspirin. Meclofenamate (like other NSAIDs) exhibits a ceiling effect for analgesia. Exceeding recommended doses results in increased toxicity without improvement in analgesia. Meclofenamate may cause gastric mucosal damage with ulceration and/or bleeding. Inhibition of prostaglandin synthesis may result in decreased uterine tone and contractility and prolonged gestation in the parturient and premature closure of the ductus arteriosus in the fetus. Unlike the irreversible effects of aspirin, meclofenamate may transiently inhibit platelet aggregation and prolong bleeding time. The drug has no uricosuric activity.

Pharmacokinetics

Onset of Action: PO, analgesic effect 30–60 minutes.

Peak Effect: PO, analgesic effect 1–2 hours; anti-inflammatory effect 1–3 weeks.
Duration of Action: PO, analgesic effect 3–7 hours.

Interactions

Risks of bleeding increased with concomitant NSAIDs, anticoagulant or heparin therapy, alcohol ingestion; decreases antihypertensive effects of β-adrenergic blocking agents; serum levels of meclofenamate decreased slightly by concomitant aspirin; increased GI toxicity with concomitant aspirin; serum levels of meclofenamate increased by concomitant probenecid; serum levels and toxic effects of salicylates, oral anti-coagulants, phenytoin, sulfonamides, sulfonylureas, methotrexate, and lithium increased by concomitant meclofenamate; GI absorption of meclofenamate delayed by food and milk; prostaglandin-mediated natriuretic effects of loop diuretics antagonized by meclofenamate.

Toxicity

Toxic Range: Not routinely monitored.
Manifestations: *Acute:* Agitation, seizures, oliguria, anuria, azotemia.
Antidote: None.
Management: Discontinue or reduce medication. Correct fluid, electrolyte, and acid-base disturbances. Support ventilation and circulation (patent airway, oxygen, IV fluids, vasopressors). Airway-protected, ipecac syrup–induced emesis (30 mL or 0.5 mL/kg ipecac syrup followed by 200 mL or 4 mL/kg of water or clear fluid) or gastric lavage (with drug ingestion) followed by administration of activated charcoal (PO

50–100 g or 1–2 g/kg). Control seizures (IV benzodiazepines or barbiturates). Dialysis to correct serious
azotemia or electrolyte problems. Symptomatic treatment.

Guidelines/Precautions

1. Use with caution in patients with active GI lesions
   (e.g., erosive gastritis, peptic ulcer), a history of
   recurrent GI lesions, hepatic or renal dysfunction,
   preexisting hypoprothrombinemia, or vitamin K
   deficiency. Meclofenamate may decrease glomerular filtration rate and cause peripheral edema. The
   drug should be used cautiously in patients with
   heart failure, hypertension, or other conditions
   associated with fluid retention.
2. Renal prostaglandins may have a supportive role in
   maintaining renal perfusion in patients with prerenal conditions. Meclofenamate should be avoided
   in such patients because it may cause a dose-
   dependent decrease in prostaglandin formation and
   thus precipitate renal decompensation.
3. Carefully observe patients with coagulation disorders and those receiving drug therapy that
   interferes with hemostasis.
4. Use with caution in pregnancy and only when the
   perceived benefits outweigh the risks.
5. Patient response to NSAIDs is variable. Patients
   who do not respond to or cannot tolerate meclofenamate may be successfully treated with another
   NSAID.
6. Meclofenamate and salicylates should not be
   administered concomitantly because there may not
   be any therapeutic advantage and the incidence of
   adverse GI side effects may be increased.

7. Contraindicated in patients with previously demonstrated hypersensitivity to meclofenamate or with the complete or partial syndrome of nasal polyps, angioedema, or bronchospastic reactivity to aspirin or other NSAIDs.
8. Signs and symptoms of infection or other diseases may be masked by the antipyretic and anti-inflammatory effects of meclofenamate.
9. Monitor stool for blood every 14 days, and monitor BUN, serum creatinine, and urinalysis every 1 to 2 months when administering meclofenamate at chronic high doses.

Principal Adverse Reactions

Cardiovascular: Peripheral edema, fluid retention, hypertension, palpitation.
Pulmonary: Dyspnea, bronchospasm.
CNS: Drowsiness, dizziness, headache, anxiety, confusion.
Gastrointestinal: Diarrhea, ulceration, bleeding, dyspepsia, nausea, vomiting, cholestatic jaundice.
Genitourinary: Renal dysfunction, acute renal failure, azotemia, cystitis, hematuria.
Dermatologic: Pruritus, urticaria.
Hematologic: Granulocytopenia, leukopenia, thrombocytopenia, aplastic anemia, hemolytic anemia.
Other: Tinnitus, blurred vision.

MEFENAMIC ACID

Class: Nonsteroidal Anti-inflammatory Drug

Use(s): Symptomatic treatment of moderate to severe inflammatory and degenerative arthritis, primary dys-

menorrhea, tension headache, postoperative and posttraumatic pain; short-term treatment for chronic pain,
cancer pain (especially with bone metastasis).

Dosing: *Pain, inflammatory disease, headache:* PO
500 mg (10 mg/kg) then 250 mg (5 mg/kg)
every 6 hours. Maximum dose 1000 mg/day.
Duration of therapy should not exceed 1
week for the relief of pain or 3 days for the
relief of primary dysmenorrhea.

Administer analgesic regularly (not as
needed). Mefenamic acid may cause
serious adverse effects, including hematologic abnormalities. It is not a drug of first
choice, and should not be used as a simple
analgesic or antipyretic. Therapy should
not exceed 1 week. Analgesia may be
enhanced by addition of opioid analgesics
(see pages xxvi–xliv for drug combinations), antidepressant agents, and use of
nondrug therapies such as transcutaneous
electrical nerve stimulation (TENS). In
rheumatoid arthritis or juvenile rheumatoid
arthritis, second-line rheumatoid agents may
include leflunomide (Arava), etanercept
(Enbrel), antimalarials, or methotrexate. In
geriatric patients and patients with decreased
renal or hepatic function, decrease doses
by one-third to one-half. The incidence of
mefenamic acid–induced gastropathy may
be decreased by administration with meals,
milk, antacids, or sucralfate (PO 1 g four
times daily). Misoprostol (PO 100–200 µg

four times daily) may be used to prevent gastric ulcers in high-risk patients.

Elimination: Hepatic, renal.

Preparations

Mefenamic acid **(Ponstel):** Capsules: 250 mg.

Pharmacology

An anthranilic acid derivative (fenamate) and potent nonsteroidal anti-inflammatory drug (NSAID), mefenamic acid is structurally and pharmacologically related to meclofenamate. As with other NSAIDs, the analgesic and anti-inflammatory activities of mefenamic acid are partly due to the inhibition of prostaglandin synthesis and/or release secondary to the inhibition of cyclooxygenase. Cyclooxygenase catalyzes the formation of prostaglandin precursors (endoperoxides) from arachidonic acid. Unlike other NSAIDs, mefenamic acid (and other fenamates) may in addition compete with prostaglandins for binding at the prostaglandin receptor site, thus potentially affecting prostaglandins that have already been formed. The antipyretic activity of mefenamic acid may occur secondary to inhibition of pyrogen-induced release of prostaglandins in the central nervous system (including the hypothalamus) and possibly to centrally mediated peripheral vasodilatation.

The analgesic and anti-inflammatory potency of mefenamic acid is similar to that of piroxicam and about three times that of ibuprofen or aspirin. Mefenamic acid (like other NSAIDs) exhibits a ceiling effect for analgesia. Exceeding recommended doses results in increased toxicity without improvement in analgesia. Mefenamic acid may cause gastric mucosal damage with ulceration and/or bleeding. Inhibition of prostaglandin synthesis may result in decreased uterine tone and contractility and prolonged gestation in the parturient and premature closure of the ductus arteriosus in the fetus. Mefenamic acid has no uricosuric activity. The drug may inhibit platelet aggregation and prolong bleeding time. Hematologic abnormalities, including decreased hematocrit, agranulocytosis, and Coombs-positive autoimmune hemolytic anemia, may occur with prolonged use. Due to the potential for serious adverse effects, therapy with mefenamic acid should be limited to 1 week; thus, the drug has limited use in patients with chronic or cancer pain.

Pharmacokinetics

Onset of Action: PO, analgesic effect 30–60 minutes.
Peak Effect: PO, analgesic effect 1–2 hours.
Duration of Action: PO, analgesic effect 3–7 hours.

Interactions

Risks of bleeding increased with concomitant NSAIDs, anticoagulant or heparin therapy, alcohol ingestion; decreases antihypertensive effects of β-adrenergic blocking agents; serum levels of mefenamic acid decreased slightly by concomitant aspirin; increased GI toxicity with concomitant aspirin; serum levels of mefenamic acid increased by concomitant probenecid; serum levels and toxic effects of salicylates, oral anticoagulants, phenytoin, sulfonamides, sulfonylureas, methotrexate, and lithium increased by concomitant mefenamic acid; GI absorption of mefenamic acid delayed by food and milk; prostaglandin-mediated natriuretic effects of loop diuretics antagonized by mefenamic acid.

Toxicity

Toxic Range: >11 μg/mL.

Manifestations: *Acute:* Agitation, seizures, muscle twitching, oliguria, anuria, azotemia, vomiting, and diarrhea.

Antidote: None.

Management: Discontinue or reduce medication. Correct fluid, electrolyte, and acid-base disturbances. Support ventilation and circulation (patent airway, oxygen, IV fluids, vasopressors). Airway-protected, ipecac syrup–induced emesis (30 mL or 0.5 mL/kg ipecac syrup followed by 200 mL or 4 mL/kg of water or clear fluid) or gastric lavage (with drug ingestion) followed by administration of activated charcoal (PO 50–100 g or 1–2 g/kg). Control seizures (IV benzodiazepines or barbiturates). Dialysis to correct serious azotemia or electrolyte problems. Symptomatic treatment.

Guidelines/Precautions

1. Use with caution in patients with active GI lesions (e.g., erosive gastritis, peptic ulcer), a history of recurrent GI lesions, hepatic or renal dysfunction, preexisting hypoprothrombinemia, or vitamin K deficiency. Mefenamic acid may cause peripheral edema and should also be used cautiously in patients with heart failure, hypertension, or other conditions associated with fluid retention.

2. Renal prostaglandins may have a supportive role in maintaining renal perfusion in patients with prerenal conditions. Mefenamic acid should be avoided

in such patients because it may cause a dose-dependent decrease in prostaglandin formation and thus precipitate renal decompensation.

3. Carefully observe patients with coagulation disorders and those receiving drug therapy that interferes with hemostasis.

4. Use with caution in pregnancy and only when the perceived benefits outweigh the risks.

5. Patient response to NSAIDs is variable. Patients who do not respond to or cannot tolerate mefenamic acid may be successfully treated with another NSAID.

6. Mefenamic acid and salicylates should not be administered concomitantly because there may not be any therapeutic advantage and the incidence of adverse GI side effects may be increased.

7. Contraindicated in patients with previously demonstrated hypersensitivity to mefenamic acid or with the complete or partial syndrome of nasal polyps, angioedema, or bronchospastic reactivity to aspirin or other NSAIDs.

8. Signs and symptoms of infection or other diseases may be masked by the antipyretic and anti-inflammatory effects of mefenamic acid.

9. Monitor stool for blood every 14 days, and monitor BUN, serum creatinine, and urinalysis every 1 to 2 months when administering mefenamic acid at chronic high doses.

Principal Adverse Reactions

Cardiovascular: Peripheral edema, fluid retention, hypertension, palpitation.

Pulmonary: Dyspnea, bronchospasm.

CNS: Drowsiness, dizziness, headache, anxiety, confusion.

Gastrointestinal: Diarrhea, ulceration, bleeding, dyspepsia, nausea, vomiting, cholestatic jaundice.

Genitourinary: Renal papillary necrosis, interstitial nephritis, acute renal failure, azotemia, cystitis, hematuria.

Dermatologic: Pruritus, urticaria.

Hematologic: Granulocytopenia, leukopenia, thrombocytopenia, aplastic anemia, hemolytic anemia, prolongation of bleeding time.

Other: Tinnitus, blurred vision.

MEPERIDINE HYDROCHLORIDE

Class: Narcotic Agonist

Use(s): Treatment of acute, chronic, and cancer pain.

Dosing: *Pain*

PO/IM/SC: 50–150 mg (1–3 mg/kg) every 3–4 hours.

Slow IV: 25–100 mg (0.5–2.0 mg/kg) every 3–4 hours.

Epidural

Bolus: 50–100 mg (1–2 mg/kg) diluted in 10 mL preservative-free normal saline or local anesthetic.

Infusion: 10–20 mg/hr (0.2–0.4 mg/kg/hr).

Spinal

Bolus: 10–50 mg (0.2–1.0 mg/kg). Use preservative-free 5% solution (50 mg/mL).

Infusion: 5–10 mg/hr (0.1–0.2 mg/kg/hr).

Patient-controlled analgesia (PCA), IV
  Bolus: 5–30 mg (0.1–0.6 mg/kg).
  Infusion: 5–40 mg/hr (0.1–0.8 mg/kg/hr).
  Lockout interval: 5–15 minutes.
Patient-controlled analgesia, epidural
  Bolus: 5–30 mg (0.1–0.6 mg/kg).
  Infusion: 5–10 mg/hr (0.1–0.2 mg/kg/hr).
  Lockout interval: 5–15 minutes.

Maximum recommended dose: 1 g/day (20 mg/kg/day). Meperidine and normeperidine serum levels should be monitored at higher doses or with prolonged administration.

Administer analgesic regularly (not as needed). Due to impaired elimination, accumulation and excess sedation may occur in patients with renal or hepatic dysfunction. Analgesia may be enhanced by addition of adjuvant drugs such as nonsteroidal anti-inflammatory drugs (NSAIDs) and antidepressant agents (see pages xxvi–xliv for drug combinations) and use of nondrug therapies such as transcutaneous electrical nerve stimulation (TENS).

Elimination: Hepatic.

Preparations

Meperidine hydrochloride **(Demerol)**
  Injection: 10 mg/mL, 25 mg/mL, 50 mg/mL, 75 mg/mL, 100 mg/mL.
  Tablets: 50 mg, 100 mg.
  Oral solution: 50 mg/5 mL.

Dilution for Infusion

IV: 100 mg in 50 mL D5W or normal saline (2 mg/mL).
Epidural
  Bolus: 50–100 mg in 10 mL local anesthetic or preservative-free normal saline.
  Infusion: 100–500 mg in 50 mL local anesthetic or preservative-free normal saline (2–10 mg/mL).

Pharmacology

This synthetic opioid agonist is approximately one-tenth as potent as morphine, with a slightly more rapid onset and shorter duration of action. Meperidine has mild vagolytic and antispasmodic effects. Compared with equipotent doses of morphine, meperidine produces less sedation and pruritus and may be more effective in neuropathic pain. Meperidine may offer a better quality of postoperative analgesia after tuboplasty surgery, ureteral surgery, or other situations involving visceral smooth muscle spasm. Meperidine may produce orthostatic hypotension at therapeutic doses and is the only opioid with a direct myocardial depressant effect at high doses. Normeperidine, the active metabolite, is a cerebral stimulant and is excreted primarily in the urine. It may accumulate with repetitive and/or prolonged administration (>3 days) of meperidine. Spinal and epidural administration of meperidine produce analgesia by specific binding and activation of opioid receptors in the substantia gelatinosa. Once activated, the opioid receptors inhibit the release of substance P from nociceptive afferent C fibers. Unlike other opiates, meperidine has potent local anesthetic activity, and epidural/spinal analgesia is accompanied by sensory, motor, and sympathetic blockade. Meperidine is not used as a topical anesthetic due to local irritation. Meperidine crosses the placental barrier and may produce depression in the neonate. Maximum placental transfer and neonatal depression occur at 2 to 3 hours following parenteral administration. The drug may appear in breast milk and should be used with caution in nursing mothers.

Pharmacokinetics

Onset: PO, 10–45 minutes. IV, <1 minute. IM, 1–5 minutes. Epidural/Spinal, 2–12 minutes.
Peak Effect: PO, <1 hour. IV, 5–20 minutes. IM, 30–50 minutes. Epidural/Spinal, 30 minutes.
Duration of Action: PO/IV/IM, 2–4 hours. Epidural/Spinal, 1–8 hours.

Interactions

Seizures, myoclonus, delirium with repeated high doses and in patients with renal and/or hepatic impairment; potentiates CNS and circulatory depression of narcotics, sedative-hypnotics, volatile anesthetics, tricyclic antidepressants; severe and sometimes fatal reaction (hyperthermia, hypertension, seizures) may occur with administration of meperidine in patients who have received monoamine oxidase (MAO) inhibitors; aggravates adverse effects of isoniazid; chemically incompatible mixture with barbiturates; analgesia enhanced and prolonged by α_2-agonists (e.g., clonidine); addition of epinephrine to intrathecal/epidural meperidine results in increased side effects (e.g., nausea).

Toxicity

Toxic Range: Meperidine, <0.55 µg/mL; normeperidine, <0.5 µg/mL.

Manifestations: Somnolence, coma, respiratory arrest, apnea, cardiac arrhythmias, combined respiratory and metabolic acidosis, circulatory collapse, cardiac arrest, death.

Antidote: Naloxone IV/IM/SC 0.4–2.0 mg. Repeat dose every 2 to 3 minutes to a maximum of 10–20 mg.

Management: Discontinue or reduce medication. Support ventilation and circulation (patent airway, oxygen, IV fluids, vasopressors). Administer antidote. Monitor blood gases, pH, and electrolytes. Correct acidosis and electrolyte disturbance (lactic acidosis may require sodium bicarbonate IV 1–2 mEq/kg). Symptomatic treatment. Airway-protected, ipecac syrup–induced emesis (30 mL or 0.5 mL/kg ipecac syrup followed by 200 mL or 4 mL/kg of water or clear fluid) or gastric lavage (with drug ingestion) followed by administration of activated charcoal (PO 50–100 g or 1–2 g/kg).

Guidelines/Precautions

1. Severe and occasionally fatal reactions in patients who are receiving or have just received MAO inhibitors. Treat with hydrocortisone IV. Use chlorpromazine IV to treat the associated hypertension.

2. Use with caution in patients with asthma, chronic obstructive pulmonary disease, increased intracranial pressure, or supraventricular tachycardia.

3. Reduce doses in elderly patients and with concomitant use of sedatives and other narcotics.

4. The narcotic antagonist naloxone is a specific antidote (IV/IM/SC 0.2–0.4 mg or higher). Reversal of narcotic effect may lead to onset of pain and release of catecholamines. The duration of rever-

sal may be shorter than the duration of narcotic effect. Naloxone may precipitate seizures, especially in patients receiving meperidine.

5. Meperidine crosses the placental barrier, and usage in labor may produce depression of respiration in the neonate. Resuscitation may be required; have naloxone available.

6. Undesirable side effects of epidural, caudal, or intrathecal meperidine include delayed respiratory depression (up to 8 hours after single dose), pruritus, nausea and vomiting, and urinary retention. Naloxone (IV/IM/SC 0.2–0.4mg as needed or infusion 5–10µg/kg/hr) is effective for prophylaxis and/or treatment of these side effects. Ventilatory support for respiratory depression must be readily available. Antihistamines, for example, diphenhydramine (IV/IM 12.5–25.0mg every 6 hours as needed) may be used in treating pruritus. Metoclopramide (IV 10mg every 6 hours) may be used in treating nausea and vomiting. Urinary retention that does not respond to naloxone may require an "in and out" bladder catheter. Bethanechol (Urecholine) PO 15–30mg three times daily or SC 2.5–5.0mg three or four times daily as required may be used as an alternative to naloxone. (Bethanechol increases the tone of the detrusor urinae muscle. It should not be given IV or IM, which may result in cholinergic overstimulation. Have atropine available [IV/SC 0.5mg].)

7. Epidural, caudal, or intrathecal meperidine should be avoided when the patient has septicemia, infection at the injection site, or coagulopathy.

8. The following infusions are incompatible with

PCA meperidine and should not be combined in the same intravenous line: aminophylline, cefaperazone, diazepam, furosemide, heparin, hydrocortisone, magnesium sulfate, prednisone, phenytoin, and sodium bicarbonate.

9. To avoid rotor problems, pH adjustment is required with use of meperidine in Medtronic implantable spinal infusion pumps.

10. Patients should be warned that meperidine may impair their ability to perform hazardous tasks requiring mental alertness or physical coordination (e.g., driving a motor vehicle, operating heavy machinery).

Principal Adverse Reactions

Cardiovascular: Hypotension, cardiac arrest.

Pulmonary: Respiratory depression, respiratory arrest, laryngospasm.

CNS: Euphoria, dysphoria, sedation, seizures, psychological dependence.

Gastrointestinal: Constipation.

Musculoskeletal: Chest wall rigidity.

Allergic: Urticaria, pruritus.

MEPIVACAINE HYDROCHLORIDE

Class: Local Anesthetic

Use(s): Regional anesthesia.

Dosing: *Infiltration:* 50–400 mg (0.5–1.5% solution).
Brachial plexus block: 300–750 mg (30–50 mL of 1.0–1.5% solution). Children, 0.5–

0.75 mL/kg. High doses (>4 mg/kg) are not recommended without addition of epinephrine 1 : 200,000 to decrease systemic toxicity (in the absence of any contraindications). Regional blockade may be potentiated by the addition of tetracaine (0.5–1.0 mg/kg) or fentanyl (1–2 µg/kg) or morphine (0.05–0.1 mg/kg).

Stellate ganglion block: 10–20 mL of 1% solution (100–200 mg) with or without epinephrine 1 : 200,000.

Lumbar sympathetic block: 10–15 mL of 1% solution (100–150 mg) with or without epinephrine 1 : 200,000.

Celiac plexus block: 20–25 mL of 1% solution (200–250 mg) with or without epinephrine 1 : 200,000.

Epidural:

Bolus: 150–400 mg (15–20 mL of 1–2% solution).

Infusion: 6–12 mL/hr (0.25–0.5% solution with or without epidural narcotics).

Rate of onset and potency of local anesthetic action may be enhanced by carbonation. (Add 1 mL of 8.4% sodium bicarbonate with 10 mL of 1–3% mepivacaine. Do not use if there is precipitation.)

Caudal: 150–400 mg (15–20 mL of 1–2% solution). Children, 0.4–0.7–1.0 mL/kg (L2-T10-T7 level of anesthesia). At higher volumes (>0.6 mL/kg), utilize lower concentrations of mepivacaine (0.5–1.0% solutions).

Maximum safe dose: 4 mg/kg without

epinephrine; 7 mg/kg with epinephrine 1:200,000. Solutions containing preservatives should not be used for epidural or caudal block. Except where contraindicated, vasoconstrictor drugs may be added to increase effect and prolong local or regional anesthesia. For dosage and route guidelines, see the "Dosing" section of Epinephrine (p. 204). Do not use vasoconstrictor drugs for local anesthesia of end organs (digits, penis, ears).

Elimination: Hepatic.

Preparations

Mepivacaine hydrochloride **(Carbocaine, Polocaine):** Injection, with or without methylparaben: 1%, 1.5%, 2%, 3%.

Pharmacology

A tertiary amine local anesthetic, mepivacaine stabilizes the neuronal membrane and prevents the initiation and transmission of impulses. The amide structure is not detoxified by plasma esterases, and metabolism occurs primarily by hepatic microsomal enzymes. Similar to lidocaine in potency and speed of onset, mepivacaine has a slightly longer duration of action and lacks vasodilator activity. High plasma levels (as occur in paracervical blocks) produce uterine vasoconstriction and decrease in uterine blood flow.

Pharmacokinetics

Onset of Action: Infiltration, 3–5 minutes. Epidural, 5–15 minutes.

Peak Effect: Infiltration/Epidural, 15–45 minutes.
Duration of Action: Infiltration, 0.75–1.5 hours; with epinephrine, 2–6 hours. Epidural, 3–5 hours (prolonged with epinephrine).

Interactions

Reduced clearance with coadministration of β-blockers, cimetidine; benzodiazepines, barbiturates, and volatile anesthetics increase seizure threshold; duration of local or regional anesthesia prolonged by vasoconstrictor agents (e.g., epinephrine) and α_2-agonists (e.g., clonidine); alkalinization increases rate of onset and potency of local or regional anesthesia.

Toxicity

Toxic Range: Not routinely monitored.
Manifestations: Hypotension, confusion, slurred speech, perioral numbness, tinnitus, seizures, arrhythmias, circulatory collapse, respiratory depression, cardiac arrest.
Antidote: No specific antidote.
Management: Discontinue or reduce medication. Support ventilation and circulation (patent airway, oxygen, IV fluids, vasopressors). Benzodiazepines (diazepam IV 0.05–0.2 mg/kg; midazolam IV/IM 0.025–0.1 mg/kg) or barbiturates (thiopental sodium IV 0.5–2.0 mg/kg) to control seizures. Prolonged cardiopulmonary resuscitation with cardiac arrest: Sodium bicarbonate IV 1–2 mEq/kg to treat cardiac toxicity (sodium channel blockade); bretylium IV 5 mg/kg; DC cardioversion/defibrillation for ventricular arrhythmias. Remove ingested drug by induced emesis followed by activated charcoal. Hypersensitivity reactions: Remove from further exposure and treat dermatitis.

Guidelines/Precautions

1. Do not use for spinal anesthesia.
2. Meperidine is not recommended for obstetrical anesthesia. High neonatal blood levels are due to placental transfer and impaired elimination.
3. Use for paracervical block may be associated with fetal bradycardia and acidosis.
4. Use with caution in patients with severe disturbance of cardiac rhythm and heart block.
5. Contraindicated in patients with hypersensitivity to amide-type local anesthetics.
6. The recommended volumes for brachial plexus block are consistent with available data on plasma levels (subtoxic) after brachial plexus block. The risks of systemic toxicity may be decreased by adding epinephrine to the local anesthetic and avoiding IV injection, which may result in an immediate toxic reaction.
7. The level of sympathetic blockade (bradycardia with block above T5) determines the degree of hypotension (often heralded by nausea and vomiting) following epidural or intrathecal mepivacaine. Fluid hydration (10–20 mL/kg normal saline or lactated Ringer's solution), vasopressor agents (e.g., ephedrine), and left uterine displacement in pregnant patients may be used for prophylaxis and/or treatment. Administer atropine to treat bradycardia.
8. Epidural motor blockade may be reversed by the epidural injection of 20 mL of 0.9% saline.
9. Epidural or caudal injections should be avoided when the patient has hypovolemic shock, septicemia, infection at the injection site, or coagulopathy.

Principal Adverse Reactions

Cardiovascular: Hypotension, bradycardia, cardiac arrest.

Pulmonary: Respiratory depression, respiratory arrest.

CNS: Tinnitus, seizures, loss of hearing, euphoria, dysphoria.

Allergic: Urticaria, pruritus, angioneurotic edema.

Epidural/Caudal: High spinal; loss of bladder and bowel control; permanent motor, sensory, and autonomic (sphincter control) deficit of lower segments.

METHADONE HYDROCHLORIDE

Class: Narcotic Agonist

Use(s): Treatment of chronic and cancer pain, treatment of severe refractory headache and migraine, detoxification treatment of narcotic addiction.

Dosing: *Pain*

Initial: IM/SC/PO 2.5–10.0 mg (0.05–0.1 mg/kg) every 3–4 hours.

Maintenance: PO 5–20 mg (0.1–0.4 mg/kg) every 6–8 hours. Once stable blood levels are achieved, dosing intervals may be increased to 12–24 hours.

Administer analgesic regularly (not as needed). Due to the long plasma half-life, accumulation of parent drug and excess sedation may occur, particularly in the elderly or in patients with renal or hepatic dysfunction. Plasma concentrations may not reach a steady state for 2

to 3 weeks, and patient response needs
to be evaluated on commencing therapy.
Epidural (bolus): 1–5 mg (0.02–0.1 mg/kg).
Dilute in 10 mL preservative-free normal
saline or local anesthetic.
Narcotic abstinence syndrome: PO 15 to 120
mg daily (highly individualized).
Patient controlled analgesia IV
Bolus: 0.5–3.0 mg (0.01–0.06 mg/kg).
Lockout interval: 10–20 minutes.
Analgesia may be enhanced by addition of
adjuvant drugs such as nonsteroidal anti-
inflammatory drugs (NSAIDs) and antidepressant agents (see pages xxvi–xliv for
drug combinations) and use of nondrug
therapies such as transcutaneous electrical
nerve stimulation (TENS).
Maintenance methadone therapy (more than
3 weeks) may be undertaken only by
approved methadone programs.

Elimination: Hepatic.

Preparations

Methadone hydrochloride **(Dolophine)**
Injection: 10 mg/mL.
Tablets: 5 mg, 10 mg, 40 mg.
Oral solution: 1 mg/mL, 2 mg/mL, 10 mg/mL.

Pharmacology

Methadone is a synthetic narcotic analgesic with multiple actions quantitatively similar to those of morphine,
mainly involving the central nervous system and organs
composed of smooth muscle. The spinal *N*-methyl D-

aspartate (NMDA) receptor is important in modulating the plasticity of the central nervous system and in aggravating chronic/neuropathic pain through the phenomenon of "wind-up." Both opioid-active (D-) and opioid-inactive (L-) isomers of methadone bind noncompetitively to the NMDA receptor and antagonize its effects. Methadone produces a concentration-dependent reduction in the neurotoxicity of exogenously applied NMDA in murine cortical cell culture. Methadone (and possibly other opioids, including morphine, fentanyl, codeine, meperidine, and dextropropoxyphene) may have neuron-protective effects that are mediated by NMDA receptors and not conventional opioid receptors.

Methadone is the analgesic of choice in severe pain. As an analgesic, methadone given in a single dose is marginally more potent than morphine. With repeated dosage, it is 3 times more potent and 1.5 to 2 times longer acting than morphine. Methadone, like morphine, has no ceiling effect. The methadone abstinence syndrome, although qualitatively similar to that of morphine, differs in that the onset is slower, the course is more prolonged, and the symptoms are less severe. Cumulative effect occurs with repeated use, resulting in a prolonged duration of action. Oral methadone is approximately one-half as potent as parenteral. Methadone crosses the placental barrier, and because of the long duration of action, the probability of neonatal respiratory depression is high. Methadone may appear in breast milk in concentrations approaching plasma levels and should be used with caution in nursing mothers.

Pharmacokinetics

Onset of Action: IV, <1 minute, IM, 1–5 minutes. PO, 30–60 minutes, Epidural, 5–10 minutes.
Peak Effect: IV, 5–20 minutes. IM, 30–60 minutes.
Duration of Action: IV/IM, 4–6 hours. PO, 22–48 hours (patients on methadone maintenance). Epidural, 6–10 hours.

Interactions

Blood concentration may be reduced by rifampin, with production of withdrawal symptoms; severe reaction with monoamine oxidase (MAO) inhibitors; withdrawal symptoms precipitated by pentazocine in heroin addicts on methadone therapy; cimetidine inhibits hepatic metabolism of methadone and may increase toxic effects; potentiates CNS and circulatory depressant effects of other narcotic analgesics, volatile anesthetics, phenothiazines, sedative-hypnotics, alcohol, and tricyclic antidepressants; analgesia enhanced and prolonged by α_2-agonists (e.g., clonidine); addition of epinephrine to epidural methadone results in increased side effects (e.g., nausea).

Toxicity

Toxic Range: Not routinely monitored.
Manifestations: Somnolence, coma, respiratory arrest, apnea, cardiac arrhythmias, combined respiratory and metabolic acidosis, circulatory collapse, cardiac arrest, death.
Antidote: Naloxone IV/IM/SC 0.4–2.0 mg. Repeat dose every 2 to 3 minutes to a maximum of 10–20 mg.
Management: Discontinue or reduce medication.

Support ventilation and circulation (patent airway, oxygen, IV fluids, vasopressors). Administer antidote. Monitor blood gases, pH, and electrolytes. Correct acidosis and electrolyte disturbance (lactic acidosis may require sodium bicarbonate IV 1–2 mEq/kg). Symptomatic treatment. Airway-protected, ipecac syrup–induced emesis (30 mL or 0.5 mL/kg ipecac syrup followed by 200 mL or 4 mL/kg of water or clear fluid) or gastric lavage (with drug ingestion) followed by administration of activated charcoal (PO 50–100 g or 1–2 g/kg).

Guidelines/Precautions

1. Do not give opioid agonist-antagonist drugs (e.g., pentazocine) to patients on long-term methadone treatment, because withdrawal symptoms may be precipitated.
2. Methadone is not appropriate for patients with rapidly changing pain levels. It is ineffective for relief of general anxiety.
3. Use with caution in patients with asthma, chronic obstructive pulmonary disease, or increased intracranial pressure.
4. Reduce dosage in elderly patients and with concomitant use of narcotics and sedative-hypnotics.
5. Methadone can produce drug dependence of the morphine type and therefore has the potential for being abused.
6. Use of doses greater than 120 mg/day requires special federal approval.
7. Undesirable side effects of epidural methadone include delayed respiratory depression, pruritus, nausea and vomiting, and urinary retention.

Naloxone (IV/IM/SC 0.2–0.4mg as needed or infusion 5–10µg/kg/hr) is effective for prophylaxis and/or treatment of these side effects. Ventilatory support for respiratory depression must be readily available. Antihistamines, for example, diphenhydramine (IV/IM 12.5–25.0mg every 6 hours as needed) may be used in treating pruritus. Metoclopramide (IV 10mg every 6 hours) may be used in treating nausea and vomiting. Urinary retention that does not respond to naloxone may require straight bladder catheterization. Bethanechol (Urecholine) PO 15–30mg three times daily or SC 2.5–5.0mg three or four times daily as required may be used as an alternative to naloxone. (Bethanechol increases the tone of the detrusor urinae muscle. It should not be given IV or IM, which may result in cholinergic overstimulation. Have atropine available [IV/SC 0.5mg].)

8. Epidural injections should be avoided when the patient has septicemia, infection at the injection site, or coagulopathy.

9. Methadone-related sedation may be treated by reducing the dose and increasing the frequency of administration. Additional measures include changing to short-acting opioids. Dextroamphetamine (PO 5–15mg/day) may be helpful if pain is well controlled but the patient is unable to function due to sedation.

10. Prescribe or supply an antiemetic (e.g., metoclopramide) for use in the event of nausea and/or vomiting.

11. Constipation may be more difficult to control than pain. Prevent and/or treat by increasing regular

exercise and oral fluids and by daily administration of stool softeners or laxatives such as Colace (docusate sodium) 100–300 mg/day. Do not administer bulk-forming agents that contain methylcellulose, psyllium, or polycarbophil. Temporary arrest in the passage through the gastrointestinal tract may lead to fecal impaction or bowel obstruction.

12. Tolerance manifests by a decrease in the duration of effect and increasing need for opioids. However, increase in pain (e.g., in cancer patients) may manifest with increasing dose requirements. Tolerance develops more rapidly following IV or spinal administration than after oral or rectal administration. Very high doses may be needed to maintain analgesia. Add adjuvant drugs (e.g., NSAIDs, antidepressant agents, dextromethorphan) or switch to alternative opioids (starting at one-half the equianalgesic dose) or supplement with nondrug therapies (e.g., TENS).

13. Abrupt discontinuation of opioids in patients with physical dependence may manifest with withdrawal symptoms. To avoid withdrawal, opioid doses should be reduced slowly (e.g., dose reduction of 75% every 2 days). When a total daily dose of IV/IM/SC 10–15 mg or PO 20 mg of methadone is reached, it should be maintained for 2 days and then discontinued. Withdrawal should be treated symptomatically.

14. Addiction occurs rarely (frequency of < 1:3000) in patients who receive opioids for legitimate medical conditions. Addiction should not be considered in deciding the proper dose and schedule of opioids. Pseudoaddiction (an iatrogenic condi-

tion with characteristics of psychological dependence) may occur as a result of inadequate pain treatment.

15. Drug combinations with adjuvant drugs enhance analgesia (see pages xxvi–xliv). NSAIDs (e.g., aspirin) potentiate analgesia, decrease inflammation, and are useful in pain related to bony metastasis and musculoskeletal inflammation. Anticonvulsants (e.g., gabapentin) are useful in cancer therapy or chronic neuralgias that complicate tumor progression (e.g., glossopharyngeal neuralgias in head and neck cancers). Phenothiazines (e.g., methotrimeprazine) minimize the constipating, respiratory depressant, and emetic effects of opioids and are useful in the treatment of opioid-tolerant patients. Antidepressant agents (e.g., paroxetine) ameliorate insomnia, potentiate analgesia, and are useful in cancer pain syndromes, neuropathies, and neuralgias. Steroids may be oncolytic for some tumors (e.g., lymphomas) and may ameliorate painful nerve or spinal compression by reducing edema in tumor or nerve tissue. Steroids may also provide euphoria and increased appetite in moribund patients. Antihistamines (e.g., hydroxyzine) provide additive analgesia with slightly more sedation and less emesis. α_2-Agonists (e.g., clonidine) enhance analgesia and suppress the adrenergic symptoms of opioid withdrawal.

16. Adjuvant drug therapies also include regional blockade, trigger-point injections (with local anesthetics and steroids), and intravenous regional anesthesia.

17. Adjuvant nondrug therapies include TENS and

modalities such as ice or heat application, ultrasound, and soft tissue mobilization.

18. Patients should be warned that methadone may
impair their ability to perform hazardous tasks
requiring mental alertness or physical coordination (e.g., driving a motor vehicle, operating
heavy machinery).

19. Methadone is subject to control under the Federal
Controlled Substances Act of 1970 as a Schedule
II (C-II) drug.

Principal Adverse Reactions

Cardiovascular: Hypotension, circulatory depression,
bradycardia, syncope.

Pulmonary: Respiratory depression.

CNS: Euphoria, dysphoria, disorientation.

Genitourinary: Urinary retention.

Gastrointestinal: Biliary tract spasm, constipation,
anorexia.

Ocular: Miosis.

Allergic: Rash, pruritus, urticaria.

METHOCARBAMOL

Class: Skeletal Muscle Relaxant

Use(s): Relief of musculoskeletal pain, adjunct treatment of tetanus.

Dosing: *Musculoskeletal pain*
Initial
PO: 1500 mg four times daily for 2–3 days.

Slow IV/IM: 1000 mg one to three times daily.

Maximum 3 g daily for 3 days. Replace with oral medication as soon as possible. IV route: Administer undiluted at a maximum rate of 3 mL/min. Patients should be recumbent during and for 10–15 minutes after IV administration. IM route: Do not inject more than 5 mL into each gluteal region. Do not administer subcutaneously.

Maintenance: PO 750 mg six times daily, or 1000 mg four times daily, or 1500 mg three times daily.

Methocarbamol should be used as an adjunct to rest, physical therapy, and analgesics for the relief of discomfort associated with acute painful musculoskeletal conditions.

Tetanus

Initial: Slow IV 1–3 g (15 mg/kg). May be repeated every 6 hours until a nasogastric tube is inserted. Tablets may then be crushed and suspended in water or saline solutions and administered through the nasogastric tube.

Maintenance: PO up to 24 g daily.

Elimination: Hepatic, renal.

Preparations

Methocarbamol **(Robaxin)**
 Tablets: 500 mg, 750 mg.
 Injection: 100 mg/mL.

Methocarbamol and aspirin **(Robaxisal):** Tablets: Methocarbamol 400 mg and aspirin 325 mg.

Pharmacology

A carbamate derivative of guaifenesin and a central-acting skeletal muscle relaxant that is structurally and pharmacologically related to chlorphenesin and mephenesin, methocarbamol is a CNS depressant with sedative and skeletal muscle relaxant effects. The precise mechanism of action is not known. However, methocarbamol does not directly relax skeletal muscle and does not depress neuronal conduction, neuromuscular transmission, or muscle excitability. Methocarbamol is ineffective in the treatment of skeletal muscle hyperactivity secondary to chronic neurologic disorders such as cerebral palsy and other dyskinesias. In the management of tetanus, methocarbamol may be less preferable to diazepam, meprobamate, barbiturates, chlorpromazine, or, in severe cases, neuromuscular blocking agents.

Pharmacokinetics

Onset of Action: PO, <30 minutes; IV, <1 minute.
Peak Effect: PO/IV, variable.
Duration of Action: Half-life 0.9–1.8 hours.

Interactions

Potentiates CNS depressant effects of alcohol, barbiturates, narcotics, volatile anesthetics; may precipitate severe weakness in patients with myasthenia gravis receiving anticholinesterase agents.

Toxicity

Toxic Range: Not routinely monitored.
Manifestations: Drowsiness, coma, CNS depression.

Antidote: No specific antidote.

Management: Discontinue or reduce medication. Support ventilation and circulation (patent airway, oxygen, IV fluids, vasopressors). Monitor urine output. Airway-protected, ipecac syrup–induced emesis (30 mL or 0.5 mL/kg ipecac syrup followed by 200 mL or 4 mL/kg of water or clear fluid) or gastric lavage (with drug ingestion) followed by administration of activated charcoal (PO 50–100 g or 1–2 g/kg). Symptomatic treatment.

Guidelines/Precautions

1. Use with caution in patients with myasthenia gravis or history of epilepsy. The polyethylene glycol vehicle may be damaging to the kidneys, and the drug should be used with caution in patients with renal impairment.
2. Patients should be warned that methocarbamol may impair their ability to perform activities requiring mental alertness or physical coordination (e.g., operating heavy machinery, driving a motor vehicle).
3. The parenteral solution is hypertonic and may cause irritation. Avoid extravasation.

Principal Adverse Reactions

Cardiovascular: Bradycardia, hypotension, syncope.
Pulmonary: Dyspnea.
CNS: Drowsiness, dizziness, blurred vision, headache, vertigo, seizures.
Gastrointestinal: Nausea and vomiting, constipation, taste disorders, abdominal pain.
Musculoskeletal: Muscle pain.
Other: Rash, pruritus, sloughing or pain at the injection site, leukopenia, hematuria.

METHYLPREDNISOLONE SODIUM SUCCINATE, METHYLPREDNISOLONE ACETATE, METHYLPREDNISOLONE

Class: Corticosteroid

Use(s): Anti-inflammatory, treatment of nerve root irritation (e.g., from herniated disk), treatment of myofascial pain with trigger points, treatment of allergic reactions, short-term management of bronchodilator-unresponsive asthma and chronic obstructive pulmonary disease, steroid replacement, organ transplantation, adjunct treatment of sympathetic mediated pain, cluster headaches.

Dosing: *Inflammatory diseases, neuritis, asthma, and steroid replacement*

Methylprednisolone (Medrol): PO 2–60 mg (0.117–1.66 mg/kg) daily in four divided doses. May be given as alternate doses to minimize side effects.

Methylprednisolone (Medrol Dosepak): For short-term use; PO 4-mg tablets.

Day 1: 24 mg (six tablets). Administer 8 mg two times daily (before breakfast and at bedtime) and 4 mg two times daily (after lunch and dinner).

Day 2: 20 mg (five tablets). Administer 4 mg three times daily (before breakfast, after lunch, and after dinner) and 8 mg at bedtime.

Day 3: 16 mg (four tablets). Administer 4 mg four times daily (before breakfast,

after lunch and after dinner, and at
bedtime).

Day 4: 12 mg (three tablets). Administer
4 mg three times daily (before breakfast, after lunch, and at bedtime).

Day 5: 8 mg (two tablets). Administer 4
mg two times daily (before breakfast
and at bedtime).

Day 6: 4 mg (one tablet). Administer 4 mg
once (before breakfast).

*Inflammatory diseases, asthma, steroid re-
placement:* Methylprednisolone sodium
succinate (Solu-Medrol) IV/IM 10.0 mg to
1.5 g (0.03–30.0 mg/kg) daily. Usual dose:
10–250 mg up to six times daily.

*Acute spinal cord injury or life-threatening
shock:* Methylprednisolone sodium succinate (Solu-Medrol) IV 30 mg/kg infused
over 10–20 minutes, then IV 5.4 mg/kg/hr
for 23 hours. Administer initial dose within
first 8 hours of injury; administer total adult
dose of 10 g within first 24 hours.

Inflammatory diseases or myofascial pain:
Methylprednisolone acetate (Depo-Medrol)
intra-articular or intratissue 4–80 mg. May
repeat at 1–5 weeks.

Sympathetic mediated pain: IV regional
block: Methylprednisolone sodium succinate (Solu-Medrol) 80 mg. Dilute in 50 mL
of normal saline or 0.5% lidocaine. May be
combined with guanethidine 20–40 mg or
bretylium (1–2 mg/kg).

Herniated disk/Back pain: Epidural methylprednisolone acetate (Depo-Medrol) 40–80 mg in 5–10 mL preservative-free normal saline or local anesthetic. (Dilute in 20–25 mL for the caudal route.) May repeat at 2–3 weeks if response is partial. Additional relief does not occur with more than three injections. Do not administer intrathecally.

Cluster headache: Methylprednisolone sodium succinate (Solu-Medrol) IV 500 mg to 1 g (10–20 mg/kg). Dilute in normal saline and infuse over 3 hours.

Elimination: Hepatic.

Preparations

Methylprednisolone **(Medrol):** Tablets: 2 mg, 4 mg, 8 mg, 16 mg, 24 mg, 32 mg.

Methylprednisolone **(Medrol Dosepak):** Tablets: 4 mg.

Methylprednisolone sodium succinate **(Solu-Medrol, A-methaPred):** Injection (IV or IM): 40 mg, 125 mg, 500 mg, 1000 mg, 2000 mg per vial.

Methylprednisolone acetate **(Depo-Medrol, Duralone, depMedalone, Depopred, Depoject, Depo-Predate, Medralone, Rep-Pred):** Parenteral suspension for IM, intra-articular, intralesional, or soft tissue injection: 20 mg/mL, 40 mg/mL, 80 mg/mL.

Pharmacology

This methyl derivative of prednisolone is a potent anti-inflammatory steroid. The anti-inflammatory potency of 4 mg of methylprednisolone is equivalent to that of 0.75 mg of dexamethasone, 5 mg of prednisolone, or 20 mg of cortisol. Methylprednisolone may decrease the number and activity of inflammatory cells, enhance the effects of β-adrenergic drugs on cyclic adenosine monophosphate (cAMP) production, and inhibit bronchoconstrictor mechanisms. Methylprednisolone is useful in the management of acute and chronic cancer pain. It may decrease nerve root edema in the presence of a herniated disk. Methylprednisolone may be oncolytic for certain tumors (e.g., lymphoma) and may ameliorate painful nerve or spinal cord compression by reducing edema in tumor and nerve tissue. Methylprednisolone is effective in the treatment of malignant spinal cord compression. In moribund patients, methylprednisolone may provide euphoria, increase appetite, and relieve tumor-related pain. In metastatic bone pain, methylprednisolone may decrease inflammation by inducing the biosynthesis of phospholipase A_2 inhibitor. Phospholipase A_2 catalyzes the release of fatty acid substrates required for the formation of prostaglandin. Prostaglandins of the E series have been shown to cause hyperalgesia. Methylprednisolone has less tendency to cause salt and water retention than prednisolone, hydrocortisone, or cortisone, and has a rapid onset but short duration of action. Prolonged therapy of pharmacologic doses may lead to hypothalamic-pituitary-adrenal (HPA) axis suppression.

Pharmacokinetics

Onset of Action: Anti-inflammatory effects: IV, almost immediate; epidural, 1–3 days.

Peak Effect: Anti-inflammatory effects: IV, <1 hour; epidural 1–2 weeks.

Duration of Action: Anti-inflammatory effects/HPA suppression: IV, 12–36 hours; epidural, variable.

Interactions

Clearance enhanced by phenytoin, phenobarbital, ephedrine, and rifampin; altered response to coumarin anticoagulants; enhanced effect in patients with hypothyroidism and cirrhosis; interacts with anticholinesterase agents (e.g., neostigmine) to produce severe weakness in patients with myasthenia gravis; potassium wasting effects enhanced with potassium-depleting diuretics (e.g., thiazides, furosemide); diminished response to toxoids and live or inactivated vaccines.

Toxicity

Toxic Range: Not defined. Acute ingestion is rarely a problem.

Manifestations: *Withdrawal after long-term use:* Acute adrenal insufficiency (fever, hypotension, dyspnea, dizziness, fainting, hypoglycemia). *Prolonged administration:* Cushingoid changes (moon face, central obesity, hypertension, osteoporosis, diabetes, peptic ulcer, increased susceptibility to infection, electrolyte and fluid imbalance).

Antidote: No specific antidote.

Management: Taper off or gradually reduce medication (alternate-day medication). Supplement medication during times of stress. Support ventilation and circulation (patent airway, oxygen, IV fluids, vasoactive drugs). Symptomatic treatment.

Guidelines/Precautions

1. Contraindicated in systemic fungal infections.
2. Use cautiously in patients with ocular herpes simplex for fear of corneal perforation.
3. Following prolonged therapy, abrupt discontinua-

tion may result in a withdrawal syndrome without evidence of adrenal insufficiency. To minimize morbidity associated with adrenal insufficiency, discontinue exogenous corticosteroid therapy gradually.

4. In patients on corticosteroid therapy subjected to any unusual stress, increased dosage of rapidly acting corticosteroid before, during, and after the stressful situation is indicated. Supplemental steroids should be empirically administered to all patients who have received daily steroid replacement for at least 1 week in the year prior to surgery.

5. May mask signs of infection. There may be decreased resistance and inability of the host defense mechanisms to prevent dissemination of infection.

6. Epidural injections should be avoided when the patient has septicemia, infection at the injection site, or coagulopathy.

7. Intra-articular methylprednisolone should not be administered more frequently than every 4 months and then only if the duration of benefit from the previous injection lasted more than 4 weeks. Short-term relief of pain does not justify the use of repeated injections.

8. Intrathecal (spinal) steroid injection of methylprednisolone and other long-acting steroids is contraindicated since polyethylene glycol, the vehicle used in depot steroid preparations, may produce meningeal inflammation. Myelographic changes of arachnoiditis may occur rapidly after such injections (within 2 to 8 weeks).

Principal Adverse Reactions

Cardiovascular: Arrhythmias, hypertension, congestive heart failure in susceptible patients.

CNS: Seizures, psychosis, increased intracranial pressure.

Gastrointestinal: Pancreatitis, peptic ulcer with perforation and hemorrhage.

Dermatologic: Impaired wound healing, petechiae, lupus erythematosus–like syndrome.

Musculoskeletal: Weakness, myopathy, osteoporosis, aseptic necrosis.

Endocrinologic: Amenorrhea, growth suppression, hyperglycemia, negative nitrogen balance.

Fluid and Electrolyte Imbalances: Sodium and water retention, hypokalemia, metabolic alkalosis, hypocalcemia.

Intraspinal: Meningitis, arachnoiditis.

Other: Thromboembolism, diminished response to toxoids and live or inactivated vaccines, increased susceptibility to infection, symptoms of infection masked.

METOCLOPRAMIDE

Class: Antiemetic

Use(s): Stimulate gastric emptying, antiemetic, treatment of symptomatic gastroesophageal reflux and diabetic gastroparesis.

Dosing: IV/IM: 10 mg (give IV injection over 1 to 2 minutes).

PO: 10 mg 30 minutes before meals and at bedtime.

Elimination: Renal.

Preparations

Metoclopramide hydrochloride **(Reglan)**
  Injection: 5 mg/mL, 10 mg/mL.
  Tablets: 5 mg, 10 mg.
  Oral solution: 5 mg/5 mL.

Pharmacology

Metoclopramide is a derivative of procainamide. It stimulates motility of the upper gastrointestinal tract and increases lower esophageal sphincter tone by 10 to 20 cm H_2O. Gastric acid secretion is not altered. The net effect is accelerated gastric emptying and intestinal transit. It sensitizes gastrointestinal smooth muscle to the effects of acetylcholine and may cause release of acetylcholine from cholinergic nerve endings. Antiemetic effects may result from its antagonism of central and peripheral dopamine receptors and inhibition of chemoreceptor trigger zone–mediated vomiting. It produces minimal sedation and, rarely, may produce extrapyramidal reactions.

Pharmacokinetics

Onset of Action: IV, 1–3 minutes; IM, 10–15 minutes; PO, 30–60 minutes.
Peak Effect: IV/IM, <1 hour; PO, 1–2 hours.
Duration of Action: IV/IM/PO, 1–2 hours.

Interactions

Effects on gastrointestinal motility antagonized by anticholinergic drugs (e.g., atropine) and narcotic analgesics; sedative effects potentiated by alcohol, sedative-hypnotics, tranquilizers, narcotics; hastens the onset of action of tetracycline, acetaminophen, levodopa, and ethanol, which are mainly absorbed in the small bowel; prolongs the duration of action of succinylcholine (by release of acetylcholine and inhibition of plasma cholinesterase); releases catecholamines in patients with essential hypertension and pheochromocytoma; intense feelings of anxiety and restlessness following rapid intravenous injection; extrapyramidal reactions.

Toxicity

Toxic Range: Not routinely monitored.

Manifestations: Drowsiness, disorientation, extrapyramidal reactions, dystonia, oculogyric crisis, agitation, motor restlessness (akathisia), parkinsonian signs and symptoms, methemoglobinemia (especially in neonates), respiratory distress, cardiac arrhythmias, convulsions.

Antidote: No specific antidote.

Management: Discontinue or reduce medication. Support ventilation and circulation (patent airway, oxygen, IV fluids, vasodilators). Maintenance of an adequate airway should be instituted if necessary. Symptomatic treatment. Treat extrapyramidal reactions with an anticholinergic antiparkinsonian agent (e.g., benztropine, trihexyphenidyl) or with diphenhydramine (IV/PO 25 mg). Airway-protected, ipecac syrup–induced emesis (30 mL or 0.5 mL/kg ipecac syrup followed by 200 mL or 4 mL/kg of water or clear fluid) or gastric lavage (with drug ingestion) followed by administration of activated charcoal (PO 50–100 g or 0.5–1.0 g/kg).

Guidelines/Precautions

1. Use cautiously in patients with hypertension or those receiving monoamine oxidase (MAO) inhibitors. Metoclopramide-induced hypertensive crisis in patients with pheochromocytoma may be controlled with phentolamine.
2. Metoclopramide is not recommended in pediatric patients because of increased incidence of extrapyramidal reactions.
3. Contraindicated in patients with pheochromocytoma; epilepsy; gastrointestinal hemorrhage, obstruction, or perforation; or those receiving other drugs likely to cause extrapyramidal reactions.
4. Extrapyramidal reactions occur in 0.2% of patients receiving 30–40 mg metoclopramide per day. In cancer chemotherapy (with patients receiving 1–2 mg/kg doses), the incidence of acute dystonic reactions is 2% in patients over 30 years of age and 25% or higher in children and young adults not premedicated with diphenhydramine. Therapy should include discontinuation of metoclopramide, or reduction in dosage, and treatment with an anticholinergic antiparkinsonian agent (e.g., benztropine, trihexyphenidyl) or with diphenhydramine (25 mg IV/PO). Maintenance of an adequate airway should be instituted if necessary.

Principal Adverse Reactions

Cardiovascular: Hypertension, hypotension, arrhythmia.

CNS: Drowsiness, extrapyramidal reactions, akathisia, insomnia, anxiety.

Gastrointestinal: Nausea, diarrhea.
Other: Galactorrhea, gynecomastia, hypoglycemia.

METOPROLOL TARTRATE

Class: β-Blocker, Antihypertensive

Use(s): Antihypertensive, treatment of supraventricular and ventricular arrhythmias and acute myocardial infarction, antianginal, symptomatic relief in thyrotoxic patients, adjunct treatment of alcohol withdrawal, prophylaxis of migraine headaches.

Dosing: *Hypertension or angina:* PO 100–450 mg daily in single or divided doses. Begin with 100 mg/day and increase at weekly intervals.
Acute myocardial infarction
Early: IV 15 mg (5 mg every 2 minutes for three doses), then PO 50 mg every 6 hrs for 48 hours, then PO 100 mg twice daily. Patients intolerant of full IV dose: PO 25–50 mg every 6 hours.
Late treatment: 100 mg PO twice daily.
Migraine prophylaxis
Initial: PO 50 mg twice daily.
Maintenance: PO 50–100 mg twice daily.

Elimination: Hepatic.

Preparations

Metoprolol tartrate **(Lopressor)**
   Tablets: 50 mg, 100 mg.
   Injection: 1 mg/mL.
Metoprolol tartrate and hydrochlorothiazide **(Lopres-**

sor HCT): Tablets: Metoprolol tartrate 50 mg and hydrochlorothiazide 25 mg; metoprolol tartrate 100 mg and hydrochlorothiazide 25 mg; metoprolol tartrate 100 mg and hydrochlorothiazide 50 mg.

Pharmacology

Metoprolol is a cardioselective β_1-blocker, but it can inhibit β_2-receptors in high doses. The mechanism for the antihypertensive effects of the drug is unknown. Reduced cardiac output, decreased renin release, or a central action may play a role. The antiarrhythmic effect is secondary to the reduction in sympathetic nervous system activity, and the antianginal effect reflects the decrease in myocardial oxygen consumption secondary to a reduction in heart rate and cardiac output. Metoprolol may prevent common migraine and reduce the number of attacks in some patients. It is not effective for a migraine attack that has already started. Compared with oral clonidine, metoprolol (even more than propranolol) may have a better migraine prophylactic effect regarding such parameters as the intensity, attack frequency, and number of migraine days. The antimigraine effect of metoprolol may be partly due to inhibition of vasodilatation. The drug may also inhibit arteriolar spasm of the pial vessels in the brain.

Pharmacokinetics

Onset of Action: Antihypertensive effects: IV, almost immediate; PO, <15 minutes.
Peak Effect: Antihypertensive effects: IV, 20 minutes. Antimigraine effects: PO, 4–6 weeks.
Duration of Action: Antihypertensive effects: IV/PO, 5–8 hours.

Interactions

Hypotensive effect potentiated by volatile anesthetics and catecholamine-depleting drugs (e.g., reserpine); may unmask negative inotropic effects of ketamine; prolongs elevation of plasma potassium following the administration of succinylcholine; potentiates depolarizing and nondepolarizing muscle relaxants (e.g., succinylcholine, tubocurarine); may mask symptoms of hypoglycemia (e.g., tachycardia); increases serum levels of digoxin and morphine; rebound hypertension with abrupt withdrawal.

Toxicity

Toxic Range: Not routinely monitored.

Manifestations: Bradycardia, hypotension, atrioventricular block, cardiogenic shock, asystole, convulsions, hypoglycemia, hyperkalemia.

Antidote: No specific antidote, but glucagon (diluted in preservative-free saline) IV 5–10 mg followed by infusion 1–5 mg/hr may be used to treat bradycardia and hypotension. Sodium bicarbonate IV 0.5–1.0 mEq/kg bolus repeated as needed may be used to treat wide complex conduction defects.

Management: Discontinue or reduce medication. Support ventilation and circulation (patent airway, oxygen, IV fluids, vasopressors). Administer antidote. Symptomatic treatment. Airway-protected, ipecac syrup–induced emesis (30 mL or 0.5 mL/kg ipecac syrup followed by 200 mL or 4 mL/kg of water or clear fluid) or gastric lavage (with drug ingestion) followed by administration of activated charcoal (PO 50–100 g or 1–2 g/kg) and cathartics.

Guidelines/Precautions

1. Excessive myocardial depression may be treated with IV atropine (1–2 mg), IV isoproterenol (0.02–0.15 µg/kg/min), IV glucagon (1–5 mg), or a transvenous cardiac pacemaker.
2. Metoprolol is contraindicated in sinus bradycardia, heart block greater than first degree, cardiogenic shock, and overt failure.
3. Use with extreme caution, if at all, in patients with bronchospastic disease.
4. Increased risk of ischemia or infarction in patients with coronary artery disease if drug is withdrawn abruptly.

Principal Adverse Reactions

Cardiovascular: Hypotension, arrhythmias, rebound angina.
Pulmonary: Bronchospasm, dyspnea, cough.
CNS: Fatigue, depression, disorientation.
Gastrointestinal: Nausea, vomiting, pancreatitis.
Hematologic: Thrombocytopenic purpura.
Musculoskeletal: Arthralgia.

MEXILETINE HYDROCHLORIDE

Class: Antiarrhythmic

Use(s): Treatment of life-threatening ventricular arrhythmias; treatment of lancinating neuropathic pain such as trigeminal neuralgia (tic douloureux) and other cranial neuralgias, postsympathectomy neuralgia, postherpetic neuralgia, diabetic neuropathy, phantom limb pain, the thalamic syndrome, or lightning tabetic pain; symptomatic treatment of carpal tunnel syndrome.

Dosing: *Pain*

Initial: PO 150–200 mg (2–3 mg/kg) one to three times daily. Titrate dose upward in 50-mg increments every 2 weeks until symptoms are controlled or side effects preclude further increases.

Maintenance: PO 150–400 mg (2–8 mg/kg) one to three times daily. Maximum dose 1800 mg/day.

Analgesia may be enhanced by combination with anticonvulsant drugs, antidepressant agents, clonidine, and use of nondrug therapies such as transcutaneous electrical nerve stimulation (TENS).

Arrhythmias: Loading dose PO 400 mg, then maintenance dose of PO 200–300 mg every 8 hours. Maximum dose 1200 mg/day. Therapeutic range: 0.5–2.0 μg/mL.

Hepatic function tests and EKGs should be determined prior to and at regular intervals during pain or antiarrhythmic therapy.

Elimination: Hepatic.

Preparations

Mexiletine hydrochloride **(Mexitil):** Capsules: 150 mg, 200 mg, 250 mg.

Pharmacology

Mexiletine is a local anesthetic class 1B antiarrhythmic agent that is structurally similar to lidocaine but orally active. The electrophysiologic properties are similar to lidocaine and different from quinidine, procainamide, and diisopyramide. Mexiletine inhibits the inward sodium current, thus reducing the rate of rise of phase 0 of the action potential. The drug is effective in induced ventricular arrhythmias (e.g., from digitalis toxicity or coronary artery ligation). Mexiletine may be used in chronic pain syndromes, primarily for suppression of the sharp lancinating and paroxysmal electrical shooting qualities common in neuropathic pain such as in idiopathic trigeminal neuralgia. Analgesic effects of mexiletine may be partly due to an antagonistic effect on *N*-methyl D-aspartate (NMDA) receptors. The activation of small diameter primary afferents is capable of producing a prolonged alteration in the excitability of neurons in the spinal cord, modifying the way these neurons respond to subsequent inputs and thereby generating a state of central sensitization. NMDA antagonists such as mexiletine block the development of central sensitization or abolish established hypersensitivity. By returning an abnormally excitable spinal cord to a normal level, NMDA antagonists return a pathologic situation where low-intensity or innocuous stimuli produce pain (allodynia) to the normal physiologic state where pain is produced by noxious stimuli. Mexiletine crosses the placenta and is distributed in breast milk. It should be avoided in pregnant and nursing mothers except in situations when discontinuation of therapy may pose a serious threat to the mother.

Pharmacokinetics

Onset of Action: Analgesic effect: PO, <5 days. Antiarrhythmic effect: PO, 30–60 minutes.

Peak Effect: Antiarrhythmic effect: PO, 2–3 hours (peak serum levels). Analgesic effect: PO, <2 weeks.
Duration of Action: 10–12 hours (half-life).

Interactions

Serum levels decreased with concomitant use of phenytoin, phenobarbital, rifampin; serum levels altered by cimetidine; theophylline serum levels and toxic effects increased by mexiletine; GI absorption decreased by narcotics, atropine, and magnesium-aluminum hydroxide.

Toxicity

Toxic Range: >2 µg/mL.
Manifestations: Nausea, hypotension, sinus bradycardia, seizures, paresthesia, intermittent left bundle branch block, asystole.
Antidote: None.
Management: Discontinue or reduce concentration of medication. Support ventilation and circulation (patent airway, oxygen, IV fluids, vasopressors). Acidification of the urine to increase excretion. Symptomatic treatment.

Guidelines/Precautions

1. Mexiletine is contraindicated in patients with cardiogenic shock or second- or third-degree atrioventricular block (without a pacemaker).
2. Use with caution in patients with hypotension, severe congestive heart failure, or abnormal liver function tests. These conditions may be exacerbated. Like other antiarrhythmics, mexiletine may occasionally trigger dangerous rhythm disturbances in patients with ventricular arrhythmias. This rarely occurs in chronic pain patients.

Principal Adverse Reactions

Cardiovascular: Arrhythmias, anginal attacks, hypotension.

Pulmonary: Shortness of breath.

CNS: Dizziness, tremor.

Gastrointestinal: Hepatic dysfunction, nausea, vomiting, diarrhea, abdominal pain.

Hematologic: Leukopenia, agranulocytosis.

Other: Rash.

MIDAZOLAM

Class: Benzodiazepine

Use(s): Premedication, conscious sedation, anticonvulsant.

Dosing: *Premedication*

IM: 2.5–10.0 mg (0.05–0.2 mg/kg).

PO, Adult: 0.25–1.0 mg/kg (20–40 mg).

PO, Children: 0.25–0.5 mg/kg (maximum dose 20 mg).

Dose should be individualized and modified based on patient age, level of anxiety, and medical need. For oral administration, use commercial oral syrup or high-potency injectate solution (5 mg/mL). Dilute injectate in 3–5 mL apple juice or carbonated cola beverage. Atropine PO 0.03 mg/kg may be added to reduce secretions.

Intranasal: 0.2–0.3 mg/kg. High-potency injectate solution (5 mg/mL) should be used.

Rectal: 15–20 mg (0.3–0.35 mg/kg). Dilute in 5 mL normal saline.

Conscious sedation: IV 0.5–5.0 mg (0.025–0.1 mg/kg). Titrate slowly to the desired effect (e.g., onset of slurred speech). Continuous monitoring of respiratory and cardiac function should occur.

Sedation: Infusion 0.5–15 mg/hr (0.15–0.5 µg/kg/min). Respiratory support and continuous monitoring are required.

Anticonvulsant: IV/IM 2–5 mg (0.025–0.1 mg/kg) every 10–15 minutes as needed.

Elimination: Renal.

Preparations

Midazolam hydrochloride **(Versed):** Injection: 1 mg/mL, 5 mg/mL.

Midazolam hydrochloride **(Versed Syrup):** Syrup: 2 mg/mL.

Pharmacology

This short-acting benzodiazepine possesses antianxiety, sedative, amnesic, anticonvulsant, and skeletal muscle relaxant properties. Neuromuscular transmission is not affected, and the action of nondepolarizing drugs is not altered. Due to the imidazole ring in its structure, midazolam is highly water soluble at a low pH (<4) with the ring opened and lipophilic at physiologic pH (>4) with the ring closed. The water solubility facilitates intravenous admixtures, and the lipophilic properties minimize venous irritation. Under the acidotic conditions required to solubilize midazolam in the oral formulation, midazolam is present in a mixture of open and closed ring forms. The amount of open ring form is dependent on the pH of the solution and may be up to 40% of the mixture. At the physiologic conditions under which the solution is absorbed, the open ring form reverts to the physiologically active and lipophilic closed ring form. The mechanism of action is unknown, but midazolam is thought to act by facilitating the effects of γ-aminobutyric acid, like other benzodiazepine drugs. Midazolam depresses ventilation and decreases peripheral vascular resistance and blood pressure, especially in the presence of narcotic premedication and/or hypovolemia. Compared with diazepam, midazolam has a more rapid onset with fewer local reactions, a shorter duration of action, greater amnesic effect, and three to four times the sedative potency. Midazolam (2 mg) has been administered intrathecally and found comparable to epidural steroids in improvement of chronic low back pain. This use, however, is still experimental.

Pharmacokinetics

Onset of Action: IV, 0.5–1.0 minute. IM, 15 minutes. PO/Rectal, <10 minutes. Intranasal, <5 minutes.
Peak Effect: IV, 3–5 minutes. IM, 15–30 minutes. PO, 30 minutes. Intranasal, 10 minutes. Rectal, 20–30 minutes.
Duration of Action: IV/IM, 15–80 minutes. PO/Rectal, 2–6 hours.

Interactions

CNS and circulatory depressant effects potentiated by alcohol, narcotics, sedatives, volatile anesthetics; effects antagonized by flumazenil.

Toxicity

Toxic Range: Not routinely monitored.
Manifestations: Respiratory depression, apnea, hypotension, confusion, coma, seizures.
Antidote: Flumazenil IV (0.2–2.0 mg).
Management: Discontinue or reduce medication. Support ventilation and circulation (patent airway, oxygen, IV fluids, vasopressors). Administer antidote. Symptomatic treatment. Airway-protected, ipecac syrup–induced emesis (30 mL or 0.5 mL/kg ipecac syrup followed by 200 mL or 4 mL/kg of water or clear fluid) or gastric lavage (with drug ingestion) followed by administration of activated charcoal (PO 50–100 g or 0.5–1.0 g/kg). Hemodialysis is not useful. Treat withdrawal hyperactivity with low-dose barbiturate.

Guidelines/Precautions

1. Reduce doses in elderly patients and with concomitant use of other sedatives or narcotics.
2. Patients with chronic obstructive pulmonary disease are unusually sensitive to the respiratory depressant effect.
3. Contraindicated in acute narrow-angle or open-angle glaucoma unless patients are receiving appropriate therapy.
4. Unexpected hypotension and respiratory depression may occur when given with opioids—consider smaller doses.
5. Respiratory depression and arrest may occur when used for conscious sedation. When used for

conscious sedation, do not administer as a bolus. Treat overdose with supportive measures and flumazenil (slow IV 0.2–1.0 mg).

6. Serious respiratory adverse effects have occurred after administration of oral midazolam, most often when it was used in combination with other central nervous system depressants. Adverse effects have included respiratory depression, airway obstruction, oxygen desaturation, and rarely respiratory or cardiac arrest. When oral midazolam is administered as the sole agent at recommended doses, respiratory depression, airway obstruction, and oxygen desaturation occur infrequently. The immediate availability of flumazenil is highly recommended.

7. Midazolam syrup is intended for use in monitored settings only and not for chronic or home use.

8. Midazolam oral formulation has not been studied in patients less than 6 months of age.

9. Reactions such as agitation, involuntary movements (including tonic/clonic movements and muscle tremor), hyperactivity and combativeness have been reported in both adult and pediatric patients. Consideration should be given to the possibility of paradoxical reaction. Should such reactions occur, the response to each dose of midazolam and all other drugs including local anesthetics should be evaluated before proceeding. Reversal of such responses with flumazenil has been reported in pediatric and adult patients.

10. Midazolam oral formulation is contraindicated in patients with known hypersensitivity to the drug

or allergies to cherries or formulation excipients (sorbitol, glycerin, citric acid anhydrous, sodium citrate, sodium benzoate, sodium saccharin, edetate disodium, FD&C red#33, artificial cough syrup flavor, artificial bitterness modifier).
11. Midazolam oral formulation is not recommended for obstetrical use. Midazolam is excreted in human milk. Caution should be exercised when midazolam is administered to a nursing woman.

Principal Adverse Reactions

Cardiovascular: Tachycardia, vasovagal episode, premature ventricular complexes, hypotension.
Pulmonary: Bronchospasm, laryngospasm, apnea, hypoventilation.
CNS: Euphoria, emergence delirium, prolonged emergence, tonic-clonic movements, agitation, hyperactivity.
Gastrointestinal: Salivation, retching, acid taste.
Dermatologic: Rash, pruritus, warmth or coldness at injection site.

MISOPROSTOL

Class: Antiulcer Agent

Use(s): Prophylaxis and treatment of peptic ulcer and NSAID-induced gastric erosions; treatment of pain and inflammatory disease in combination with diclofenac.

Dosing: *Prophylaxis/Treatment:* PO 100–200µg four times daily.

Elimination: Hepatic.

Preparations

Misoprostol **(Cytotec):** Tablets: 100μg, 200μg.
Misoprostol and diclofenac sodium **(Arthrotec 50):**
   Tablets: Misoprostol 200μg and diclofenac 50mg.
Misoprostol and diclofenac sodium **(Arthrotec 75):**
   Tablets: Misoprostol 200μg and diclofenac 75mg.

Pharmacology

A synthetic analogue of prostaglandin E_1, misoprostol inhibits gastric acid secretion and has cytoprotective effects on the gastroduodenal mucosa. Misoprostol may protect the mucosa from irritant effects of certain drugs, including nonsteroidal anti-inflammatory drugs (NSAIDs). Endogenous prostaglandins have complex effects in the GI tract and may decrease acid secretion, increase mucus and bicarbonate secretion, prevent disruption of the gastric mucosal barrier, inhibit or reduce back diffusion of hydrogen ions, regulate mucosal blood flow, prevent microvascular stasis, and preserve mucosal capacity to regenerate cells. Misoprostol may have beneficial effects on renal function (increased renal blood flow, sodium excretion, and glomerular filtration rate) in patients with cyclosporine-induced nephrotoxicity.

Pharmacokinetics

Onset: Inhibition of gastric acid secretion: PO, <30 minutes.
Peak Effect: Inhibition of gastric acid secretion: PO, 60–90 minutes.
Duration of Action: Inhibition of gastric acid secretion: PO, 3 hours.

Interactions

GI absorption of misoprostol decreased by food and antacids; may reverse cyclosporine nephrotoxicity.

Toxicity

Toxic Range: Not routinely monitored.
Manifestations: Sedation, tremor, seizures, dyspnea, abdominal pain, chest pain, arrhythmia, increased serum concentration of cardiac enzymes, diarrhea, constipation, bradycardia, spontaneous abortions.
Antidote: No specific antidote.
Management: Discontinue or reduce medication. Support ventilation and circulation (patent airway, oxygen, IV fluids). Symptomatic treatment.

Guidelines/Precautions

1. Use with caution in patients with inflammatory bowel disease. Misoprostol may exacerbate intestinal inflammation and produce severe diarrhea and secondary dehydration.
2. Contraindicated in patients with known hypersensitivity to prostaglandins.
3. Due to abortifacient effects, misoprostol therapy should not be initiated in women of childbearing potential until the possibility of pregnancy has been excluded.

Principal Adverse Reactions

Cardiovascular: Chest pain, hypotension, hypertension, arrhythmia, increased serum concentration of cardiac enzymes.
CNS: Headache, depression, dizziness.

Gastrointestinal: Diarrhea, constipation, nausea, vomiting, abdominal pain.
Dermatologic: Rash, pruritus.
Genitourinary: Dysmenorrhea, hypermenorrhea, spotting, dysuria, polyuria, hematuria, spontaneous abortions.
Other: Anemia, thrombocytopenia.

MORPHINE SULFATE

Class: Narcotic Agonist

Use(s): Treatment of acute, chronic, and cancer pain; relief of air hunger and dyspnea in terminal patients.

Dosing: *Pain*

> PO: 10–60 mg every 4 hours. Administer regularly (not as needed). Titrate upward in increments of 25% to 50% every 8–24 hours until adequate analgesia is obtained. Doses of more than 500 mg every 4 hours have been used. Dosing intervals should be adjusted up or down to provide continuous analgesia with minimal sedation. Bedtime doses may be 1.5 to 2 times the daytime dose. Once adequate analgesia is obtained with short-acting preparations, substitute with an equianalgesic dose (see Appendix 4) of the extended-release preparation

or a long-acting opioid for patient convenience.

PO, extended release: 15–200 mg every 12 hours (some patients may require 8-hour dosing intervals). Patients taking the extended-release preparation should be given a supply of the short-acting preparation or other short-acting opioid (e.g., hydromorphone) to control breakthrough pain.

Rectal: 10–20 mg every 4 hours.

Slow IV: 2.5–15.0 mg (children 0.05–0.2 mg/kg; maximum 15 mg). Administer over 4–5 minutes.

IM/SC: 2.5–20.0 mg every 4 hours (children 0.05–0.2 mg/kg; maximum 15 mg).

Intra-articular: 0.5–1.0 mg. Dilute in 40 mL normal saline or 0.0625–0.25% bupivacaine.

Epidural bolus (acute pain): 2–5 mg daily (40–100 µg/kg/day). Use preservative-free morphine. Dilute in 10 mL preservative-free normal saline or local anesthetic.

Spinal bolus: 0.1–1.0 mg (2–20 µg/kg).

Chronic malignant pain

Epidural bolus: 2–10 mg once or twice daily (40–200 µg/kg/day). Use preservative-free morphine. Dilute in preservative-free normal saline or local anesthetic. Titrate upward by 20–30% every 24–48 hours until satisfactory pain relief is achieved.

Epidural infusion: 2–30 mg/day (0.083–1.25 mg/hr). Titrate upward by 20–30% every 24–48 hours until satisfactory pain relief is achieved. Higher doses of epidural morphine may be required (up to 0.25–0.33% of 24-hour IV dose). Use preservative-free solution. Epidural morphine may be combined with local anesthetic (e.g., 0.0625–0.125% bupivacaine) for additive analgesia.

Spinal infusion

Initial: 0.2–2.0 mg/day (0.008–0.083 mg/hr). Titrate upward by 20–30% every 24–48 hours until satisfactory pain relief is achieved.

Maintenance: 0.1–10.0 mg/day (0.004–0.417 mg/hr). Higher doses of intrathecal morphine may be required (up to 25 mg/day or 10% of the 24-hour epidural dose) in chronic malignant pain. Average infusion volume of 0.5–1.5 mL/day. Infusion pump (Medtronic) may not be run at less than 0.1 mL/day or greater than 0.9 mL/hr. To determine concentration of morphine for the infusion pump:

$$\text{Drug Concentration} = \frac{\text{Daily Dose (mg/day)}}{\text{Pump Flow Rate (mL/day)}}$$

Use preservative-free solution. To determine the refill interval:

$$\text{Max. Refill Interval (days)} = \frac{\text{Pump Volume (mL)}}{\text{Flow Rate (mL/day)}}$$

For rate accuracy and to ensure that adequate pain relief is maintained, refill the pump before the reservoir volume decreases below 2 mL.

Intrathecal morphine may be combined with local anesthetic (e.g., 0.25–0.75% bupivacaine 1–5 mg/day) for additive analgesia or in patients with muscle spasm in whom temporary motor blockade is desired. Use of this local anesthetic–opioid combination is limited with chronic infusions due to occurrence of tachyphylaxis. Intrathecal morphine may also be combined with intrathecal clonidine or baclofen to provide synergistic pain relief (baclofen/clonidine) and decreased spasticity (baclofen).

Patient-controlled analgesia (PCA) IV
    Bolus: 0.5–3.0 mg (10–60 µg/kg).
    Infusion: 0.5–10.0 mg/hr (15–200 µg/kg/hr).
    Lockout interval: 5–20 minutes.

Patient-controlled analgesia epidural
    Bolus: 0.05–0.2 mg (1–4 µg/kg).
    Infusion: 0.1–0.4 mg/hr (2–8 µg/kg/hr).
    Lockout interval: 10 minutes.

Analgesia may be enhanced by addition of adjuvant drugs such as nonsteroidal anti-inflammatory drugs (NSAIDs) and antidepressant agents (see pages xxvi–xliv for drug combinations) and use of nondrug therapies such as transcutaneous electrical nerve stimulation (TENS).

When the level of pain is significantly altered by other measures (e.g., regional blockade), lower doses are required, especially in patients with limited respiratory reserve. Initial doses should be lower in patients with renal and/or hepatic dysfunction.

Relief of air hunger (terminal patients): Inhalation: Administer 2.5–10.0 mg morphine diluted in 2 mL sterile water in mistometer.

Conversion from conventional oral morphine to MS Contin: Administer one-half the patient's 24-hour requirement as MS Contin on an every-12-hour schedule.

Conversion from parenteral morphine to MS Contin: Utilize a dose of oral morphine 3 times the 24-hour parenteral morphine, in two divided doses.

Conversion from MS Contin to parenteral morphine: Utilize a dose of IM 1 mg morphine for every 6 mg of morphine as MS Contin. Divide the IM 24-hour dose by 6 and administer on an every-4-hour regimen.

Elimination: Hepatic.

Preparations

Morphine sulfate **(Morphine Sulfate, MSIR):** Tablets: 10 mg, 15 mg, 30 mg.

Morphine sulfate **(Oramorph SR):** Tablets, extended release: 30 mg, 60 mg, 100 mg.

Morphine sulfate **(MS Contin):** Tablets, extended release, film coated: 15 mg, 30 mg, 60 mg, 100 mg,

200 mg (200-mg tablets are for use in opioid-tolerant patients only).

Morphine sulfate **(Morphine Sulfate Oral Solution, Roxanol, MSIR Oral Solution):** Oral solution: 4 mg/mL, 10 mg/5 mL, 20 mg/mL, 20 mg/5 mL, 100 mg/5 mL.

Morphine sulfate **(Morphine Sulfate):** Injection: 0.5 mg/mL, 1 mg/mL, 2 mg/mL, 3 mg/mL, 4 mg/mL, 5 mg/mL, 8 mg/mL, 10 mg/mL, 15 mg/mL.

Morphine sulfate **(Morphine Sulfate Suppositories, Roxanol, RMS):** Rectal suppositories: 5 mg, 10 mg, 20 mg, 30 mg.

Morphine sulfate **(Duramorph, Astramorph):** Preservative-free injection for epidural, intrathecal, or IV use: 0.5 mg/mL, 1 mg/mL.

Morphine sulfate **(Infumorph):** Preservative-free injection for epidural or intrathecal use via continuous microinfusion device only: 10 mg/mL, 25 mg/mL.

Dilution for Infusion

IV: 20 mg in 100 mL normal saline (0.2 mg/mL).

Epidural bolus: 2–5 mg in 10 mL local anesthetic or preservative-free normal saline.

Epidural infusion: 10 mg in 100 mL local anesthetic or preservative-free normal saline (0.1 mg/mL).

Spinal: 1–10 mg/mL. Use undiluted solution or dilute to desired concentration with preservative-free normal saline. Drug Concentration (mg/mL) = Daily Dose (mg/day)/Pump Flow Rate (mL/day). Concentrations greater than 10 mg/mL are rarely required and may produce a dyesthetic reaction with paradoxical hyperalgesia.

Pharmacology

This alkaloid of opium exerts its primary effects on the central nervous system and organs containing smooth muscle. Excitatory synaptic pain transmission is decreased by opioid receptor–mediated inhibition of neurotransmitter release (e.g., bradykinin at site of tissue injury, substance P in the dorsal horn, and dopamine in the basal ganglia). In addition, morphine (and other opioids) may alter cognitive and emotional processing of painful input by acting on limbic and cortical opioid receptors. Morphine is a potent analgesic and has no ceiling effect for analgesia. Compared with meperidine or nalbuphine, morphine is significantly better at controlling pain associated with motion or deep breathing but may have a higher incidence of side effects (e.g., sedation, pruritus). Oral doses are one-third as potent as parenteral doses. In the liver, morphine undergoes conjugation with glucoronic acid to form metabolites, including morphine-6-glucuronide. Morphine-6-glucuronide is more potent than morphine and may accumulate in patients with renal insufficiency.

Spinal or epidural administration of morphine produces intensive analgesia by specific binding and activation of opioid receptors in the substantia gelatinosa. Once activated, the opioid receptors inhibit the release of substance P from nociceptive afferent C fibers. Analgesia is achieved without sensory, motor, or sympathetic blockade. Drowsiness, euphoria, depression of the cough reflex, dose-dependent respiratory depression, and reduction in peripheral resistance (arteriolar and venous dilatation) may occur. Clinically important respiratory depression is rarely seen in patients with severe pain due to malignant disease even with large doses, because pain and emotional stress are powerful antagonists to narcotic-induced respiratory depression. The reduction in respiratory rate may actually be beneficial in patients distressed with tachypnea. The constipating effects of morphine result from induction of nonpropulsive contractions through the GI tract. Emetic effects are due to opioid-induced stimulation of the chemoreceptor trigger zone in the floor of the fourth ventricle. Morphine activates opioid receptors on mast cells, resulting in peripheral histamine release and localized to generalized pruritus. Altered sensory modulation secondary to direct binding of morphine (and other opioids) to opiate receptors in the medulla oblongata may be the mechanism for late-onset pruritus (2–3 hours) after epidural/intrathecal administration.

Epidural morphine partitions itself preferentially into the cerebrospinal fluid (CSF). Rostral spread enables saturation of the entire length of the spinal cord. Thus, epidural morphine (more than epidural fentanyl or sufentanil) may be infused or bolused at lower lumbar interspaces and still provide analgesia for the upper abdomen and thorax (as long as it is diluted in an adequate volume). Rostral spread and delivery of morphine molecules to the brainstem respiratory centers may lead to late-onset respiratory depression (occurring at 8 to 12 hours). The early phase of respiratory depression observed shortly after epidural administration reflects rapid systemic absorption and is of similar magnitude to that noted after parenteral administration. Intra-articular analgesia occurs secondary to binding of morphine to opiate receptors in synovial tissue.

Morphine crosses the placental barrier and may produce depression in the neonate. The drug may appear in breast milk and should be used with caution in nursing mothers. In terminal patients (e.g., with end-stage lung disease or congestive heart failure), nebulized morphine relieves air hunger and dyspnea. This may be due to a central action after absorption across the respiratory mucosa or binding to opioid receptors in lung tissue.

Pharmacokinetics

Onset of Action: IV, <1 minute. IM, 1–5 minutes. SC, 15–30 minutes. PO, 15–60 minutes. PO (slow release), 60–90 minutes. Epidural/Spinal, 15–60 minutes.
Peak Effect: IV, 5–20 minutes. IM, 30–60 minutes. SC, 50–90 minutes. PO, 30–60 minutes. PO (slow release), 1–4 hours. Rectal, 20–60 minutes. Epidural/Spinal, 90 minutes.
Duration of Action: IV/IM/SC/PO, 2–7 hours. PO (slow release), 6–12 hours. Epidural/Spinal, 6–24 hours.

Interactions

CNS and circulatory depressant effects potentiated by alcohol, sedatives, narcotics, antihistamines, phenothiazines, butyrophenones, monoamine oxidase (MAO) inhibitors, and tricyclic antidepressants; may decrease the effect of diuretics in patients with congestive heart failure; analgesia enhanced and prolonged by NSAIDs, α_2-agonists (e.g., clonidine, epinephrine); addition of epinephrine to intrathecal/epidural morphine results in increased side effects (e.g., nausea).

Toxicity

Toxic Range: Not routinely monitored.

Manifestations: Somnolence, coma, respiratory arrest, apnea, cardiac arrhythmias, combined respiratory and metabolic acidosis, circulatory collapse, cardiac arrest, death.

Antidote: Naloxone IV/IM/SC 0.4–2.0 mg. Repeat dose every 2 to 3 minutes to a maximum of 10–20 mg.

Management: Discontinue or reduce medication. Support ventilation and circulation (patent airway, oxygen, IV fluids, vasopressors). Administer antidote. Monitor blood gases, pH, and electrolytes. Correct acidosis and electrolyte disturbance (lactic acidosis may require sodium bicarbonate IV 1–2 mEq/kg). Symptomatic treatment. Airway-protected, ipecac syrup–induced emesis (30 mL or 0.5 mL/kg ipecac syrup followed by 200 mL or 4 mL/kg of water or clear fluid) or gastric lavage (with drug ingestion) followed by administration of activated charcoal (PO 50–100 g or 1–2 g/kg).

Guidelines/Precautions

1. Reduce dose in elderly patients and with concomitant use of sedatives and other narcotics.
2. The narcotic antagonist naloxone is a specific antidote (IV/IM/SC 0.2–0.4 mg or higher). Reversal of narcotic effect may lead to onset of pain and release of catecholamines.
3. Opioid-induced biliary tract spasm may be reversed with naloxone or glucagon (IV/IM 0.2–0.25 mg). Reversal of analgesia may occur with naloxone but not glucagon.
4. Morphine crosses the placental barrier, and usage

in labor may produce depression of respiration in the neonate. Resuscitation may be required; have naloxone available.

5. Incidences of reactivation of herpes simplex have occurred following administration of epidural or spinal morphine. The herpes virus may be reactivated directly by mechanical irritation of the sensory nerves when patients scratch (in response to itching) or by opioid activity in the medulla.

6. Undesirable side effects of epidural, caudal, or intrathecal morphine include delayed respiratory depression (up to 24 hours after single dose), pruritus, nausea and vomiting, and urinary retention. Naloxone (IV/IM/SC 0.2–0.4 mg as needed or infusion 5–10 µg/kg/hr) is effective for prophylaxis and/or treatment of these side effects. Ventilatory support for respiratory depression must be readily available. Antihistamines, for example, diphenhydramine (IV/IM 12.5–25.0 mg every 6 hours as needed) may be used in treating pruritus. Metoclopramide (IV 10 mg every 6 hours as needed) may be used in treating nausea and vomiting. Urinary retention that does not respond to naloxone may require straight bladder catheterization. Bethanechol (Urecholine) PO 15–30 mg three times daily or SC 2.5–5.0 mg three or four times daily as required may be used as an alternative to naloxone. (Bethanechol increases the tone of the detrusor urinae muscle. It should not be given IV or IM, which may result in cholinergic overstimulation. Have atropine available [IV/SC 0.5 mg].)

7. Epidural, caudal, or intrathecal morphine should

be avoided when the patient has septicemia, infection at the injection site, or coagulopathy.

8. Narcotic-related sedation may be treated by reducing the dose and increasing the frequency of administration. This avoids high peak concentration of the drug in the brain. Additional measures include changing to shorter-acting preparations or using other short-acting opioids. Dextroamphetamine (PO 5–15 mg/day) or Ritalin (methylphenidate) PO 5–10 mg (with breakfast) may be helpful if pain is well controlled but the patient is unable to function due to sedation.

9. Prescribe or supply an antiemetic (e.g., metoclopramide) for use in the event of nausea and/or vomiting.

10. Constipation may be more difficult to control than pain. Prevent and/or treat by increasing regular exercise and oral fluids and by daily administration of stool softeners or laxatives, for example, Colace (docusate sodium) 100–300 mg/day. Do not administer bulk-forming agents that contain methylcellulose, psyllium, or polycarbophil. Temporary arrest in the passage through the gastrointestinal tract may lead to fecal impaction or bowel obstruction.

11. With long-term administration, tolerance may develop to both the desired and unwanted effects of the drug. Very high doses may be needed to maintain analgesia. In cancer patients, increase in dose requirements is often due to progression of the disease.

12. Tolerance develops more rapidly following IV or spinal administration than after oral or rectal

administration. Add adjuvant drugs (e.g., NSAIDs, antidepressant agents, dextromethorphan) or switch to alternative opioids (starting at one-half the equianalgesic dose) or supplement with nondrug therapies (e.g., TENS).

13. Abrupt discontinuation of opioids in patients with physical dependence may manifest with withdrawal symptoms. To avoid withdrawal, opioid doses should be reduced slowly (e.g., dose reduction of 75% every 2 days). When a total daily dose of IV/IM/SC 10–15 mg or PO 60 mg of morphine is reached, it should be maintained for 2 days and then discontinued. Withdrawal should be treated symptomatically.

14. Achievement of pain relief with neuroaxial morphine (or other opioids) may place the patient at high risk for systemic withdrawal if parenteral opioids are not tapered or substitution therapy is not initiated (e.g., transdermal clonidine 0.1–0.3 mg/24 hr).

15. Addiction occurs rarely (frequency of less than 1 : 3000) in patients who receive opioids for legitimate medical conditions. Addiction should not be considered in deciding the proper dose and schedule of opioids. Pseudoaddiction (an iatrogenic condition with characteristics of psychological dependence) may occur as a result of inadequate pain treatment.

16. Drug combinations with adjuvant drugs enhance analgesia (see pages xxvi–xliv). NSAIDs (e.g., aspirin) potentiate narcotic analgesia, decrease inflammation, and are useful in pain related to bony metastasis and musculoskeletal inflamma-

tion. Anticonvulsants (e.g., gabapentin) are useful in cancer therapy or chronic neuralgias that complicate tumor progression (e.g., glossopharyngeal neuralgias in head and neck cancers). Phenothiazines minimize the constipating and emetic effects of opioids and are useful in the treatment of opioid-tolerant patients. Antidepressant agents (e.g., paroxetine) ameliorate insomnia, potentiate analgesia, and are useful in cancer pain syndromes, neuropathies, and neuralgias. Steroids may be oncolytic for some tumors (e.g., lymphomas) and may ameliorate painful nerve or spinal compression by reducing edema in tumor or nerve tissue. Steroids may also provide euphoria and increased appetite in moribund patients. Antihistamines (e.g., hydroxyzine) provide additive analgesia with slightly more sedation and less emesis. α_2-Agonists (e.g., clonidine) enhance analgesia and suppress the adrenergic symptoms of opioid withdrawal.

17. Adjuvant drug therapies also include regional blockade, trigger-point injections (with local anesthetics and steroids), and intravenous regional anesthesia.

18. Adjuvant nondrug therapies include TENS and modalities such as ice or heat application, ultrasound, and soft tissue mobilization.

19. The following infusions are incompatible with PCA morphine and should not be combined in the same intravenous line: aminophylline, heparin, sodium bicarbonate, magnesium sulfate, methicillin, phenobarbital, phenytoin, and ranitidine.

20. Patients should be warned that morphine may impair their ability to perform hazardous tasks requiring mental alertness or physical coordination (e.g., driving a motor vehicle, operating heavy machinery).

21. Development of new catheter materials and placement techniques has allowed long-term delivery of epidural/spinal morphine for months to years. This is accomplished by placement of long-term subcutaneously tunneled exteriorized catheters or by the use of implantable drug delivery systems (e.g., Medtronic). The implantable systems feature either a drug reservoir or an implanted infusion device. Some of these devices may allow for external programming. Complications of these long-term delivery systems include superficial and deep infection, catheter malfunction (migration, leak, occlusion, dislodgment), and pain on injection (possibly due to formation of a fibrous sheath around the catheter). In one study (*Anesthesiology* 1990;73:905–909), there was an infection rate of 5% with long-term externalized catheters and of 6.7% with Port-a-Cath implanted epidural access systems, and a 16% incidence of catheter malfunction. Long-term sequelae of implantable pumps may include edema, polyarthralgia, amenorrhea, and granuloma at the tip of the catheter.

22. Long-term therapy with neuroaxial (doses >5 mg/day) and oral opioids may result in a decrease in the sex hormones and sexual dysfunction, including impotence, decreased libido, delayed ejaculation, and amenorrhea. In males,

the effect on testosterone may be treated with intramuscular injections of Depo-Testosterone 200 mg every 2 to 3 weeks or by use of a testosterone patch.

23. Morphine is subject to control under the Federal Controlled Substances Act of 1970 as a Schedule II (C-II) drug.

24. MS Contin tablets are to be taken whole and are not to be broken, chewed, or crushed because so doing could lead to the rapid release and absorption of a potentially toxic dose of morphine.

Principal Adverse Reactions

Cardiovascular: Hypotension, hypertension, bradycardia, arrhythmias, chest wall rigidity.

Pulmonary: Bronchospasm, laryngospasm.

CNS: Blurred vision, syncope, euphoria, dysphoria.

Genitourinary: Urinary retention, antidiuretic effect, ureteral spasm.

Gastrointestinal: Biliary tract spasm, constipation, anorexia, nausea, vomiting, delayed gastric emptying.

Ocular: Miosis.

Musculoskeletal: Chest wall rigidity.

Allergic: Pruritus, urticaria.

NABUMETONE

Class: Medium-Potency Anti-inflammatory Drug

Use(s): Symptomatic treatment of moderate to severe inflammatory and degenerative arthritis, primary dysmenorrhea, migraine, ankylosing spondylitis, posttraumatic pain, chronic pain, and cancer pain (especially with bone metastasis).

Dosing: *Pain or inflammatory diseases:* PO 1000–2000 mg daily (20–40 mg/kg/day). Administer once daily or in two divided doses. Maximum dose 2000 mg/day. Nabumetone may be administered orally without regard to meals.

Administer analgesic regularly (not as needed). Addition of opioid analgesics and antidepressant agents and use of nondrug therapies such as transcutaneous electrical nerve stimulation (TENS) may enhance analgesia (see pages xxvi–xliv for drug combinations). In rheumatoid arthritis or juvenile rheumatoid arthritis, second-line rheumatoid agents may include leflunomide (Arava), etanercept (Enbrel), antimalarials, or methotrexate. In geriatric patients and patients with decreased renal or hepatic function, decrease doses by one-third to one-half. The incidence of nabumetone-induced gastropathy may be decreased by administration with antacids or sucralfate (PO 1 g four times daily). Misoprostol (PO 100–200 µg four times daily) may be used to prevent gastric ulcers in high-risk patients.

Elimination: Hepatic, renal.

Preparations

Nabumetone **(Relafen):** Tablets: 500 mg, 750 mg.

Pharmacology

A naphthylacetic acid derivative and nonsteroidal anti-inflammatory drug (NSAID), nabumetone is a prodrug that undergoes hepatic biotransformation to the active component, 6-methoxy-2-naphthyl acetic acid (6-MNA). The analgesic and anti-inflammatory activities of nabumetone are similar to that of naproxen sodium and are partly due to the inhibition of prostaglandin synthesis and/or release secondary to the inhibition of cyclooxygenase. Cyclooxygenase enzyme catalyzes the formation of prostaglandin precursors (endoperoxides) from arachidonic acid. Nabumetone may cause gastric mucosal damage that may result in ulceration or bleeding. However, nabumetone is better tolerated than aspirin, naproxen, or ibuprofen, and equipotent doses are associated with less gastric mucosal abnormalities. The antipyretic activity of nabumetone may occur secondary to inhibition of pyrogen-induced release of prostaglandins in the central nervous system (including the hypothalamus) and possibly to centrally mediated peripheral vasodilatation.

Nabumetone (like other NSAIDs) exhibits a ceiling effect for analgesia. Exceeding recommended doses results in increased toxicity without improvement in analgesia. Inhibition of prostaglandin synthesis may result in decreased uterine tone and contractility and prolonged gestation in the parturient and premature closure of the ductus arteriosus in the fetus. Nabumetone minimally inhibits platelet aggregation and prolongs bleeding time. The drug has no uricosuric activity.

Pharmacokinetics

Onset of Action: PO, analgesic effect 15–30 minutes.
Peak Effect: PO, analgesic effect 1–2 hours.
Duration of Action: PO, analgesic effect 4–6 hours.

Interactions

Risks of bleeding increased with concomitant NSAIDs, anticoagulant or heparin therapy, alcohol ingestion; decreases antihypertensive effects of β-adrenergic blocking agents; serum levels of nabumetone decreased slightly by concomitant aspirin; serum levels of nabumetone increased by concomitant probenecid; serum levels and toxic effects of phenytoin, oral anticoagulants, salicylates, sulfonamides, sulfonylureas (e.g., tolbutamide), methotrexate, and lithium increased by concomitant nabumetone; GI absorption of nabumetone increased by food and milk, but total amount of 6-MNA in the plasma is unchanged.

Toxicity

Toxic Range: Not routinely monitored.
Manifestations: *Acute:* Drowsiness, nausea, vomiting, lethargy, paresthesia, disorientation, abdominal pain, GI bleeding, thrombocytopenia.
Antidote: None.
Management: Discontinue or reduce medication. Correct fluid, electrolyte, and acid-base disturbances. Support ventilation and circulation (patent airway, oxygen, IV fluids, vasopressors). Airway-protected, ipecac syrup–induced emesis (30 mL or 0.5 mL/kg ipecac syrup followed by 200 mL or 4 mL/kg of water or clear fluid) or gastric lavage (with drug ingestion)

followed by administration of activated charcoal (PO 50–100 g or 1–2 g/kg). Forced alkaline diuresis with IV sodium bicarbonate (IV furosemide if necessary) after correction of dehydration. Symptomatic treatment.

Guidelines/Precautions

1. Use with caution in patients with active GI lesions (e.g., erosive gastritis, peptic ulcer), a history of recurrent GI lesions, hepatic or renal dysfunction, preexisting hypoprothrombinemia, or vitamin K deficiency. Nabumetone may cause peripheral edema and should be used cautiously in patients with heart failure, hypertension, and conditions associated with fluid retention.

2. Renal prostaglandins may have a supportive role in maintaining renal perfusion in patients with pre-renal conditions. Nabumetone should be avoided in such patients because it may cause a dose-dependent decrease in prostaglandin formation and thus precipitate renal decompensation.

3. Carefully observe patients with coagulation disorders and those receiving drug therapy that interferes with hemostasis.

4. Avoid the use of nabumetone during pregnancy. In the third trimester, the drug may produce adverse fetal effects, including constriction of the ductus arteriosus, neonatal primary pulmonary hypertension, and fetal death.

5. Nabumetone and salicylates should not be administered concomitantly because there may not be any therapeutic advantage and incidences of adverse GI side effects may be increased.

6. Patient response to NSAIDs is variable. Patients

who do not respond to or cannot tolerate nabumetone may be successfully treated with another NSAID.

7. Contraindicated in patients with previously demonstrated hypersensitivity to nabumetone or with the complete or partial syndrome of nasal polyps, angioedema, or bronchospastic reactivity to aspirin or other NSAIDs.

8. Signs and symptoms of infection or other diseases may be masked by the antipyretic and anti-inflammatory effects of nabumetone.

9. Monitor stool for blood every 14 days, and monitor BUN, serum creatinine, and urinalysis every 1 to 2 months when administering nabumetone at chronic high doses.

Principal Adverse Reactions

Cardiovascular: Congestive heart failure, peripheral edema, fluid retention, hypertension, tachycardia, arrhythmias.

Pulmonary: Dyspnea, bronchospasm.

CNS: Drowsiness, dizziness, headache, anxiety, confusion.

Gastrointestinal: Ulceration, bleeding, dyspepsia, nausea, vomiting, diarrhea, hepatic dysfunction, jaundice.

Genitourinary: Renal dysfunction, acute renal failure, azotemia, cystitis, hematuria.

Dermatologic: Pruritus, urticaria.

Hematologic: Prolongation of bleeding time, leukopenia, thrombocytopenia, aplastic anemia, hemolytic anemia.

Other: Tinnitus, blurred vision, optic neuropathy.

NALBUPHINE HYDROCHLORIDE

Class: Narcotic Agonist-Antagonist

Use(s): Treatment of acute and chronic pain.

Dosing: *Pain:*   IV/IM/SC   5–10 mg   (0.1–0.3 mg/kg)
            every 3–6 hours.
            Patient-controlled analgesia IV
              Bolus: 1–5 mg (0.02–0.1 mg/kg).
              Infusion: 1–8 mg/hr (0.02–0.15 mg/kg/hr).
              Lockout interval: 5–15 minutes.
         Administer   analgesic   regularly   (not   as
            needed). Due to impaired elimination,
            accumulation and excess sedation may
            occur in patients with hepatic dysfunction.
            Analgesia may be enhanced by addition of
            adjuvant drugs such as NSAIDs and anti-
            depressant agents (see pages xxvi–xliv for
            drug combinations) and use of nondrug
            therapies such as transcutaneous electrical
            nerve stimulation (TENS).

Elimination: Hepatic.

Preparations

Nalbuphine hydrochloride **(Nubain):** Injection: 10 mg/
   mL, 20 mg/mL.

Pharmacology

A synthetic opioid agonist-antagonist and a potent analgesic, nalbuphine is related chemically to oxymorphone
and naloxone. Nalbuphine is equal in potency as an
analgesic to morphine and one-fourth as potent as
nalorphine as an antagonist. It exhibits ceiling effect at

high doses (greater than 30 mg) for respiratory depression and analgesia. It is effective in reversing the ventilatory depression of agonist opioids (e.g., fentanyl) while maintaining reasonable analgesia. In patients who are not opiate dependent, the analgesic effects of nalbuphine and morphine are additive, but in patients tolerant to opiates, nalbuphine may produce a dose-related reduction in the analgesic effects of morphine. Nalbuphine is not recommended for patients with cancer pain and patients who have received opioids on a long-term basis. Naloxone reverses the respiratory depressant, analgesic, and sedative effects of nalbuphine.

Pharmacokinetics

Onset of Action: IV, 2–3 minutes; IM/SC, <15 minutes.
Peak Effect: IV, 5–15 minutes.
Duration of Action: IV/IM/SC, 3–6 hours.

Interactions

Potentiates CNS and circulatory depressant effects of other narcotic analgesics, volatile anesthetics, phenothiazines, sedative-hypnotics, alcohol, and tricyclic antidepressants; analgesia enhanced and prolonged by narcotic and non-narcotic analgesics (e.g., aspirin, acetaminophen) and α_2-agonists (e.g., clonidine).

Toxicity

Toxic Range: Not routinely monitored.
Manifestations: Somnolence, coma, respiratory arrest, apnea, cardiac arrhythmias, combined respiratory and metabolic acidosis, precipitation of withdrawal symptoms from opioids (abdominal cramps, vomiting, skin

crawling, piloerection, nasal stuffiness, lacrimation, yawning, sweating, tremor, myalgia), circulatory collapse, cardiac arrest, death.

Antidote: Naloxone IV/IM/SC 0.4–2.0 mg. Repeat dose every 2 to 3 minutes to a maximum of 10–20 mg. Do not administer naloxone if withdrawal symptoms are present. Conversely, administer opioid agonists and benzodiazepines and treat withdrawal symptomatically.

Management: Discontinue or reduce medication. Support ventilation and circulation (patent airway, oxygen, IV fluids, vasopressors). Administer antidote. Monitor blood gases, pH, and electrolytes. Correct acidosis and electrolyte disturbance (lactic acidosis may require sodium bicarbonate IV 1–2 mEq/kg). Symptomatic treatment. Airway-protected, ipecac syrup–induced emesis (30 mL or 0.5 mL/kg ipecac syrup followed by 200 mL or 4 mL/kg of water or clear fluid) or gastric lavage (with drug ingestion) followed by administration of activated charcoal (PO 50–100 g or 1–2 g/kg).

Guidelines/Precautions

1. Reduce dosage in elderly patients and with concomitant use of narcotics and sedative-hypnotics.
2. Prescribe or supply an antiemetic (e.g., metoclopramide) for use in the event of nausea and/or vomiting.
3. Constipation may be more difficult to control than pain. Prevent and/or treat by daily administration of laxatives and stool softeners, for example, Colace (docusate sodium) 100–300 mg/day. Do not administer bulk-forming agents that contain methylcellulose, psyllium, or polycarbophil.

Temporary arrest in the passage through the gastrointestinal tract may lead to fecal impaction or bowel obstruction.

4. Tolerance may develop in all patients taking narcotic analgesics for more than a couple of weeks. It may be a function of dose, frequency, and route of administration, since IV and spinal infusions of narcotics are associated with rapid development of tolerance. The first sign is a decrease in duration of effective analgesia. To delay the development of tolerance, add adjuvant drugs (e.g., NSAIDs, antidepressant agents, dextromethorphan) or switch to alternative opioids (starting at one-half the equianalgesic dose) or supplement with nondrug therapies (e.g., TENS).

5. Nalbuphine should be used with caution in patients who have been chronically receiving opiate agonists, because nalbuphine does not suppress the abstinence syndrome in these patients and high doses may precipitate withdrawal symptoms. Titrated doses of benzodiazepines or opioid agonists may be used in the management of acute withdrawal.

6. Drug combinations with adjuvant drugs enhance analgesia (see pages xxvi–xliv).

7. Adjuvant drug therapies also include regional blockade, trigger-point injections (with local anesthetics and steroids), and intravenous regional anesthesia.

8. Adjuvant nondrug therapies include TENS and modalities such as ice or heat application, ultrasound, and soft tissue mobilization.

9. Patients should be warned that nalbuphine may

impair their ability to perform hazardous tasks requiring mental alertness or physical coordination (e.g., driving a motor vehicle, operating heavy machinery).

10. The drug formulation may contain sodium metabisulfite, which may cause allergic reactions or anaphylaxis in susceptible individuals.

Principal Adverse Reactions

Cardiovascular: Hypertension, hypotension, tachycardia, bradycardia.

Pulmonary: Respiratory depression, dyspnea, asthma.

CNS: Sedation, dizziness, vertigo, headache, euphoria, confusion, hallucinations.

Gastrointestinal: Nausea, vomiting, dry mouth.

Ocular: Miosis.

Dermatologic: Urticaria, itching, burning.

Other: Flushing, speech difficulty, urinary urgency.

NALOXONE HYDROCHLORIDE

Class: Narcotic Antagonist

Use(s): Reversal of narcotic depression and biliary tract spasm; adjunct treatment of captopril, clonidine, codeine, dextromethorphan, diphenoxylate, or propoxyphene overdose; prophylaxis and treatment of narcotic side effects (e.g., pruritus, nausea); adjunct therapy of septic and cardiogenic shock.

Dosing: *Narcotic depression or drug overdose*
IV/IM/SC: 0.1–2.0 mg (neonates/children, 10–100 µg/kg). Titrate to patient re-

sponse. May repeat at 2- to 3-minute
intervals. Response should occur with a
maximum dose of 10 mg.

Infusion: 5–15 µg/kg/hr (children, 10–150
µg/kg/hr). Titrate to patient response.

*Prophylaxis and treatment of narcotic side
effects*

IV/IM/SC: 0.1–0.8 mg.

Infusion: 50–250 µg/hr (1–5 µg/kg/hr). Infusion rate of <125 mL/hr if one to two
ampules of naloxone are diluted in 1000
mL of patient's maintenance intravenous
fluid.

Septic shock

IV: 30 µg/kg.

Infusion: 30–200 µg/kg/hr (for 1–16 hours).

Elimination: Hepatic.

Preparations

Naloxone hydrochloride **(Narcan):** Injection: 0.4 mg/
mL, 1 mg/mL. Neonatal injection: 0.02 mg/mL.

Dilution for Infusion

Narcotic depression or drug overdose: IV 1 mg in
100 mL D5W or normal saline (10 µg/mL).

Narcotic side effects: IV 0.4–0.8 mg (one to two
ampules) in 1000 mL of maintenance IV fluid.

Pharmacology

This drug is a pure opioid antagonist with no agonist
activity. It competitively inhibits opiate agonists at µ-,
δ-, and κ-receptor sites and prevents or reverses the

effects of opioids, including respiratory depression, sedation, hypotension, analgesia, and biliary tract spasm. Naloxone can also reverse the psychotomimetic and dysphoric effects of agonists-antagonists such as pentazocine. CNS and respiratory depression secondary to captopril, clonidine, codeine, dextromethorphan, diphenoxylate, or propoxyphene overdose may be reversed with naloxone. Naloxone may reverse the hypotension and cardiovascular instability secondary to endogenous endorphins (potent vasodilators) released in patients with septic or cardiogenic shock. It does not produce respiratory depression, psychotomimetic effects, or pupillary constriction. It shows no pharmacologic activity in the absence of narcotics and produces withdrawal symptoms in the presence of physical dependence.

Pharmacokinetics

Onset of Action: IV, 1–2 minutes; IM/SC, 2–5 minutes.
Peak Effect: IV/IM/SC, 5–15 minutes.
Duration of Action: IV/IM/SC, 1–4 hours.

Interactions

Reversal of analgesia; increased sympathetic nervous system activity, including tachycardia, hypertension, pulmonary edema, and cardiac arrhythmias; nausea and vomiting related to dose and speed of injection.

Toxicity

Toxic Range: Not routinely monitored.
Manifestations: Excitement, reversal of analgesia, hypertension/hypotension, sweating, tachycardia, pulmonary edema, precipitation of acute abstinence syn-

drome (in patients who have been receiving opiate agonists chronically).

Antidote: No specific antidote.

Management: Discontinue or reduce medication. Support ventilation and circulation (patent airway, oxygen, IV fluids, vasopressors). Symptomatic treatment. Titrated doses of benzodiazepines or opioid agonists may be used in the management of acute withdrawal.

Guidelines/Precautions

1. Use with caution in patients with preexisting cardiac disease or who have received potentially cardiotoxic drugs.
2. Titrate slowly to desired effect. Excessive dosage of naloxone may result in reversal of analgesia and other significant side effects (hypertension, excitement, acute pulmonary edema, cardiac arrhythmias).
3. Patients who have responded to naloxone should be carefully monitored because the duration of action of some opiates may exceed that of naloxone. Repeated doses of naloxone should be administered to those patients when necessary.
4. If intravenous access is not available, the drug may be diluted 1:1 in sterile normal saline and injected via an endotracheal tube. The absorption rate, duration, and pharmacologic effects of endotracheal drug administration compare favorably with the IV route.
5. Administer cautiously to persons who are known or suspected to be physically dependent on opioids, including newborns of mothers with nar-

cotic dependence. Reversal of narcotic effects will precipitate acute abstinence syndrome.

Principal Adverse Reactions

Cardiovascular: Tachycardia, hypertension, hypotension, arrhythmias.
Pulmonary: Pulmonary edema.
CNS: Tremulousness, reversal of analgesia, seizures.
Gastrointestinal: Nausea, vomiting.
Other: Sweating.

NALTREXONE HYDROCHLORIDE

Class: Narcotic Antagonist

Use(s): Prophylaxis and treatment of opioid side effects (e.g., pruritus, nausea); induction and maintenance therapy for opiate cessation; treatment of alcohol dependence.

Dosing: *Prophylaxis and treatment of opioid side effects:* PO 12.5–50.0 mg daily as necessary.
Alcohol dependence: PO 50 mg once daily.
Opiate cessation
   Initial: PO 12.5–25.0 mg daily. Dose should be increased in increments of 12.5–25.0 mg daily until the maintenance dose has been achieved.
   Maintenance: PO 50 mg daily.
To avoid precipitating withdrawal, naltrexone therapy should not be attempted in opiate-dependent patients until detoxification is complete and the naloxone challenge test

is negative (naloxone IV 0.2–2.0 mg and observe for evidence of withdrawal, such as abdominal cramps, vomiting, skin crawling, piloerection, nasal stuffiness, lacrimation, yawning, sweating, tremor, myalgia).

Elimination: Hepatic.

Preparations

Naltrexone hydrochloride **(ReVia, formerly Trexan):** Tablet: 50 mg.

Pharmacology

This thebaine derivative is a pure opioid antagonist with no agonist activity. It competitively inhibits opiate agonists at μ-, δ-, and κ-receptor sites and prevents or reverses the effects of opioids, including respiratory depression, sedation, hypotension analgesia, and biliary tract spasm. Naltrexone differs structurally from naloxone in replacement of the allyl group on the nitrogen atom by a cyclopropylmethyl group. The structural modification results in increased oral activity and a longer duration of action for naltrexone compared with naloxone. Like naloxone, naltrexone reverses the psychotomimetic and dysphoric effects of opiate agonist-antagonists such as pentazocine. CNS and respiratory depression secondary to captopril, clonidine, codeine, dextromethorphan, diphenoxylate, or propoxyphene overdose may be reversed with naltrexone. Naltrexone may reverse the hypotension and cardiovascular instability secondary to endogenous endorphins (potent vasodilators) released in patients with septic or cardiogenic shock. It does not produce respiratory depression, psychotomimetic effects, or physical or psychological dependence. It shows no pharmacologic activity in the absence of narcotics and may precipitate withdrawal symptoms in individuals physically dependent on opiates or pentazocine. Naltrexone decreases alcohol craving and reduces alcohol consumption in patients with alcohol dependence. The mechanism of action may involve the endogenous opioid system. The drug must be used in conjunction with a behavior modification program. Naltrexone is not aversive therapy and does not cause a disulfiram-like reaction as a result of either opiate use or alcohol ingestion.

Pharmacokinetics

Onset of Action: PO, 15–30 minutes.
Peak Effect: PO, 6–12 hours.
Duration of Action: PO, 24–72 hours (dose dependent).

Interactions

Reversal of analgesia; increased sympathetic nervous system activity, including tachycardia, hypertension, pulmonary edema, and cardiac arrhythmias; precipitation of withdrawal symptoms in patients who are opiate dependent; decreased effectiveness of opiate-containing preparations (e.g., cough, cold, diarrhea, and pain preparations); increased lethargy and somnolence in patients receiving phenothiazines.

Toxicity

Toxic Range: Not routinely monitored.
Manifestations: Excitement, reversal of analgesia, hypertension/hypotension, sweating, tachycardia, pulmonary edema, precipitation of acute abstinence syn-

drome (in patients who have chronically been receiving opiate agonists).

Antidote: No specific antidote. If withdrawal symptoms are precipitated by naltrexone, administer opioid agonists or benzodiazepines and treat withdrawal symptomatically.

Management: Discontinue or reduce medication. Support ventilation and circulation (patent airway, oxygen, IV fluids, vasopressors). Symptomatic treatment. Titrated doses of benzodiazepines or opioid agonists may be used in the management of acute withdrawal.

Guidelines/Precautions

1. Naltrexone may precipitate severe withdrawal and is contraindicated in patients who are physically dependent on opiates and who fail a naloxone challenge test. Withdrawal symptoms should be treated symptomatically.
2. Naltrexone is embryocidal in rats and rabbits. It should be used in pregnancy only if the potential benefit justifies the potential risk to the fetus. Whether naltrexone is excreted in human milk is unknown; therefore, it should be used with caution in nursing mothers.

Principal Adverse Reactions

Cardiovascular: Tachycardia, hypertension, arrhythmias.

Pulmonary: Nasal congestion, cough, shortness of breath.

CNS: Tremulousness, reversal of analgesia, seizures.

Gastrointestinal: Nausea, vomiting, hepatotoxicity.

Other: Sweating, skin rash, increased thirst.

NAPROXEN, NAPROXEN SODIUM

Class: Nonsteroidal Anti-inflammatory Drug

Use(s): Symptomatic treatment of mild to moderate inflammatory and degenerative arthritis, primary dysmenorrhea, migraine, postoperative and posttraumatic pain, chronic pain, cancer pain (especially with bone metastasis).

Dosing: *Pain*

Naproxen: PO 500 mg (10 mg/kg) then 250 mg (5 mg/kg) three or four times daily. Maximum dose 1.25 g daily.

Naproxen sodium: PO 550 mg (11 mg/kg) then 275 mg (5 mg/kg) three or four times daily. Maximum dose 1.375 g daily.

Naproxen sodium, controlled release: PO 750 mg to 1 g (20 mg/kg) once daily.

Inflammatory disease or headache

Naproxen: PO 250–500 mg (5–10 mg/kg) twice daily. It is not necessary to administer the medication more frequently than twice daily. Morning and evening doses do not have to be equal in size.

Naproxen, delayed release: PO 375 or 500 mg (5–10 mg/kg) twice daily.

Naproxen sodium: PO 275–550 mg (5–11 mg/kg) twice daily.

Naproxen sodium, controlled release: PO 750 mg to 1 g (15–20 mg/kg) once daily.

Acute gouty arthritis

Naproxen: PO 750 mg (12 mg/kg) then 250 mg (5 mg/kg) three times daily.

Naproxen sodium: PO 825 mg (16 mg/kg) then 275 mg (5 mg/kg) three times daily. Naproxen sodium, controlled release: PO 750 mg to 1 g (20 mg/kg) once daily.

Administer analgesic regularly (not as needed). Addition of opioid analgesics, antidepressant agents, and use of nondrug therapies such as transcutaneous electrical nerve stimulation (TENS) may enhance analgesia (see pages xxvi–xliv for drug combinations). In rheumatoid arthritis or juvenile rheumatoid arthritis, second-line rheumatoid agents may include leflunomide (Arava), etanercept (Enbrel), antimalarials, or methotrexate. In geriatric patients and patients with decreased renal or hepatic function, decrease doses by one-third to one-half. The incidence of naproxen-induced gastropathy may be decreased by administration with meals, milk, antacids, or sucralfate (PO 1 g four times daily). Misoprostol (PO 100–200 μg four times daily) may be used to prevent gastric ulcers in high-risk patients.

Elimination: Hepatic, renal.

Preparations

Naproxen **(Naprosyn)**
  Tablets: 250 mg, 375 mg, 500 mg.
  Oral suspension: 125 mg/5 mL.
Naproxen, delayed release **(EC-Naprosyn):** Tablets: 375 mg, 500 mg.
Naproxen sodium **(Aleve):** Tablets or caplets: 220 mg
Naproxen sodium **(Anaprox):** Tablets, film coated: 275 mg, 550 mg.

Naproxen sodium, controlled release **(Naprelan):**
Tablets: 375 mg, 500 mg.

Pharmacology

A propionic acid derivative and nonsteroidal anti-inflammatory drug (NSAID), naproxen is structurally and pharmacologically related to ibuprofen and ketoprofen. Naproxen is unique in that the longer elimination half-life makes twice-daily administration effective. Naproxen is commercially available as the acid (naproxen) or the sodium salt (naproxen sodium). The sodium salt is more rapidly absorbed following oral administration and produces higher peak plasma levels (275 mg of naproxen sodium is equivalent to 250 mg naproxen). As with other NSAIDs, the analgesic and anti-inflammatory activities of naproxen are partly due to the inhibition of prostaglandin and leukotriene synthesis and to antibradykinin and lysosomal membrane stabilizing activity. The antipyretic activity may occur secondary to inhibition of pyrogen-induced release of prostaglandins in the central nervous system (including the hypothalamus) and possibly to centrally mediated peripheral vasodilatation. The analgesic potency of naproxen is similar to that of ketoprofen or piroxicam and about three times that of ibuprofen or aspirin.

Naproxen (like other NSAIDs) exhibits a ceiling effect for analgesia. Exceeding recommended doses results in increased toxicity without improvement in analgesia. Naproxen may be better tolerated than aspirin, and equipotent doses are associated with less gastric mucosal abnormalities. Inhibition of prostaglandin synthesis may result in decreased uterine tone and contractility and prolonged gestation in the parturient and premature closure of the ductus arteriosus in the fetus. Naproxen inhibits platelet aggregation and prolongs bleeding time (to a greater extent than indomethacin). However, unlike the irreversible effects of aspirin, these effects are transient and platelet function and aggregation return to normal within 24 hours. The drug has no uricosuric activity.

Pharmacokinetics

Onset of Action: PO: analgesic effect, 30–60 minutes; anti-inflammatory effect, <14 days.
Peak Effect: PO: analgesic effect, 1–2 hours; anti-inflammatory effect, 2–4 weeks.
Duration of Action: PO: analgesic effect, 3–7 hours.

Interactions

Risks of bleeding increased with concomitant NSAIDs, anticoagulant or heparin therapy, alcohol ingestion; decreases antihypertensive effects of β-adrenergic blocking agents; serum levels of naproxen decreased slightly by concomitant aspirin; serum levels of naproxen increased by concomitant probenecid; renal elimination decreased and serum levels and toxic effects of methotrexate and lithium increased by concomitant naproxen; GI absorption of naproxen delayed by food and milk; prostaglandin-mediated natriuretic effects of loop diuretics antagonized by naproxen.

Toxicity

Toxic Range: Not routinely monitored.
Manifestations: *Acute:* Drowsiness, vomiting, abdominal pain.
Antidote: None.

Management: Discontinue or reduce medication. Correct fluid, electrolyte, and acid-base disturbances. Support ventilation and circulation (patent airway, oxygen, IV fluids, vasopressors). Airway-protected, ipecac syrup–induced emesis (30 mL or 0.5 mL/kg ipecac syrup followed by 200 mL or 4 mL/kg of water or clear fluid) or gastric lavage (with drug ingestion) followed by administration of activated charcoal (PO 50–100 g or 1–2 g/kg). Forced alkaline diuresis with IV sodium bicarbonate (IV furosemide if necessary) after correction of dehydration. Symptomatic treatment.

Guidelines/Precautions

1. Use with caution in patients with active GI lesions (e.g., erosive gastritis, peptic ulcer), a history of recurrent GI lesions, hepatic or renal dysfunction, preexisting hypoprothrombinemia, or vitamin K deficiency. Naproxen may cause peripheral edema and should be used cautiously in patients with heart failure, hypertension, or conditions associated with fluid retention.
2. Renal prostaglandins may have a supportive role in maintaining renal perfusion in patients with pre-renal conditions. Naproxen should be avoided in such patients because it may cause a dose-dependent decrease in prostaglandin formation and thus precipitate renal decompensation.
3. Carefully observe patients with coagulation disorders and those receiving drug therapy that interferes with hemostasis.
4. Use with caution in pregnancy and only when the perceived benefits outweigh the potential risks.

5. Patient response to NSAIDs is variable. Patients who do not respond to or cannot tolerate naproxen may be successfully treated with another NSAID.
6. Naproxen and salicylates should not be administered concomitantly because there may not be any therapeutic advantage and incidences of adverse GI side effects may be increased.
7. Contraindicated in patients with previously demonstrated hypersensitivity to naproxen or with the complete or partial syndrome of nasal polyps, angioedema, or bronchospastic reactivity to aspirin or other NSAIDs.
8. Signs and symptoms of infection or other diseases may be masked by the antipyretic and anti-inflammatory effects of naproxen.
9. Monitor stool for blood every 14 days, and monitor BUN, serum creatinine, and urinalysis every 1 to 2 months when administering naproxen at chronic high doses.

Principal Adverse Reactions

Cardiovascular: Peripheral edema, fluid retention, hypertension, palpitation.
Pulmonary: Dyspnea, bronchospasm.
CNS: Drowsiness, dizziness, headache, anxiety, confusion.
Gastrointestinal: Ulceration, bleeding, dyspepsia, nausea, vomiting, diarrhea, hepatic dysfunction.
Genitourinary: Renal dysfunction, acute renal failure, azotemia, cystitis, hematuria.
Dermatologic: Pruritus, urticaria.
Hematologic: Prolongation of bleeding time, leuko-

penia, thrombocytopenia, aplastic anemia, hemolytic anemia.

Other: Tinnitus, blurred vision.

NIFEDIPINE

Class: Calcium Channel Blocker

Use(s): Antianginal, antihypertensive, migraine pro-phylaxis, suppression of preterm labor.

Dosing: *Angina or hypertension*

PO: 10–20 mg three times daily. Maximum 180 mg/day.

PO, sustained release (PO-SR): 30–60 mg once daily.

Other routes: Sublingual (puncture capsule and apply contents sublingually) or intra-buccal (puncture capsule 10 times and chew). *Note:* The sublingual route is not approved by the Food and Drug Admin-istration. See the "Guidelines/Precau-tions" section.

Migraine prophylaxis: PO 10 mg three times daily.

Preterm labor: 10 mg sublingually every 20 minutes until cessation of contractions (maximum dose: 40 mg in 1 hour), then PO 20 mg every 8 hours for 3 days.

Elimination: Hepatic, renal.

Preparations

Nifedipine **(Procardia, Adalat):** Capsules: 10 mg, 20 mg.

Nifedipine **(Procardia XL, Adalat CC):** Tablets, extended release: 30 mg, 60 mg, 90 mg.

Pharmacology

Nifedipine is a dihydropyridine calcium channel blocker. It inhibits the transmembrane influx of calcium ions into cardiac muscle and smooth muscle. It possesses greater coronary and peripheral arterial vasodilator properties than verapamil and minimal effects on venous capacitance. It has little or no direct depressant effect on sinoatrial node or atrioventricular node activity and consequently may be safely used in patients with low heart rates. The antihypertensive effects are probably due to decreased peripheral vascular resistance. A reflex increase in heart rate, cardiac output, and fluid retention from peripheral vasodilatation may offset the antihypertensive effect. Nifedipine improves myocardial oxygen supply-and-demand balance, which accounts for its effectiveness in the treatment of angina pectoris. Nifedipine may alter excessive vasomotor reactivity and thus is useful for the prophylaxis of migraine and symptomatic relief of ischemic pain. Nifedipine may increase the pain threshold and enhance analgesia when combined with opiates. This may be a central effect resulting from modulation of opiate effects and pain transmission secondary to calcium channel blockade.

Pharmacokinetics

Onset of Action: PO, 20 minutes; SL, 5 minutes.
Peak Effect: PO, 30 minutes; PO-SR, 6 hours; SL, 20–45 minutes.

Duration of Action: PO/SL, 4–12 hours; PO-SR, 24 hours.

Interactions

Potentiates effects of depolarizing and nondepolarizing muscle relaxants; additive cardiovascular depressant effects with use of volatile anesthetics and other anti-hypertensives, such as diuretics, angiotensin-converting enzyme inhibitors, vasodilators; increases toxicity of digoxin, benzodiazepines, carbamazepine, oral hypo-glycemics, and possibly quinidine and theophylline; cardiac failure, atrioventricular conduction disturbances, and sinus bradycardia with concurrent use of β-blockers; potentiates myocardial depressant effects (hypotension and bradycardia) of bupivacaine and local anesthetics; concomitant use of IV verapamil and IV dantrolene may result in cardiovascular collapse; decreases lithium effect and neurotoxicity; decreased clearance with cimetidine; chemically incompatible with solutions of bicarbonate or nafcillin; other highly protein-bound drugs (e.g., oral anticoagulants, hydan-toins, salicylates, sulfonamides, and sulfonylureas) may be displaced from binding sites by nifedipine or may displace nifedipine from binding sites.

Toxicity

Toxic Range: Not routinely monitored.
Manifestations: Tachycardia, respiratory failure, head-ache, delirium, psychosis.
Antidote: No specific antidote.
Management: Discontinue or reduce medication. Support ventilation and circulation (patent airway,

oxygen, IV fluids, vasopressors). Treat reflex tachycardia with a β-blocker (e.g., esmolol IV 10–40 mg or propranolol IV 0.5–3.0 mg). Remove ingested drug by induced emesis. Symptomatic treatment.

Guidelines/Precautions

1. Carefully monitor blood pressure during initial administration and titration of nifedipine.
2. Use with caution in the elderly and in those with acute myocardial infarction, unstable angina, or increased intracranial pressure.
3. Do not chew or divide sustained-release tablets.
4. Despite its popularity, the use of sublingual nifedipine in the management of hypertensive emergencies and urgencies cannot be recommended because the fall in blood pressure is both unpredictable and uncontrolled, with the consequent and unacceptable risk of organ ischemia. For hypertensive emergencies (e.g., associated with aortic dissection) in which irreversible damage would occur within hours if left untreated, patients should probably be admitted to the Intensive Care Unit and given vasodilators (e.g., nitroprusside). If the risk to the patient is measured in days rather than hours, then oral therapy (e.g., with nifedipine slow release or atenolol) will be sufficient. Furthermore, the sublingual delivery method may actually delay the attainment of peak plasma concentrations of the drug. Peak nifedipine serum concentrations have been shown to be lesser following sublingual administration than following oral administration.

Principal Adverse Reactions

Cardiovascular: Hypotension, palpitations, peripheral edema.

Pulmonary: Bronchospasm, shortness of breath, nasal and chest congestion.

CNS: Headache, dizziness, nervousness.

Gastrointestinal: Nausea, diarrhea, constipation.

Musculoskeletal: Inflammation, joint stiffness, peripheral edema.

Dermatologic: Pruritus, urticaria.

Other: Fever, chills, sweating.

NORTRIPTYLINE HYDROCHLORIDE

Class: Tricyclic Antidepressant

Use(s): Treatment of neurotic and endogenous depression; adjunct treatment of neuropathic pain syndromes, including diabetic neuropathy, postherpetic neuralgia, tic douloureux, and cancer pain; anxiety disorders; migraine; phobias; panic disorders; enuresis; eating disorders.

Dosing: *Pain syndromes*

        Initial: PO 10–50 mg (0.5–1.0 mg/kg) daily at bedtime. Titrate dose upward every 3–4 weeks by increments of 10–25 mg as necessary.

        Maintenance: PO 10–150 mg (0.2–3.0 mg/kg) daily at bedtime. Doses should be decreased if unacceptable side effects occur. Serum levels should be determined if there are signs of toxicity. The higher

end of the dose range may be required in
the management of painful diabetic neuropathy. Lower doses should be used in
geriatric and adolescent patients.

Depression

Initial: PO 50–100 mg (1–2 mg/kg) daily in
one to four divided doses.

Maintenance: PO 50–150 mg (1–3 mg/kg)
daily in one to four divided doses.
Monitor serum levels with doses that
exceed 100 mg daily.

Doses for pain are generally smaller than
those used for treatment of affective disorders. Medication should be administered
on a fixed schedule and not as needed.
Administration of the entire daily dose at
bedtime may reduce daytime sedation.
After symptoms are controlled, dosage
should be gradually reduced to the lowest
level that will maintain relief of symptoms.
Analgesia may be enhanced by addition
of opioid analgesics (see pages xxvi–xliv
for drug combinations), nonsteroidal anti-
inflammatory drugs (NSAIDs), and use of
nondrug therapies such as transcutaneous
electrical nerve stimulation (TENS). In geriatric patients and patients with decreased
renal or hepatic function, decrease doses
by one-third to one-half. The possibility for
suicide is inherent in depression and may
persist until significant remission occurs.
The quantity of drug dispensed should
reflect this consideration.

Elimination: Hepatic, renal.

Preparations

Nortriptyline hydrochloride **(Pamelor, Aventyl)**
    Capsules: 10 mg, 25 mg, 50 mg, 75 mg.
    Oral solution: 2 mg/mL.

Pharmacology

A dibenzocycloheptene derivative and a secondary amine tricyclic antidepressant, nortriptyline is the active metabolite of amitriptyline. Antidepressant activity may be partly due to inhibition of the amine-pump uptake of neurotransmitters (e.g., norepinephrine and serotonin) at the presynaptic neuron, down-regulation of β-receptor sensitivity, and peripheral/central anticholinergic effects. Although blockade of neurotransmitter uptake may occur immediately, antidepressant response may take days to weeks. Patients with low norepinephrine levels may respond better to nortriptyline compared with serotonin-deficient patients. Nortriptyline does not inhibit the monoamine oxidase (MAO) system.

The analgesic effects of nortriptyline (and other antidepressants) may occur partly through the alleviation of depression, which may be responsible for increased pain suffering, but also by mechanisms that are independent of mood effects. Serotonin and norepinephrine activity may be increased in descending pain inhibitory pathways. Activation of these pathways decreases the transmission of nociceptive impulses from primary afferent neurons to first-order cells in laminae I and V of the spinal cord dorsal horn. Nortriptyline may also potentiate the analgesic effect of opioids by increasing their binding efficacy to opioid receptors. Nortriptyline (and other tricyclic antidepressants) may have an antagonistic effect on spinal *N*-methyl D-aspartate (NMDA) receptors, and inhibit NMDA receptor activation–induced neuroplasticity. Spinal NMDA receptor activation is believed to be central to the generation and maintenance of hyperalgesic pain. Nortriptyline has varying degrees of efficacy in different pain syndromes and may be better at relieving the burning, aching, and dyesthetic component of neuropathic pain. The drug is seldom useful in the management of lancinating, shooting paroxysmal pain.

Compared with the parent drug, amitriptyline, nortriptyline has fewer side effects. The sedative, anticholinergic, and antihistaminic effects are mild. Nortriptyline is the only tricyclic antidepressant with a therapeutic window for serum levels (50–150 ng/mL). Abnormal EEG patterns may be produced, and the seizure threshold may be lowered. Therapeutic doses do not affect respiration, but toxic doses may lead to respiratory depression. The direct quinidine-like effects may manifest at toxic doses and produce cardiovascular disturbances (e.g., conduction blockade). Nortriptyline does not have addiction liability and its use is not associated with drug-seeking behavior. Withdrawal symptoms may be precipitated by acute withdrawal. Tolerance develops to the sedative and anticholinergic effects, but there are no reports of tolerance to the analgesic effects. Nortriptyline crosses the placenta, and use in pregnancy may be associated with fetal malformations. The drug is excreted in breast milk and has a potential for serious adverse effects in nursing infants.

Pharmacokinetics

Onset of Action: Analgesic effect: PO, <5 days. Antidepressant effect: PO, 1–2 weeks.
Peak Effect: Antidepressant effect: PO, 2–4 weeks.
Duration of Action: Antidepressant effect: PO, variable.

Interactions

Increased risk of hyperthermia with concomitant administration of anticholinergics (e.g., atropine), phenothiazines, thyroid medications; serum levels and toxic effects of nortriptyline increased by concomitant methylphenidate, fluoxetine, cimetidine, quinidine, phenothiazines, and haloperidol; ventilatory and circulatory depressant effects of CNS depressant drugs and alcohol potentiated by nortriptyline; increases the pressor and cardiac effects of sympathomimetics (e.g., isoproterenol, phenylephrine, norepinephrine, epinephrine, amphetamine); decreases serum levels and pharmacologic effects of levodopa and phenylbutazone; increases serum levels and toxic effects of dicumarol; onset of therapeutic effects shortened and adverse cardiac effects of nortriptyline increased with concomitant administration of levothyroxine and liothyronine; fatal hyperpyretic crisis or seizures with concomitant use of MAO inhibitors; uptake-dependent efficacy of IV regional bretylium decreased by nortriptyline.

Toxicity

Toxic Range: >150 ng/mL.
Manifestations: *Chronic:* Dream and sleep disturbances, akathisia, anxiety, chills, coryza, malaise,

myalgia, headache, dizziness, nausea and vomiting.
Acute: In addition to the previously listed symptoms,
CNS stimulation with excitement, delirium, hallucinations, hyperreflexia, myoclonus, choreiform movements, parkinsonian symptoms, seizures, hyperpyrexia,
then CNS depression with drowsiness, areflexia,
hypothermia, respiratory depression, cyanosis, hypotension, coma; peripheral anticholinergic symptoms,
including urinary retention, dry mucous membranes,
mydriasis, constipation, adynamic ileus; cardiac irregularities, including tachycardia, QRS prolongation;
metabolic and/or respiratory acidosis; polyradiculoneuropathy; renal failure; vomiting; ataxia; dysarthria;
bullous cutaneous lesions; pulmonary consolidation.

Antidote: None.

Management: Discontinue or reduce medication.
Correct fluid, electrolyte, and acid-base disturbances.
Airway-protected, ipecac syrup–induced emesis (30 mL
or 0.5 mL/kg ipecac syrup) or gastric lavage (with drug
ingestion) followed by administration of activated charcoal (PO 50–100 g or 1–2 g/kg). These purging actions
should be performed even if several hours have elapsed
after ingestion because the anticholinergic effects may
delay gastric emptying, and the drug may also be
secreted into the stomach. Control seizures: Intravenous
benzodiazepines are the first choice because IV barbiturates may enhance respiratory depression; however,
IV barbiturates may be useful in refractory seizures.
Control hyperpyrexia with ice packs and cooling
sponge baths. Support ventilation and circulation
(patent airway, oxygen, IV fluids, vasopressors). Continuous EKG monitoring. Treat cardiac arrhythmias with
IV lidocaine or propranolol. Digoxin, quinidine, pro-

cainamide, and diisopyramide should be avoided because they may further depress myocardial conduction and/or contractility. Temporary pacemakers may be necessary in patients with advanced atrioventricular block, severe bradycardia, and/or life-threatening ventricular arrhythmias unresponsive to drug therapy. Physostigmine (slow IV 1–3 mg) may be used in the treatment of life-threatening anticholinergic toxicity. Routine use of physostigmine is not advisable due to its serious adverse effects (e.g., seizures, bronchospasm, and severe bradyarrhythmias). Hemodialysis or peritoneal dialysis is ineffective because the drug is highly protein bound. Symptomatic treatment. Consider the possibility of multiple drug involvement. Counseling prior to and after discharge for patients who attempted suicide.

Guidelines/Precautions

1. To avoid withdrawal symptoms, the medication should be tapered down over a couple of weeks and not discontinued abruptly.
2. Use with caution in patients with cardiovascular disease, thyroid disease, seizure disorders, and in those in whom excessive anticholinergic activity may be harmful (e.g., patients with benign prostatic hypertrophy, a history of urinary retention, or increased intraocular pressure). The drug should be used in close-angle glaucoma only when the glaucoma is adequately controlled by drugs and closely monitored.
3. Contraindicated in patients receiving MAO inhibitors (concurrently or within the past 2 weeks), patients in the acute recovery phase fol-

lowing myocardial infarction, and those with demonstrated hypersensitivity to nortriptyline. Cross-sensitivity with other tricyclic antidepressants may occur.
4. Patients should be warned of the possibility of drowsiness that may impair performance of potentially hazardous tasks such as driving an automobile or operating machinery. Persisting daytime drowsiness may be decreased by administering a lower dose, administering the dose earlier in the evening, or substituting a less sedating alternative.

Principal Adverse Reactions

Cardiovascular: Postural hypotension, arrhythmias, conduction disturbances, hypertension, sudden death.
Pulmonary: Respiratory depression.
CNS: Confusion, disorientation, extrapyramidal symptoms.
Gastrointestinal: Hepatic dysfunction, jaundice, nausea, vomiting, constipation, decrease in lower esophageal sphincter tone.
Genitourinary: Urinary retention, paradoxical nocturia, urinary frequency.
Ocular: Blurred vision, mydriasis, increased intraocular pressure.
Dermatologic: Pruritus, urticaria, petechiae, photosensitivity.
Hematologic: Leukopenia, thrombocytopenia, eosinophilia, agranulocytosis, purpura.
Endocrinologic: Increased or decreased libido, impotence, gynecomastia, SIADH.
Other: Hyperthermia.

ONDANSETRON

Class: Serotonin Antagonist

Use(s): Prevention and treatment of chemotherapy-induced and postoperative nausea and vomiting.

Dosing: *Chemotherapy- or radiotherapy-induced nausea*

> PO: Adults, 8 mg two or three times daily. Children, 4 mg three times daily. Administer first dose 30 minutes to 2 hours before start of chemotherapy or radiotherapy and for 1 to 2 days afterward.
>
> IV: 32 mg in one dose. Dilute in 50 mL D5W and infuse over 15 minutes, beginning a half hour before the start of chemotherapy or radiotherapy.
>
> IV (alternative regimen): 0.15 mg/kg in three doses. Dilute each dose in 50 mL D5W and infuse over 15 minutes. Give dose a half hour before the start of chemotherapy or radiotherapy and repeat dose 4 hours and 8 hours afterward.

Dosage should be reduced (maximum daily dose of 8 mg) in patients with hepatic impairment.

Postoperative nausea

> PO: 8–16 mg administered as premedication 1 hour before induction of anesthesia.
>
> Slow IV: 4 mg. Give undiluted over 1–5 minutes immediately before induction of

anesthesia or postoperatively. Dose may
be repeated if necessary.

Elimination: Hepatic.

Preparations

Ondansetron hydrochloride **(Zofran)**
  Injection: 2mg/mL.
  Injection, premixed: 32mg/50mL in 5% dextrose.
  Tablets: 4mg, 8mg.
  Oral solution: 4mg/5mL.

Pharmacology

Ondansetron is a selective serotonin 5-HT$_3$ receptor
antagonist. 5-HT$_3$ receptors are present both peripherally on vagal nerve terminals and centrally in the
chemoreceptor trigger zone of the area postrema.
Ondansetron may antagonize the emetic effects of serotonin at either or both receptor sites. Ondansetron does
not antagonize dopamine receptors. Transient increases
in hepatic transaminase levels may occur following
therapy. The drug may cross the placenta and may be
excreted in breast milk. It should be used with caution
in pregnant and nursing mothers.

Pharmacokinetics

Onset of Action: IV, <30 minutes.
Peak Effect: IV, variable.
Duration of Action: IV, 12–24 hours.

Interactions

Serum levels may be altered with concomitant administration of phenytoin, phenobarbital, or rifampin.

Toxicity

Toxic Range: Not routinely monitored.
Manifestations: Hypotension, sudden blindness (amaurosis), vasovagal episodes.
Antidote: No specific antidote.
Management: Discontinue or reduce medication. Support ventilation and circulation (patent airway, oxygen, IV fluids, vasopressors). Symptomatic treatment.

Guidelines/Precautions

1. Ondansetron does not stimulate gastric or intestinal peristalsis. It should not be used in place of a nasogastric tube. As with other antiemetics, the use of ondansetron in abdominal surgery may mask a progressive ileus and/or gastric distention.

Principal Adverse Reactions

Cardiovascular: Hypotension, bradycardia, tachycardia, angina, second-degree heart block.
Pulmonary: Bronchospasm, shortness of breath.
CNS: Extrapyramidal reactions, seizures.
Gastrointestinal: Constipation, hepatic dysfunction.
Other: Blurred vision, hypokalemia, pain and redness at site of injection.

OXYCODONE HYDROCHLORIDE

Class: Narcotic Agonist

Use(s): Treatment of acute, chronic, and cancer pain; treatment of severe refractory headache and migraine.

Dosing: *Analgesia*

> PO, immediate release: 5–10 mg every 4–6 hours.
>
> PO, sustained release (OxyContin): 10–80 mg every 12 hours. Titrate dose to maintain adequate analgesia with acceptable side effects. Opioid-tolerant patients with severe pain may require up to 240 mg every 12 hours. Combinations with adjuvant drugs (e.g., NSAIDs), antidepressant agents, and use of nondrug therapies enhance analgesia and reduce opioid requirements.
>
> Maximum daily dose of nonopioid ingredient in fixed-combination preparations (e.g., Percocet): Acetaminophen, 4 g; aspirin, 6 g.
>
> Administer sustained release preparation regularly (i.e., around the clock). Administer immediate release preparation as necessary for breakthrough pain. Due to impaired elimination, dose should be modified depending on clinical response in patients with renal or hepatic dysfunction.

Elimination: Hepatic, renal.

Preparations

Oxycodone hydrochloride **(Roxicodone)**
   Tablets: 5 mg.
   Oral solution: 5 mg/5 mL.
Oxycodone hydrochloride **(OxyFast Oral Concentrate, Roxicodone Intensol):** Concentrated oral solution: 20 mg/mL.

Oxycodone hydrochloride **(OxyIR):** Capsules, immediate release: 5 mg.

Oxycodone hydrochloride **(OxyContin):** Tablets, sustained release: 10 mg, 20 mg, 40 mg, 80 mg (80 mg tablets are for use only in opioid-tolerant patients requiring daily oxycodone equivalent dosages of 160 mg or more.

Oxycodone hydrochloride and acetaminophen **(Tylox, Roxilox):** Capsules: Oxycodone 5 mg and acetaminophen 500 mg.

Oxycodone hydrochloride and acetaminophen **(Percocet, Oxycet, Roxicet):** Tablets: Oxycodone 5 mg and acetaminophen 325 mg; oxycodone 5 mg and acetaminophen 500 mg.

Oxycodone hydrochloride and acetaminophen **(Roxicet):** Solution: Oxycodone 5 mg/5 mL and acetaminophen 325 mg/5 mL.

Oxycodone hydrochloride, oxycodone terephthalate, and aspirin **(Percodan-Demi):** Tablets: Oxycodone HCL 2.25 mg, oxycodone terephthalate 0.19 mg, and aspirin 325 mg.

Oxycodone hydrochloride, oxycodone terephthalate, and aspirin **(Percodan, Roxiprin):** Tablets: Oxycodone HCL 4.5 mg, oxycodone terephthalate 0.38 mg, and aspirin 325 mg.

Pharmacology

A synthetic phenanthrene-derivative opiate agonist, oxycodone differs from hydrocodone by the attachment of a hydroxyl group on the phenanthrene nucleus. Oxycodone exerts its primary effects on the central nervous system and organs containing smooth muscle. Excitatory synaptic pain transmission is decreased by opioid-receptor–mediated inhibition of neurotransmitter release (e.g., bradykinin at site of tissue injury, substance P in the dorsal horn, and dopamine in the basal ganglia). Also, oxycodone (and other opioids) may alter cognitive and emotional processing of painful input by acting on limbic and cortical opioid receptors. Oxycodone is a potent analgesic with no ceiling effect for analgesia. Drowsiness, euphoria, depression of cough reflex, and dose-dependent respiratory depression may occur. Clinically important respiratory depression is rarely seen in patients with severe pain due to malignant disease even with large doses, because pain and emotional stress are powerful antagonists to narcotic-induced respiratory depression. Constipating effects of oxycodone result from induction of nonpropulsive contractions through the GI tract. Emetic effects are due to opioid-induced stimulation of the chemoreceptor trigger zone in the floor of the fourth ventricle. Adverse effects are generally milder than those of morphine. The analgesic efficacy of 10 mg of orally administered oxycodone is equivalent to that of 20 mg of oral morphine sulfate, 70 mg of oral codeine, 5 mg of intramuscular oxycodone, or 3.3 mg of intramuscular morphine sulfate. Antitussive effects may occur with doses lower than those usually required for analgesia. The drug has no antipyretic effects. Physical dependence and tolerance may develop with repeated administration. Abuse liability is similar to that of codeine. Oxycodone will only partially suppress the withdrawal syndrome in patients physically dependent on other narcotics. Oxycodone crosses the placenta and low levels may be detected in breast milk; however, no adverse effects have been noted in nursing infants.

Pharmacokinetics

Onset of Action: PO, 10–15 minutes.
Peak Effect: PO, 30–60 minutes.
Duration of Action: PO, 3–6 hours; PO, slow release, 12 hours.

Interactions

Potentiates CNS and circulatory depressant effects of other narcotic analgesics, volatile anesthetics, phenothiazines, sedative-hypnotics, alcohol, tricyclic antidepressants; analgesia enhanced and prolonged by narcotic and non-narcotic analgesics (e.g., aspirin, acetaminophen), α_2-agonists (e.g., clonidine); increases serum levels and toxic effects of carbamazepine; hepatic metabolism increased and efficacy of oxycodone decreased in cigarette smokers; hypoprothrombinemic effects of warfarin increased by oxycodone–acetaminophen combination.

Toxicity

Toxic Range: 0.6–10.0 µg/mL.
Manifestations: Somnolence, coma, respiratory arrest, apnea, cardiac arrhythmias, combined respiratory and metabolic acidosis, circulatory collapse, cardiac arrest, death.
Antidote: Naloxone IV/IM/SC 0.4–2.0 mg. Repeat dose every 2 to 3 minutes to a maximum of 10–20 mg.
Management: Discontinue or reduce medication. Support ventilation and circulation (patent airway, oxygen, IV fluids, vasopressors). Administer antidote. Monitor blood gases, pH, and electrolytes. Correct acidosis and electrolyte disturbance (lactic acidosis may require sodium bicarbonate IV 1–2 mEq/kg). Symptomatic treatment. Airway-protected, ipecac syrup–

induced emesis (30 mL or 0.5 mL/kg ipecac syrup followed by 200 mL or 4 mL/kg of water or clear fluid) or gastric lavage (with drug ingestion) followed by administration of activated charcoal (PO 50–100 g or 1–2 g/kg).

Guidelines/Precautions

1. Reduce dosage in elderly patients and with concomitant use of narcotics and sedative-hypnotics.
2. The drug formulation may contain sodium metabisulfite, which may cause allergic reactions or anaphylaxis in susceptible individuals.
3. Prescribe or supply an antiemetic (e.g., metoclopramide) for use in the event of nausea and/or vomiting.
4. Constipation may be more difficult to control than pain. Prevent and/or treat by daily administration of stool softeners or laxatives, for example, Colace (docusate sodium) 100–300 mg/day. Do not administer bulk-forming agents that contain methylcellulose, psyllium, or polycarbophil. Temporary arrest in the passage through the gastrointestinal tract may lead to fecal impaction or bowel obstruction.
5. Tolerance is manifested by decreased duration of effect and increasing need for the drug. In these cases, add adjuvant drugs (e.g., NSAIDs, antidepressant agents) or switch to alternative opioids (starting at one-half the equianalgesic dose) or supplement with nondrug therapies (e.g., TENS).
6. Abrupt discontinuation of opioids in patients with physical dependence may manifest with withdrawal symptoms. To avoid withdrawal, doses should be reduced slowly (e.g., dose reduction of

75% every 2 days). Withdrawal should be treated symptomatically.

7. Addiction occurs rarely (frequency of < 1:3000) and should not be considered in deciding the proper dose and schedule of oxycodone.

8. Drug combinations with adjuvant drugs enhance analgesia (see pages xxvi–xliv).

9. Adjuvant drug therapies also include regional blockade, trigger-point injections (with local anesthetics and steroids), and intravenous regional anesthesia.

10. Adjuvant nondrug therapies include TENS and modalities such as ice or heat application, ultrasound, and soft tissue mobilization.

11. Patients should be warned that oxycodone may impair their ability to perform hazardous tasks requiring mental alertness or physical coordination (e.g., driving a motor vehicle, operating heavy machinery).

12. OxyContin sustained-release 80mg tablets are for use only in opioid-tolerant patients requiring daily oxycodone equivalent dosages of 160mg or more. Patients should be instructed against use by individuals other than the patient for whom it was prescribed, as such inappropriate use may have severe medical consequences.

13. Oxycodone is subject to control under the Federal Controlled Substances Act of 1970 as a Schedule II (C-II) drug.

Principal Adverse Reactions

Cardiovascular: Hypotension, circulatory depression, bradycardia, syncope.

Pulmonary: Respiratory depression.
CNS: Sedation, somnolence, euphoria, dysphoria, disorientation.
Genitourinary: Urinary retention.
Gastrointestinal: Nausea, vomiting, abdominal pain, biliary tract spasm, constipation, anorexia, hepatic dysfunction.
Ocular: Miosis.
Allergic: Rash, pruritus, urticaria.

OXYMORPHONE HYDROCHLORIDE

Class: Narcotic Agonist

Use(s): Teatment of acute, chronic, and cancer pain.

Dosing: *Analgesia*
SC/IM: 0.5–1.5 mg every 4–6 hours.
IV: 0.5 mg every 4–6 hours.
Rectal: 5 mg every 4–6 hours.
Patient-controlled analgesia IV
Bolus: 0.3 mg (0.006 mg/kg).
Lockout interval: 5–10 minutes.
Administer analgesic regularly (not as needed). Due to impaired elimination, accumulation and excess sedation may occur in patients with renal or hepatic dysfunction. Analgesia may be enhanced by addition of adjuvant drugs such as nonsteroidal anti-inflammatory drugs (NSAIDs) and antidepressant agents (see pages xxvi–xliv for drug combinations) and use of nondrug therapies such as transcutaneous electrical nerve stimulation (TENS).

Elimination: Hepatic, renal.

Preparations

Oxymorphone hydrochloride **(Numorphan)**
  Suppositories: 5 mg.
  Injection: 1 mg/mL, 1.5 mg/mL.

Pharmacology

A synthetic phenanthrene-derivative opiate agonist, oxymorphone differs from hydromorphone by the addition of a hydroxyl group. It exerts its potent analgesic actions on the central nervous system. Oxymorphone has little antitussive activity and may be less constipating than morphine. However, oxymorphone may be associated with more nausea, vomiting, and euphoria than morphine. The analgesic efficacy of 1 mg of IM oxymorphone is equivalent to that of 10 mg of IM morphine sulfate. Oxymorphone crosses the placental barrier and may produce depression in the neonate. The drug may appear in breast milk and should be used with caution in nursing mothers.

Pharmacokinetics

Onset of Action: IV, 5–10 minutes. SC/IM, 10–15 minutes. Rectal, 15–30 minutes.
Peak Effect: IV/IM, 30–60 minutes.
Duration of Action: IV/IM/SC/Rectal, 3–6 hours.

Interactions

Potentiates CNS and circulatory depressant effects of other narcotic analgesics, volatile anesthetics, phenothiazines, sedative-hypnotics, alcohol, tricyclic antidepressants; analgesia enhanced and prolonged by narcotic and non-narcotic analgesics (e.g., aspirin, acetaminophen), α_2-agonists (e.g., clonidine); hepatic metabolism increased and efficacy of oxymorphone decreased in cigarette smokers.

Toxicity

Toxic Range: Not routinely monitored.

Manifestations: Somnolence, coma, respiratory arrest, apnea, cardiac arrhythmias, combined respiratory and metabolic acidosis, circulatory collapse, cardiac arrest, death.

Antidote: Naloxone IV/IM/SC 0.4–2.0 mg. Repeat dose every 2 to 3 minutes to a maximum of 10–20 mg.

Management: Discontinue or reduce medication. Support ventilation and circulation (patent airway, oxygen, IV fluids, vasopressors). Administer antidote. Monitor blood gases, pH, and electrolytes. Correct acidosis and electrolyte disturbance (lactic acidosis may require sodium bicarbonate IV 1–2 mEq/kg). Symptomatic treatment. Airway-protected, ipecac syrup–induced emesis (30 mL or 0.5 mL/kg ipecac syrup followed by 200 mL or 4 mL/kg of water or clear fluid) or gastric lavage (with drug ingestion) followed by administration of activated charcoal (PO 50–100 g or 1–2 g/kg).

Guidelines/Precautions

1. Abuse liability is similar to that of morphine. Tolerance and addiction may develop with repeated administration. Oxymorphone is subject to control under the Federal Controlled Substances Act as a Schedule II (C-II) drug.
2. Reduce dosage in elderly patients and with concomitant use of narcotics and sedative-hypnotics.

3. May contain sodium hydrosulfite, which may cause allergic reactions or anaphylaxis in susceptible individuals.

4. Prescribe or supply an antiemetic (e.g., metoclopramide) for use in the event of nausea and/or vomiting.

5. Constipation may be more difficult to control than pain. Prevent and/or treat by daily administration of stool softeners or laxatives, for example, Colace (docusate sodium) 100–300 mg/day. Do not administer bulk-forming agents that contain methylcellulose, psyllium, or polycarbophil. Temporary arrest in the passage through the gastrointestinal tract may lead to fecal impaction or bowel obstruction.

6. Tolerance is manifested by decreased duration of effect and increasing need for the drug. In these cases, add adjuvant drugs (e.g., NSAIDs, antidepressant agents) or switch to alternative opioids (starting at one-half the equianalgesic dose) or supplement with nondrug therapies (e.g., TENS).

7. Abrupt discontinuation of opioids in patients with physical dependence may manifest with withdrawal symptoms. To avoid withdrawal, doses should be reduced slowly (e.g., dose reduction of 75% every 2 days). Withdrawal should be treated symptomatically.

8. Addiction occurs rarely (frequency of < 1:3000) and should not be considered in deciding the proper dose and schedule of oxymorphone.

9. Drug combinations with adjuvant drugs enhance analgesia (see pages xxvi–xliv).

10. Adjuvant drug therapies also include regional blockade, trigger-point injections (with local anesthetics and steroids), and intravenous regional anesthesia.
11. Adjuvant nondrug therapies include TENS and modalities such as ice or heat application, ultrasound, and soft tissue mobilization.
12. Patients should be warned that oxymorphone may impair their ability to perform hazardous tasks requiring mental alertness or physical coordination (e.g., driving a motor vehicle, operating heavy machinery).

Principal Adverse Reactions

Cardiovascular: Hypotension, circulatory depression, bradycardia, syncope.
Pulmonary: Respiratory depression.
CNS: Sedation, somnolence, euphoria, dysphoria, disorientation.
Genitourinary: Urinary retention.
Gastrointestinal: Nausea, vomiting, abdominal pain, biliary tract spasm, constipation, anorexia, hepatic dysfunction.
Ocular: Miosis.
Allergic: Rash, pruritus, urticaria.

PAMIDRONATE DISODIUM

Class: Aminobisphosphonate

Use(s): Treatment of hypercalcemia of malignancy; treatment of osteolytic bone metastasis of breast cancer and osteolytic bone lesions of multiple myeloma; slowing of bone disease progression and reduction of tumor-associated metastatic bone pain; treatment of osteoporosis and bone pain associated with reflex sympathetic dystrophy (RSD).

Dosing: *Hypercalcemia* (serum calcium 12.0–13.5 mg/dL): IV infusion, 60–90 mg. Administer 60-mg dose over at least 4 hours and 90-mg dose over 24 hours. Dilute dose in 1000 mL normal saline or D5W.

Severe hypercalcemia (serum calcium >13.5 mg/dL): IV infusion, 90 mg. Administer over 24 hours. Dilute dose in 1000 mL normal saline or D5W.

Retreatment may be carried out after a minimum of 7 days if serum calcium does not return to normal after initial treatment.

Paget's disease: IV infusion, 30 mg daily for 3 days. Administer as a 4-hour infusion over 3 consecutive days for a total dose of 90 mg. Dilute dose in 500 mL normal saline or D5W.

Osteolytic bone lesions of multiple myeloma: IV infusion, 90 mg monthly. Administer as a 4-hour infusion. Dilute dose in 500 mL normal saline or D5W. Patients with marked Bence-Jones proteinuria and dehydration should receive adequate hydration prior to infusion.

Osteolytic bone metastasis of breast cancer: IV infusion, 90 mg every 3–4 weeks. Administer as a 2-hour infusion. Pamidronate disodium may be used in combination with chemotherapeutic agents (e.g., doxorubicin, fluorouracil).

Elimination: Renal.

Preparations

Pamidronate disodium **(Aredia):** Vials: 30 mg, 60 mg, or 90 mg of sterile lyophilized pamidronate disodium and 470 mg, 400 mg, or 375 mg mannitol, respectively.

Dilution for Infusion: IV: Add 10 mL sterile water to each vial (30 mg/10 mL, 60 mg/10 mL, 90 mg/10 mL). The drug should be completely dissolved before the solution is withdrawn. Dilute further as follows.

Hypercalcemia of malignancy: 60 or 90 mg pamidronate in 1000 mL normal saline or D5W.

Paget's disease: 30 mg pamidronate in 500 mL normal saline or D5W.

Osteolytic bone metastasis of breast cancer: 90 mg pamidronate in 250 mL normal saline or D5W.

Osteolytic bone lesions of multiple myeloma: 90 mg pamidronate in 500 mL normal saline or D5W.

Pamidronate reconstituted with sterile water for injection may be stored under refrigeration at 2°C to 8°C for up to 24 hours. Pamidronate must not be mixed with calcium-containing infusion solutions, such as Ringer's solution, and should be given in a single intravenous solution and line separate from all other drugs. Parenteral products must be inspected visually for particulate matter and discoloration prior to administration, whenever solution and container permit.

Pharmacology

This second-generation aminobisphosphonate binds to bone hydroxyapatite and specifically inhibits the activity of osteoclasts, the bone-resorbing cells. Pamidronate reduces bone resorption with no direct effect on bone formation, although the latter process is ultimately reduced because bone resorption and formation are coupled during bone turnover. Pamidronate thus reduces elevated rates of bone turnover. Osteoclastic activity resulting in excessive bone resorption is the underlying pathophysiologic derangement in metastatic bone disease and hypercalcemia of malignancy. Excessive release of calcium into the blood as bone is resorbed results in polyuria and gastrointestinal disturbances with progressive dehydration and decreasing glomerular filtration rate. This results in increased renal absorption of calcium, setting up a cycle of worsening systemic hypercalcemia. Correction of excessive bone resorption and adequate fluid administration to correct fluid deficits are therefore essential to the management of hypercalcemia. Pamidronate shows preferential localization to sites of bone resorption specifically under osteoclasts. The drug inhibits osteoclast activity but does not interfere with osteoclast recruitment or attachment. The osteoclasts adhere normally to the bone surface but lack the ruffled border that is indicative of active resorption. Dose-dependent inhibition of resorption is manifested by decreases in serum phosphate levels. This is presumably due to decreased release of phosphate from bone and increased renal excretion as parathyroid hormone levels (which are usually suppressed in hypercalcemia of malignancy) return toward normal. Phosphate therapy may be administered in response to a decrease in serum phosphate levels. However, phosphate levels usually return toward normal within 7 to 10 days.

In treatment of metastatic bone disease, pamidronate

and other bisphosphonates (e.g., alendronate) treat hypercalcemia, reduce tumor-associated pain, reduce the incidence of pathologic fractures, and also slow bone disease progression. Administration of bisphosphonates shortly after adjuvant chemotherapy can preserve bone density in female patients with chemotherapy-induced menopause. A related bisphosphonate, clodronate, has been shown to reduce the incidence of bone metastasis in patients with early-stage breast cancer. There was no difference in the incidence of nonskeletal metastatic disease. Pamidronate may reduce bone resorption and relieve bone pain in patients with RSD. Osteoporosis and bone resorption in RSD may be partly due to increased deep tissue blood flow secondary to surface or capillary vasoconstriction.

Pharmacokinetics

Onset of Action: 4 weeks.
Peak Effect: 3–6 months.
Duration of Action: 7 months.

Interactions

There is no effect on the calcium-lowering action of pamidronate with concomitant administration of a loop diuretic.

Toxicity

Toxic Range: Not routinely monitored.
Manifestations: Hypocalcemia, hypophosphatemia, fever, hypotension.
Antidote: None.
Management: Discontinue or reduce medication. Administer intravenous or oral calcium to correct hypocal-

cemia. Support ventilation and circulation (patent airway, oxygen, IV fluids, vasopressors). Symptomatic treatment.

Guidelines/Precautions

1. Standard hypercalcemia-related metabolic parameters, such as serum levels of calcium, phosphate, magnesium, and potassium, should be carefully monitored following the initiation of therapy with pamidronate. Patients should also have periodic evaluations of standard laboratory and clinical parameters of renal function.
2. Pamidronate is contraindicated in patients with clinically significant hypersensitivity to pamidronate or other bisphosphonates.

Principal Adverse Reactions

Cardiovascular: Hypertension.
Ocular: Uveitis, iritis, scleritis and episcleritis.
Gastrointestinal: Abdominal pain, anorexia, constipation, nausea, vomiting.
Genitourinary: Urinary tract infection.
Musculoskeletal: Bone, muscle, or joint pain.
Metabolic: Hypokalemia, hypomagnesemia, hypophosphatemia.
Other: Transient elevation of temperature (>1°C), anemia, fluid overload, generalized pain.

PAROXETINE HYDROCHLORIDE

Class: Selective Serotonin Reuptake Inhibitor—Antidepressant

Use(s): Treatment of neurotic and endogenous depression; adjunct treatment of neuropathic pain syndromes, including diabetic neuropathy, postherpetic neuralgia, tic douloureux, and cancer pain; anxiety disorders; phobias; panic disorders; alcohol dependency; enuresis; eating disorders.

Dosing: *Pain syndromes*

Initial: PO 10–20 mg daily, preferably in the morning.

Maintenance: PO 10–50 mg daily in the morning. Doses may be titrated upward in increments of 10 mg/day at 1-week intervals. Doses should be decreased if unacceptable side effects occur. Serum levels should be determined if there are signs of toxicity. The higher end of the dose range may be required in the management of painful diabetic neuropathy.

Depression

Initial: PO 20 mg daily, preferably in one dose in the morning.

Maintenance: PO 20–50 mg daily in one dose in the morning. Doses may be titrated upward in increments of 10 mg/day at 1-week intervals.

Doses for pain are generally smaller than those used for treatment of affective disorders. Medication should be administered on a fixed schedule and not as needed. After symptoms are controlled, dosage should be gradually reduced to the lowest level that will maintain relief of symptoms.

Analgesia may be enhanced by addition of opioid analgesics (see pages xxvi–xliv for drug combinations), nonsteroidal anti-inflammatory drugs (NSAIDs), and use of nondrug therapies such as transcutaneous electrical nerve stimulation (TENS). In geriatric patients and patients with decreased renal or hepatic function, decrease doses by one-third to one-half. The possibility for suicide is inherent in depression and may persist until significant remission occurs. The quantity of drug dispensed should reflect this consideration.

Elimination: Hepatic, renal.

Preparations

Paroxetine hydrochloride **(Paxil):** Tablets: 10 mg, 20 mg, 30 mg.

Pharmacology

A phenylpiperidine-derivative antidepressant agent, paroxetine differs structurally and pharmacologically from currently available antidepressant agents, including other selective serotonin reuptake inhibitors (e.g., fluoxetine) and tricyclic/tetracyclic agents. Antidepressant activity is comparable with fluoxetine or imipramine and superior to doxepin or trazodone, with fewer adverse effects, and may be partly due to highly selective reuptake inhibition of serotonin. Paroxetine has little or no effect on norepinephrine and dopamine neuronal uptake. Synaptic concentrations of serotonin are increased, with enhanced serotonergic neurotransmission and numerous CNS effects (e.g., appetite suppression). Paroxetine may be associated with some anxiety and activation of mania/hypomania. Unlike with the tricyclics, sedating and cardiovascular effects are minimal due to the lack of substantial antihistaminic, anticholinergic, α_1-adrenergic-blocking, catecholamine-potentiating, and quinidine-like cardiotoxic effects. Paroxetine undergoes hepatic metabolism to inactive metabolites. Paroxetine does not appear to affect cardiac conduction and is not arrhythmogenic. It does not inhibit the reuptake of tyramine and has no effect on the pressor response to tyramine. Paroxetine does not inhibit the monoamine oxidase (MAO) system. Onset of action and relief of associated anxiety symptoms occurs earlier compared with fluoxetine and the tricyclic antidepressants. Although blockade of neurotransmitter uptake may occur immediately, antidepressant response may take days to weeks.

The analgesic effects of paroxetine may occur partly through the alleviation of depression, which may be responsible for increased pain suffering, but also by mechanisms that are independent of mood effects. Paroxetine may potentiate the analgesic effect of opiate agonists, possibly by enhancing serotonergic transmission. The drug may produce abnormal EEG patterns and lower the seizure threshold. Therapeutic doses do not affect respiration, but the effects of higher doses remain to be established. Paroxetine does not appear to have addiction liability. Paroxetine crosses the placenta and is excreted in breast milk. It should be used with caution in pregnant and nursing mothers.

Pharmacokinetics

Onset of Action: Analgesic effect: PO, <5 days. Antidepressant effect: PO, 1–2 weeks.
Peak Effect: Antidepressant effect: PO, 3–4 weeks.

Duration of Action: Antidepressant effect: PO, variable.

Interactions

Increased risk of serotonin syndrome (myoclonus, rigidity, hyperreflexia, seizures, hyperthermia, hypertension, restlessness, diaphoresis, shivering, diarrhea, and tremor) with concomitant administration of serotonergics (e.g., clomipramine), tryptophan, pseudoephedrine, tricyclic antidepressant agents, cocaine, lithium, and MAO inhibitors; serum levels and toxic effects of paroxetine increased by cimetidine; serum levels of paroxetine decreased by enzyme inducers (e.g., phenytoin, phenobarbital, rifampin); extrapyramidal effects of antipsychotic drugs may be potentiated by paroxetine; may increase the risks of bleeding in patients receiving warfarin.

Toxicity

Toxic Range: Not routinely monitored.

Manifestations: Serotonin syndrome (myoclonus, rigidity, hyperreflexia, seizures, hyperthermia, hypertension, restlessness, diaphoresis, shivering, diarrhea, and tremor), nausea and vomiting, drowsiness, sinus tachycardia, dilated pupils.

Antidote: Serotonin antagonists: Cyproheptadine PO 4–12 mg stat *or* methysergide PO 2 mg twice daily (three doses may be sufficient).

Management: Discontinue medication. Administer antidote. Correct fluid, electrolyte, and acid-base disturbances. Airway-protected, ipecac syrup–induced emesis (30 mL or 0.5 mL/kg ipecac syrup) or gastric lavage (with drug ingestion) followed by administration of activated charcoal (PO 50–100g or 1–2g/kg). Activated charcoal may be administered every 4 to 6 hours during the first 24 to 48 hours after ingestion. Control seizures: Intravenous benzodiazepines are the first choice; however, IV barbiturates or phenytoin may be useful in refractory seizures. Support ventilation and circulation (patent airway, oxygen, IV fluids, vasopressors). Control hyperpyrexia with ice packs and cooling sponge baths. Hemodialysis or peritoneal dialysis is ineffective because the drug is highly protein bound. Symptomatic treatment. Consider the possibility of multiple drug involvement. Counseling prior to and after discharge for patients who attempted suicide.

Guidelines/Precautions

1. To avoid withdrawal symptoms, the medication should be tapered down over a couple of weeks and not discontinued abruptly.
2. Use with caution in patients with cardiovascular disease, diabetes mellitus, anorexia nervosa, thyroid disease, or seizure disorders.
3. Paroxetine is contraindicated in patients receiving MAO inhibitors (concurrently or within the past 2 weeks), patients in the acute recovery phase following myocardial infarction, and those with demonstrated hypersensitivity to paroxetine. The combination of paroxetine and MAO inhibitors may result in the serotonin syndrome (see "Interactions").
4. Loss of libido and significant sexual dysfunction may occur in patients on paroxetine (and other SSRI antidepressants). In late stages of chronic regional pain syndrome and in patients treated

with morphine or hydromorphone pumps, serum levels of estrogen and testosterone are at or below the lower limits of normal. The low sex hormones are often accompanied by edema, fatigue, hot flashes in women, and tendency for inactivity. SSRI antidepressants may aggravate these symptoms and preclude their continued use. Supplemental estrogen or testosterone may counteract the chronic fatigue and cold extremities and improve the level of analgesia.

5. Patients should be warned of the possibility of drowsiness that may impair performance of potentially hazardous tasks such as driving an automobile or operating machinery. Persisting daytime drowsiness may be decreased by administering a lower dose, administering the dose earlier in the evening, or substituting a less sedating alternative.

Principal Adverse Reactions

Cardiovascular: Tachycardia, bradycardia, hypertension.

Pulmonary: Respiratory depression.

CNS: Amnesia, CNS stimulation, emotional lability, vertigo, ataxia, seizures, extrapyramidal symptoms, activation of mania/hypomania.

Gastrointestinal: Hepatic dysfunction, jaundice, nausea, vomiting, diarrhea.

Genitourinary: Amenorrhea, dysmenorrhea, dysuria, urinary urgency, urinary retention.

Ocular: Blurred vision, mydriasis, increased intraocular pressure.

Dermatologic: Pruritus, urticaria, petechiae, photosensitivity.

Hematologic: Anemia, thrombocytopenia, eosinophilia, agranulocytosis.
Endocrinologic: Increased or decreased libido, impotence, gynecomastia, SIADH.
Other: Hyperthermia.

PENTAZOCINE HYDROCHLORIDE

Class: Narcotic Agonist-Antagonist

Use(s): Treatment of acute and chronic pain.

Dosing: *Analgesia*

> PO: 50–100 mg (1–2 mg/kg) every 3–4 hours. Maximum oral daily dose 600 mg.
>
> IV: 15–30 mg (0.3–0.5 mg/kg) every 3–4 hours.
>
> IM/SC: 30–60 mg (0.5–1.0 mg/kg) every 3–4 hours.
>
> Maximum parenteral daily dose 360 mg.

Administer analgesic regularly (not as needed). Due to impaired elimination, accumulation and excess sedation may occur in patients with renal or hepatic dysfunction. Analgesia may be enhanced by addition of adjuvant drugs such as nonsteroidal anti-inflammatory drugs (NSAIDs) and antidepressant agents (see pages xxvi–xliv for drug combinations) and use of nondrug therapies such as transcutaneous electrical nerve stimulation (TENS).

Elimination: Hepatic, renal.

Preparations

Pentazocine lactate **(Talwin):** Injection: 30 mg/mL.

Pentazocine hydrochloride with aspirin **(Talwin Compound Caplets):** Caplets: Pentazocine 12.5 mg with aspirin 325 mg.

Pentazocine hydrochloride with acetaminophen **(Talacen Caplets):** Caplets: Pentazocine 25 mg with acetaminophen 650 mg.

Pentazocine hydrochloride and naloxone hydrochloride **(Talwin Nx Caplets):** Caplets: Pentazocine 50 mg with naloxone 0.5 mg.

Pharmacology

A benzomorphan derivative and potent analgesic, pentazocine is a competitive antagonist at μ-receptors and an agonist at δ- and κ-receptors. Opioid antagonist activity is weak, being only one-fifth as potent as nalorphine. The analgesic efficacy of 30 mg pentazocine is equivalent to that of 10 mg morphine. Pentazocine incompletely reverses morphine-induced cardiovascular and respiratory depression, but it may precipitate withdrawal symptoms in patients who have received opiates regularly. In patients who are not opiate dependent, the analgesic effects of pentazocine and morphine are additive, but in patients tolerant to opiates, pentazocine may produce a dose-related reduction in the analgesic effects of morphine. Pentazocine is not recommended for patients with cancer pain and patients who have received opioids on a long-term basis. Pentazocine produces respiratory depression, sedation, miosis, and antitussive effects. Psychotomimetic effects (hallucinations, dysphoria, delirium) may result from agonist effects at σ-receptors. Naloxone reverses the respiratory depressant and psychotomimetic effects of pentazocine. There is no histamine release. Pentazocine crosses the placental barrier and may produce depression in the neonate. The drug may appear in breast milk and should be used with caution in nursing mothers.

Pharmacokinetics

Onset of Action: PO, 1–30 minutes. IM/SC, 15–20 minutes. IV, 2–3 minutes.
Peak Effect: PO, 1–3 hours. IM, 1 hour. IV, 15 minutes.
Duration of Action: PO, 3–6 hours. IM, 2 hours. IV, 1 hour.

Interactions

Potentiates CNS and circulatory depressant effects of other narcotic analgesics, volatile anesthetics, phenothiazines, sedative-hypnotics, alcohol, tricyclic antidepressants; analgesia enhanced and prolonged by narcotic and non-narcotic analgesics (e.g., aspirin, acetaminophen), α_2-agonists (e.g., clonidine).

Toxicity

Toxic Range: Not routinely monitored.
Manifestations: Somnolence, coma, respiratory arrest, apnea, cardiac arrhythmias, combined respiratory and metabolic acidosis, precipitation of withdrawal symptoms from opioids (abdominal cramps, vomiting, skin crawling, piloerection, nasal stuffiness, lacrimation, yawning, sweating, tremor, myalgia), circulatory collapse, cardiac arrest, death.
Antidote: Naloxone IV/IM/SC 0.4–2.0 mg. Repeat dose every 2 to 3 minutes to a maximum of 10–20 mg. If withdrawal symptoms are precipitated by pentazocine,

administer opioid agonists or benzodiazepines and treat
withdrawal symptomatically.

Management: Discontinue or reduce medication. Support ventilation and circulation (patent airway, oxygen,
IV fluids, vasopressors). Administer antidote. Monitor
blood gases, pH, and electrolytes. Correct acidosis and
electrolyte disturbance (lactic acidosis may require
sodium bicarbonate IV 1–2 mEq/kg). Symptomatic treatment. Airway-protected, ipecac syrup–induced emesis
(30 mL or 0.5 mL/kg ipecac syrup followed by 200 mL or
4 mL/kg of water or clear fluid) or gastric lavage (with
drug ingestion) followed by administration of activated
charcoal (PO 50–100 g or 1–2 g/kg).

Guidelines/Precautions

1. Reduce dosage in elderly patients and with
   concomitant use of narcotics and sedative-
   hypnotics.
2. Prescribe or supply an antiemetic (e.g., metoclopramide) for use in the event of nausea and/or
   vomiting.
3. Constipation may be more difficult to control than
   pain. Prevent and/or treat by daily administration
   of laxatives and stool softeners, for example,
   Colace (docusate sodium) 100–300 mg/day. Do
   not administer bulk-forming agents that contain
   methylcellulose, psyllium, or polycarbophil. Temporary arrest in the passage through the gastrointestinal tract may lead to fecal impaction or
   bowel obstruction.
4. Pentazocine has been abused in combination with
   tripelennamine (T's and blues) by drug abusers in
   an attempt to provide effects similar to IV heroin.

Potentially lethal side effects of this combination
and a lack of sterile technique include pulmonary
emboli, pulmonary edema, renal granulomas, vascular occlusion, ulcerations, abscesses, cellulitis,
bacterial endocarditis, and precipitation of acute
withdrawal in opiate-dependent patients.

5. Signs and symptoms of acute withdrawal following discontinuance of pentazocine and tripelennamine include shaking, chills, nausea, vomiting,
hallucinations, psychosis, restlessness, insomnia,
and drug craving. Benzodiazepines, hydroxyzine,
and/or pentazocine may be used in the management of acute withdrawal.

6. Addiction (psychological dependence) is characterized by a continued craving for a narcotic and
the need to use the narcotic for effects other than
for pain relief. The patient exhibits drug-seeking
behavior. Most patients with psychological dependence are also physically dependent, but the
reverse is rare in patients using narcotics for the
management of pain.

7. Drug combinations with adjuvant drugs enhance
analgesia (see pages xxvi–xliv).

8. Adjuvant drug therapies also include regional
blockade, trigger-point injections (with local anesthetics and steroids), and intravenous regional
anesthesia.

9. Adjuvant nondrug therapies include TENS and
modalities such as ice or heat application, ultrasound, and soft tissue mobilization.

10. Patients should be warned that pentazocine may
impair their ability to perform hazardous tasks
requiring mental alertness or physical coordina-

tion (e.g., driving a motor vehicle, operating heavy machinery).

11. The drug formulation may contain sodium metabisulfite, which may cause allergic reactions or anaphylaxis in susceptible individuals.

12. Abuse liability for pentazocine is reported to be less than that for codeine or propoxyphene. The oral dosage form has been reformulated to contain a small amount of naloxone that is inactive when administered orally in the amount present. However, if the tablets are ground up and solubilized for parenteral administration, the naloxone will antagonize the effects of pentazocine and precipitate withdrawal in opiate-dependent patients.

13. Pentazocine should be used with caution in patients who have been chronically receiving opiate agonists, because it does not suppress the abstinence syndrome in these patients and high doses may precipitate withdrawal symptoms. Titrated doses of benzodiazepines or opioid agonists may be used in the management of acute withdrawal.

14. Pentazocine is subject to control under the Federal Controlled Substances Act of 1970 as a Schedule IV (C-IV) drug.

Principal Adverse Reactions

Cardiovascular: Hypotension, tachycardia, circulatory depression, hypertension.

Pulmonary: Respiratory depression, dyspnea.

CNS: Sedation, euphoria, headache, disorientation, hallucinations, syncope.

Gastrointestinal: Nausea, vomiting, constipation, cramps, diarrhea.

Ocular: Miosis, blurred vision, nystagmus, diplopia.

Allergic: Rash, urticaria, facial edema.

Dermatologic: Pruritus; skin sloughing; injection site sclerosis of skin, subcutaneous tissue, and (rarely) underlying muscle.

Hematologic: Depression of white blood cells (reversible), eosinophilia.

Other: Urinary retention, muscle tremors, dry mouth.

PENTOSAN POLYSULFATE SODIUM

Class: Carbohydrate Derivative

Use(s): Treatment of interstitial cystitis.

Dosing: PO 100 mg three times daily. Take on an empty stomach—at least 1 hour before or 2 hours after meals. Reassess patient after 3 months. If there is no improvement and no limiting adverse effects, pentosan may be continued for another 3 months. After 6 months, patients who have failed to respond to pentosan are unlikely to receive any benefit from the drug.

Elimination: Hepatic, renal.

Preparations

Pentosan polysulfate sodium **(Elmiron):** Capsules: 100 mg.

Pharmacology

Pentosan polysulfate sodium is a low-molecular-weight heparin-like compound. Pentosan has anticoagulant and fibrinolytic effects with one-fifteenth the anticoagulant activity of heparin. Upon absorption, pentosan is mainly distributed to the uroepithelium of the genitourinary tract (with lesser amounts found in the liver, spleen, lung, skin, periosteum, and bone marrow) and adheres to the bladder wall mucosal membrane. In interstitial cystitis, the drug may act as a buffer to control cell permeability, preventing irritating solutes in the urine from reaching the cells. Clinical improvement of bladder pain (>50%) occurs within 6 months in 40% of patients.

Pharmacokinetics

Onset of Action: Few weeks.
Peak Effect: Within 3 months.
Duration of Action: Variable.

Interactions

Increased risk of bleeding with concomitant administration of coumarin anticoagulants, heparin, tissue-type plasminogen activator (tPA), streptokinase, or high-dose aspirin.

Toxicity

Toxic Range: Not routinely monitored.
Manifestations: Anticoagulation, bleeding, thrombocytopenia, liver function abnormalities, gastric distress.
Antidote: None.
Management: Discontinue or reduce medication. Support ventilation and circulation (patent airway, oxygen,

IV fluids, vasopressors). Administer antidote. Symptomatic treatment. Airway-protected, ipecac syrup–induced emesis (30 mL or 0.5 mL/kg ipecac syrup followed by 200 mL or 4 mL/kg of water or clear fluid) or gastric lavage followed by administration of activated charcoal (PO 50–100 g or 1–2 g/kg).

Guidelines/Precautions

1. Use with caution in patients undergoing invasive procedures or having signs/symptoms of underlying coagulopathy or other risk of bleeding (due to other therapies such as coumarin anticoagulants, heparin, tPA, streptokinase, or high-dose aspirin).
2. Use with caution in patients with liver insufficiency or those who have a history of heparin-induced thrombocytopenia.

Principal Adverse Reactions

CNS: Insomnia.
Gastrointestinal: Elevated liver enzymes, abdominal pain, diarrhea, dehydration.
Hematologic: Increased bleeding time, ecchymosis, epistaxis, gum hemorrhage.
Other: Alopecia.

PERPHENAZINE HYDROCHLORIDE

Class: Phenothiazine

Use(s): Antipsychotic, antiemetic, relief of hiccups, adjunct treatment of neuropathic pain syndromes (e.g., diabetic neuropathy, postherpetic neuralgia).

Dosing: *Pain:* PO 4–12 mg (0.08–0.24 mg/kg) once daily at bedtime. Titrate dose to effect. Monitor for akathisia, cogwheel rigidity, and orthostatic hypotension.

Medication should be administered on a fixed schedule (not as needed). After symptoms are controlled, dosage should be gradually reduced to the lowest level that will maintain relief of symptoms. Due to the risk of serious adverse effects (e.g., permanent tardive dyskinesia), perphenazine is not a drug of first choice for neuropathic pain. It should be used after initial therapy with antidepressants, narcotics, and/or nonsteroidal anti-inflammatory agents. It is advisable to obtain informed consent before instituting perphenazine therapy for chronic pain management.

Psychosis

PO: 4–16 mg (0.08–0.32 mg/kg) three times daily. Maximum daily dosage 64 mg.

IM: 5–10 mg (0.1–0.2 mg/kg) every 6 hours as needed.

Hiccups or nausea

PO: 8–24 mg (0.16–0.5 mg/kg) daily in divided doses.

IM: 5–10 mg (0.1–0.2 mg/kg) every 6 hours as needed.

Slow IV: 1–5 mg titrated (0.02–0.1 mg/kg). Dilute to 1 mg/mL with normal saline. Titrate in increments of 1 mg/min. Observe for hypotension.

Elimination: Hepatic.

Preparations

Perphenazine **(Trilafon)**
  Oral solution: 16mg/5mL.
  Tablets: 2mg, 4mg, 8mg, 16mg.
  Injection: 5mg/mL.
Perphenazine and amitriptyline hydrochloride **(various; previously Triavil):** Tablets, film coated: Perphenazine 2mg and amitriptyline hydrochloride 10mg; perphenazine 2mg and amitriptyline hydrochloride 25mg; perphenazine 4mg and amitriptyline hydrochloride 10mg; perphenazine 4mg and amitriptyline hydrochloride 25mg.

Pharmacology

Perphenazine is a phenothiazine tranquilizer with antiemetic, antiadrenergic, anticholinergic, and antiserotonergic actions. The neuroleptic actions are most likely due to antagonism of dopamine as a synaptic neurotransmitter in the basal ganglia and limbic portions of the forebrain. Strong extrapyramidal side effects are evidence of interference with the normal actions of dopamine. The significant antiemetic effects are mediated by dopamine receptor blockade in the medullary chemoreceptor trigger zone. At high doses, the antiarrhythmic effects may be evident and caused by the direct quinidine-like property or a local anesthetic effect.

Perphenazine may lower the seizure threshold and cause EEG changes. Therapeutic doses have little effect on respiration, but the drug may enhance respiratory depression produced by other CNS depressants. Perphenazine is relatively nonsedating and may be useful in chronic pain syndromes by altering the perception of pain and, where applicable, relieving psychosis and/or anxiety. Perphenazine is occasionally useful in postherpetic neuralgia and other neuropathies in which burning dyesthetic pain and lancinating sensations are prominent features. Unlike the anticonvulsant drugs, perphenazine appears to be helpful in the management of both qualities of pain.

Pharmacokinetics

Onset of Action: Antiemetic effects: PO, 30–60 minutes; IV/IM, within 30 minutes.
Peak Effect: Antiemetic effects: PO, 2–3 hours. Antipsychotic effects: PO, variable.
Duration of Action: Antiemetic/Antipsychotic effects: PO, 4–6 hours; IM, 3–4 hours.

Interactions

Potentiates depressant effects of barbiturates, narcotics, anesthetics; additive anticholinergic effects with atropine, glycopyrrolate, and other anticholinergics; decreased hepatic metabolism and increased serum levels and pharmacologic/toxic effects of tricyclic antidepressants; neuronal uptake and antihypertensive effects of guanethidine inhibited; α-adrenergic effects of epinephrine blocked, leaving unopposed β activity; may potentiate neuromuscular blockade in conjunction with polypeptide antibiotics; interferes with metabolism of phenytoin and may precipitate toxicity; lithium reduces bioavailability; mephentermine, epinephrine, thiazide diuretics potentiate perphenazine-induced hypotension; concomitant administration of propranolol increases plasma levels of both drugs.

Toxicity

Toxic Range: Not routinely monitored.

Manifestations: Hypotension, tardive dyskinesia (rhythmic involuntary movement of the tongue, face, mouth, or jaw), extrapyramidal symptoms (akathisia, cogwheel rigidity, oculogyric crisis), neuroleptic malignant syndrome (hyperpyrexia, muscle rigidity, altered mental status, autonomic instability).

Antidote: No specific antidote.

Management: Discontinue or reduce medication. Support ventilation and circulation (patent airway, oxygen, IV fluids, vasopressors). Phenylephrine or norepinephrine should be used to treat hypotension. Epinephrine should not be used because it may paradoxically further lower the blood pressure. Treat extrapyramidal symptoms with anticholinergic antiparkinsonian agents (e.g., benztropine IV/PO 1–2 mg two or three times daily, or trihexyphenidyl PO 5–15 mg daily) or with H_1 receptor antagonists such as diphenhydramine (IV/PO 25 mg). Treat neuroleptic malignant syndrome symptomatically and with dantrolene (IV 1.0–2.5 mg/kg every 6 hours for up to 2 days). Symptomatic treatment.

Guidelines/Precautions

1. Perphenazine may suppress laryngeal reflex, with possible aspiration of vomitus.
2. The drug may lower seizure threshold.
3. Use cautiously in geriatric patients; patients with glaucoma, prostatic hypertrophy, or seizure dis-

orders; and children with acute illnesses (e.g., chickenpox, measles).

4. Neuroleptic malignant syndrome, a rare but potentially fatal side effect, may manifest with hyperpyrexia, muscle rigidity, altered mental status, and evidence of autonomic instability (irregular pulse or blood pressure, tachycardia, diaphoresis, arrhythmias). Discontinue perphenazine; treat symptomatically and with dantrolene or bromocriptine (PO 2.5–10.0 mg three times daily).

5. Extrapyramidal reactions may consist of dystonic reactions, feelings of motor restlessness (akathisia), and parkinsonian signs and symptoms. Dystonic reactions occur more frequently in children, especially those with acute infections, whereas parkinsonian symptoms predominate in geriatric patients. Therapy should include discontinuation or reduction in dosage of perphenazine and treatment with an anticholinergic antiparkinsonian agent (e.g., benztropine, trihexyphenidyl) or with diphenhydramine (IV/PO 25 mg). Maintenance of an adequate airway should be instituted if necessary.

6. Do not use epinephrine to treat perphenazine-associated hypotension. Phenothiazines cause a reversal of epinephrine's vasopressor effects and a further lowering of blood pressure. Treat the drug-induced hypotension with norepinephrine or phenylephrine.

Principal Adverse Reactions

Cardiovascular: Hypotension, tachycardia, bradycardia.

CNS: Extrapyramidal reactions, seizures, syncope, drowsiness, exacerbation of psychosis.

Allergic: Urticaria, photosensitivity.
Hematologic: Agranulocytosis, hemolytic anemia.
Other: Neuroleptic malignant syndrome.

PHENYTOIN SODIUM

Class: Anticonvulsant, Antiarrhythmic

Use(s): Anticonvulsant; treatment of lancinating neuropathic pain, such as trigeminal neuralgia (tic douloureux) and other cranial neuralgias, postsympathectomy neuralgia, postherpetic neuralgia, diabetic neuropathy, phantom limb pain, the thalamic syndrome, or lightning tabetic pain; migraine; treatment of digitalis toxic arrhythmias, lidocaine-resistant ventricular arrhythmias, congenital prolonged QT syndrome, and ventricular arrhythmias occurring after congenital heart surgery.

Dosing: *Pain:* PO 100–150 mg (2–3 mg/kg) two to four times daily. It is advisable to obtain informed consent before institution of phenytoin for chronic pain management, given the potential for side effects. Analgesia may be enhanced by combination with other anticonvulsants (e.g., gabapentin), benzodiazepines (e.g., diazepam), and antidepressant agents (e.g., paroxetine) and by the use of nondrug therapies (e.g., transcutaneous electrical nerve stimulation [TENS]).

Anticonvulsant

Loading: IV/PO 1 g (10–15 mg/kg) in three divided doses over 6 hours.

Maintenance: IV/PO 100 mg three times
daily. (Children, 5 mg/kg/day. Do not
exceed IV rate of 50 mg/min or 0.5–
1.5 mg/kg/min in children.)

Therapeutic range: 10–20 µg/mL.

Antiarrhythmic

IV: 1.5 mg/kg every 5 minutes until arrhythmia is controlled (maximum dose 10–
15 mg/kg).

PO: 200–400 mg once daily (2–4 mg/kg/
day).

Elimination: Hepatic.

Preparations

Phenytoin sodium **(Dilantin, Phenytoin Sodium)**
Oral suspension: 25 mg/mL.
Injection: 50 mg/mL.

Phenytoin sodium **(Dilantin Infatabs, Phenytoin
Sodium):** Tablets, chewable: 50 mg.

Phenytoin sodium prompt **(Diphenylan Sodium):**
Capsules: 30 mg, 100 mg.

Phenytoin sodium extended **(Dilantin Kapseals):** Capsules, extended release: 30 mg, 100 mg.

Pharmacology

Phenytoin (also called diphenylhydantoin) is an anticonvulsant with primary site of action in the motor
cortex, where it stabilizes the neuronal membranes and
prevents the spread of activity through neuronal nets.
It stabilizes cellular electrical activity by either preventing influx or enhancing efflux of sodium ions. Phenytoin may be used for treatment of all kinds of epilepsy
except petit mal epilepsy. It is also a class 1b anti-

arrhythmic that decreases automaticity, duration of action potential, velocity of conduction, and the effective refractory period of cardiac fibers. Phenytoin use in chronic pain syndromes is primarily for suppression of the sharp lancinating and paroxysmal electrical shooting qualities common in neuropathic pain, such as in idiopathic trigeminal neuralgia. It is less effective than carbamazepine. Phenytoin is not as effective with the more chronic aching pains (e.g., in posttraumatic trigeminal pain). Phenytoin crosses the placenta and may result in birth defects. It should be avoided in pregnancy except in situations when discontinuation of therapy may pose a serious threat to the mother. The drug is distributed in breast milk and should be used in nursing mothers only if the benefits to the mother outweigh the risks to the infant.

Pharmacokinetics

Onset of Action: Anticonvulsant effects: IV, few minutes. Analgesic effects: 3–5 days.
Peak Effect: Anticonvulsant effects: IV, 1–2 hours; PO, 4–12 hours.
Duration of Action: Anticonvulsant effects: 10–15 hours (half-life).

Interactions

Serum level increased by diazepam, chloramphenicol, dicumarol, disulfiram, tolbutamide, salicylates, halothane, cimetidine, acute alcohol intake, sulfonamides, chlordiazepoxide; serum levels decreased by chronic alcohol abuse, reserpine, carbamazepine; oral absorption decreased by antacids containing calcium; seizures precipitated with use of tricyclic antidepressants;

decreases effects of corticosteroids, coumarin anticoagulants, quinidine, digitoxin, and furosemide.

Toxicity

Toxic Range: Toxicity is usually observed at levels
above 20 µg/mL.

Manifestations: Nystagmus, ataxia, dysarthria, nausea
and vomiting, diplopia, hyperglycemia, agitation, irritability, coma, respiratory arrest.

Antidote: No specific antidote.

Management: Discontinue or reduce medication. Support ventilation and circulation (patent airway, oxygen,
IV fluids, vasopressors). Symptomatic treatment. Airway-protected, ipecac syrup–induced emesis (30 mL or
0.5 mL/kg ipecac syrup followed by 200 mL or 4 mL/kg
of water or clear fluid) or gastric lavage (with drug
ingestion) followed by administration of activated charcoal (PO 50–100 g or 1–2 g/kg). Hemodialysis may be
useful. Total exchange transfusion has been used in the
treatment of severe intoxication in children.

Guidelines/Precautions

1. A trial of withdrawal of phenytoin therapy in
   chronic pain may be attempted after 4 to 6 months
   of therapy. Patients occasionally may maintain pain
   relief once they are off the medication.
2. Monitor serum blood levels to achieve optimal therapeutic effect. Blood counts should be determined
   prior to and at regular intervals during therapy.
3. Phenytoin may be associated with exfoliative dermatitis and the Stevens-Johnson syndrome as a
   non–dose-related hypersensitivity reaction. Discontinue the drug if a rash occurs.

4. Patients should be advised to maintain good oral hygiene and inform their dentist of the medication usage. They should be warned that phenytoin may impair their ability to perform activities requiring mental alertness or physical coordination (e.g., operating heavy machinery, driving a motor vehicle).

5. Because of its effect on ventricular automaticity, do not use IV phenytoin in sinus bradycardia, sinoatrial block, second- and third-degree atrioventricular block, or in patients with Adams-Stokes syndrome.

6. Use with caution in hypotension and severe myocardial insufficiency.

7. Abrupt withdrawal in epileptic patients may precipitate status epilepticus. Reduce dosage, discontinue phenytoin, or substitute other anticonvulsant medications gradually.

8. Administration of phenytoin during pregnancy may result in the fetal hydantoin syndrome. This may manifest as wide-set eyes, broad mandible, and finger deformities.

Principal Adverse Reactions

Cardiovascular: Hypotension, cardiovascular collapse, atrial and ventricular conduction depression, ventricular fibrillation.

CNS: Ataxia, confusion, dizziness, tremors, headaches, peripheral neuropathy.

Gastrointestinal: Nausea, vomiting, constipation.

Dermatologic: Stevens-Johnson syndrome, lupus erythematosus, rash, hypertrichosis.

Hematologic: Thrombocytopenia, leukopenia, megaloblastic anemia.

Other: Hyperglycemia, gingival hyperplasia.

PIROXICAM

Class: Nonsteroidal Anti-inflammatory Drug

Use(s): Symptomatic treatment of moderate to severe inflammatory and degenerative arthritis, primary dysmenorrhea, postoperative and posttraumatic pain, chronic pain, and cancer pain (especially with bone metastasis).

Dosing: *Pain or inflammatory disease:* PO 20–40 mg (0.4–0.8 mg/kg) daily, in one or two divided doses. Doses greater than 20 mg for over 3 weeks are associated with increased frequency of GI side effects, especially in the elderly. Therapeutic efficacy should not be assessed for at least 2 weeks after initiation of therapy or adjustment of dosage.

Administer analgesic regularly (not as needed). Addition of opioid analgesics, antidepressant agents, and use of nondrug therapies such as transcutaneous electrical nerve stimulation (TENS) may enhance analgesia (see pages xxvi–xliv for drug combinations). In rheumatoid arthritis or juvenile rheumatoid arthritis, second-line rheumatoid agents may include leflunomide (Arava), etanercept (Enbrel), antimalarials, or methotrexate. In geriatric patients and patients with decreased renal or hepatic function, decrease doses by one-third to one-half. The incidence of piroxicam-induced gastropathy may be decreased by administration with meals, milk, antacids, or sucralfate (PO 1g four times daily). Misoprostol (PO 100–200µg four times daily) may be used to prevent gastric ulcers in high-risk patients.

Elimination: Hepatic, renal.

Preparations

Piroxicam **(Feldene):** Capsules: 10mg, 20mg.

Pharmacology

An oxicam derivative and nonsteroidal anti-inflammatory drug (NSAID), piroxicam is structurally unrelated to other NSAIDs. The analgesic and anti-inflammatory activities of piroxicam are partly due to the inhibition of prostaglandin and leukotriene synthesis and to anti-bradykinin and lysosomal membrane stabilizing activity. Unlike with other NSAIDs, the antipyretic activity of piroxicam may occur secondary to inhibition of pyrogen-induced release of prostaglandins in the central nervous system (including the hypothalamus) and possibly to centrally mediated peripheral vasodilatation.

The analgesic and anti-inflammatory potency of piroxicam is similar to that of naproxen and about three times that of ibuprofen or aspirin. Piroxicam (like other NSAIDs) exhibits a ceiling effect for analgesia. Exceeding recommended doses results in increased toxicity without improvement in analgesia. Piroxicam may cause gastric mucosal damage with ulceration and/or bleeding. This may be due to inhibition of synthesis of prostaglandins (e.g., prostacyclin, prostaglandins of the E series) that have cytoprotective effects on GI mucosa. Inhibition of prostaglandin synthesis may also result in decreased uterine tone and contractility and prolonged gestation in the parturient and premature closure of the ductus arteriosus in the fetus. Piroxicam may inhibit platelet aggregation and prolong bleeding time. Uricosuric activity is undetermined.

Pharmacokinetics

Onset of Action: PO, analgesic effect 30–60 minutes; anti-inflammatory effect 7–12 days.
Peak Effect: PO, analgesic effect 1–2 hours; anti-inflammatory effect 2–3 weeks.
Duration of Action: PO, analgesic effect 48–72 hours.

Interactions

Risks of bleeding increased with concomitant NSAIDs, anticoagulant or heparin therapy, alcohol ingestion; decreases antihypertensive effects of β-adrenergic blocking agents; serum levels of piroxicam decreased slightly by concomitant aspirin; increased GI toxicity with concomitant aspirin; serum levels of piroxicam increased by concomitant probenecid; serum levels and toxic effects of salicylates, oral anticoagulants, phenytoin, sulfonamides, sulfonylureas, methotrexate, and lithium increased by concomitant piroxicam; GI absorption of piroxicam delayed by food and milk;

prostaglandin-mediated natriuretic effects of loop diuretics antagonized by piroxicam.

Toxicity

Toxic Range: Not routinely monitored.
Manifestations: *Acute:* Vomiting, diarrhea, acidosis, dehydration, pancytopenia, GI bleeding, hyponatremia, seizures.
Antidote: None.
Management: Discontinue or reduce medication. Correct fluid, electrolyte, and acid-base disturbances. Support ventilation and circulation (patent airway, oxygen, IV fluids, vasopressors). Airway-protected, ipecac syrup–induced emesis (30 mL or 0.5 mL/kg ipecac syrup followed by 200 mL or 4 mL/kg of water or clear fluid) or gastric lavage (with drug ingestion) followed by administration of activated charcoal (PO 50–100 g or 1–2 g/kg). Control seizures (IV benzodiazepines or barbiturates). Symptomatic treatment.

Guidelines/Precautions

1. Use with caution in patients with active GI lesions (e.g., erosive gastritis, peptic ulcer), a history of recurrent GI lesions, hepatic or renal dysfunction, preexisting hypoprothrombinemia, or vitamin K deficiency. Piroxicam may cause peripheral edema and should be used cautiously in patients with heart failure, hypertension, or other conditions associated with fluid retention.

2. Renal prostaglandins may have a supportive role in maintaining renal perfusion in patients with prerenal conditions. Piroxicam should be avoided in

such patients because it may cause a dose-dependent decrease in prostaglandin formation and thus precipitate renal decompensation.

3. Carefully observe patients with coagulation disorders and those receiving drug therapy that interferes with hemostasis.

4. Use with caution in pregnancy and only when the perceived benefits outweigh the risks.

5. Patient response to NSAIDs is variable. Patients who do not respond to or cannot tolerate piroxicam may be successfully treated with another NSAID.

6. Piroxicam and salicylates should not be administered concomitantly because there may not be any therapeutic advantage and incidences of adverse GI side effects may be increased.

7. Contraindicated in patients with previously demonstrated hypersensitivity to piroxicam or with the complete or partial syndrome of nasal polyps, angioedema, or bronchospastic reactivity to aspirin or other NSAIDs.

8. Signs and symptoms of infection or other diseases may be masked by the antipyretic and anti-inflammatory effects of piroxicam.

9. Monitor stool for blood every 14 days, and monitor BUN, serum creatinine, and urinalysis every 1 to 2 months when administering piroxicam at chronic high doses.

Principal Adverse Reactions

Cardiovascular: Peripheral edema, fluid retention, hypertension, palpitation.
Pulmonary: Dyspnea, bronchospasm.

CNS: Drowsiness, dizziness, headache, anxiety, confusion.

Gastrointestinal: Diarrhea, ulceration, bleeding, dyspepsia, nausea, vomiting, cholestatic jaundice.

Genitourinary: Renal papillary necrosis, interstitial nephritis, acute renal failure, azotemia, cystitis, hematuria.

Dermatologic: Pruritus, urticaria.

Hematologic: Granulocytopenia, leukopenia, thrombocytopenia, aplastic anemia, hemolytic anemia, prolongation of bleeding time.

Other: Tinnitus, blurred vision.

PREDNISONE

Class: Corticosteroid

Use(s): Treatment of refractory bone pain; treatment of aching, burning, lancinating neuropathic pain and pain caused by malignant lesions of the brachial and lumbosacral plexus; prophylaxis of postherpetic neuralgia; treatment of inflammatory disease (e.g., systemic lupus erythematosus); treatment of aspiration pneumonitis, bronchial asthma, allergic reactions; prevention of cluster headache; prevention of rejection in organ transplantation.

Dosing: *Bone pain, neuropathic pain, plexus pain:* PO 30–100 mg daily in two to four divided doses.

Prophylaxis of cluster headache: PO 40 mg daily in two to four divided doses.

Prophylaxis of postherpetic neuralgia: PO 60–80 mg daily in two to four divided doses.

Inflammatory diseases: PO 5–60 mg daily in two to four divided doses.

Taper off prednisone dose if used for more than a few days. Avoid concomitant NSAID use.

Elimination: Hepatic.

Preparations

Prednisone **(Meticorten, Prednisone, Deltasone, Cortan, Orasone, Panasol):** Tablets: 1 mg, 2.5 mg, 5 mg, 10 mg, 20 mg, 50 mg.

Prednisone **(Prednicen-M):** Tablets, film coated: 5 mg.

Prednisone **(Prednisone Oral Solution, Liquid Pred):** Oral solution: 1 mg/mL.

Prednisone **(Prednisone Intensol):** Oral solution, concentrate: 5 mg/mL.

Pharmacology

Prednisone is a synthetic glucocorticoid with potent anti-inflammatory effect: 5 mg prednisone is equivalent to 0.75 mg dexamethasone, 4 mg methylprednisolone, or 20 mg cortisol. Prednisone may decrease the number and activity of inflammatory cells, decrease capillary wall permeability and edema formation, enhance the effects of β-adrenergic drugs on cyclic AMP production, and inhibit bronchoconstrictor mechanisms. Like other glucocorticoids, prednisone promotes protein catabolism, gluconeogenesis, renal excretion of calcium, and redistribution of fat from peripheral to central areas of the body. Prednisone has half of the sodium-retaining property of hydrocortisone. It may suppress the hypothalamic-pituitary-adrenal (HPA) axis.

Prednisone is useful in the management of acute and chronic cancer pain. In metastatic bone pain, prednisone may interfere with the formation of prostaglandin E by inhibiting tumor-secreted phospho-lipase A_2, which catalyzes the release of arachidonic acid from plasma membranes. Prednisone may ameliorate painful nerve or spinal cord compression by reducing edema in tumor and nerve tissue. Short-term therapy (1–2 weeks) may be useful in the management of pain caused by malignant lesions of the brachial or lumbosacral plexus. In patients with cluster headache, prednisone enhances the vasoconstrictor and prophylactic effects of methysergide. In moribund patients, prednisone may provide a sense of well-being, increase appetite, and relieve tumor-related pain.

Pharmacokinetics

Onset of Action: Anti-inflammatory effects: PO, few minutes.
Peak Effect: Anti-inflammatory effects: PO, 12–24 hours.
Duration of Action: Anti-inflammatory effects/HPA suppression: PO, 30–36 hours.

Interactions

Clearance enhanced by phenytoin, phenobarbital, rifampin, ephedrine; alters response to coumarin anticoagulants; increases insulin requirements; interacts with anticholinesterase agents (e.g., neostigmine) to produce severe weakness in patients with myasthenia gravis; potassium-wasting effects enhanced with potassium-depleting diuretics (e.g., thiazides, furosemide); diminishes response to toxoids and live or inactivated vaccines; increased risks of GI bleeding with concomitant NSAIDs.

Toxicity

Toxic Range: Not defined.

Manifestations: *Withdrawal after long-term use:* Acute adrenal insufficiency (fever, hypotension, dyspnea, dizziness, fainting, hypoglycemia). *Prolonged administration:* Cushingoid changes (moon face, central obesity, hypertension, osteoporosis, diabetes, peptic ulcer, increased susceptibility to infection, electrolyte and fluid imbalance).

Antidote: No specific antidote.

Management: Taper off or gradually reduce medication (alternate-day medication). Supplement medication during times of stress. Support ventilation and circulation (patent airway, oxygen, IV fluids, vasoactive drugs). Symptomatic treatment.

Guidelines/Precautions

1. Adrenocortical insufficiency may occur with rapid withdrawal of prednisone.
2. Use with caution in patients with hypertension, congestive heart failure, thromboembolytic tendencies, hypothyroidism, cirrhosis, myasthenia gravis, peptic ulcer, diverticulitis, nonspecific ulcerative colitis, fresh intestinal anastomosis, psychosis, seizure disorders, or systemic fungal and viral infections.
3. Administration of live virus vaccines (e.g., small-

pox) is contraindicated in patients receiving immunosuppressive doses.

4. Avoid rapid withdrawal, which may exacerbate pain independent of progression of systemic cancer (pseudorheumatoid syndrome).

5. Patients with inflammatory disease (e.g., rheumatoid arthritis, systemic lupus erythematosus) on long-term low-dose prednisone therapy should be placed on calcium supplements (1000 mg elemental calcium daily) to prevent the development of osteoporosis.

Principal Adverse Reactions

Cardiovascular: Arrhythmias, hypertension, congestive heart failure in susceptible patients.

CNS: Seizures, increased intracranial pressure, steroid psychosis.

Gastrointestinal: Ulceration, bleeding.

Dermatologic: Impaired wound healing, petechiae, erythema.

Ocular: Increased intraocular pressure, subcapsular cataracts.

Metabolic: Fluid retention, sodium retention, potassium depletion.

Endocrinologic: Secondary adrenocortical and pituitary unresponsiveness during stress, growth suppression, increased requirements for insulin.

Musculoskeletal: Myopathy, weakness, osteoporosis, aseptic necrosis.

Other: Thromboembolism, diminished response to toxoids and live or inactivated vaccines, increased susceptibility to infection and masking of symptoms of infection.

PRILOCAINE HYDROCHLORIDE

Class: Local Anesthetic

Use(s): Regional anesthesia.

Dosing: *Intravenous regional*

Upper extremities: 200–250 mg (40–50 mL of 0.5% solution).

Lower extremities: 250–300 mg (100–120 mL of 0.25% solution).

Do not add epinephrine for intravenous regional block. If desired, add fentanyl 50 µg to enhance the block and/or a muscle relaxant (pretreatment doses only), for example, pancuronium 0.5 mg. Rate of onset and potency of local anesthetic action may be enhanced by carbonation. (Add 5 mL of 8.4% sodium bicarbonate with 40 mL of 0.5% prilocaine. Do not use if there is precipitation.)

Topical: See dosing information for EMLA (Eutectic mixture of lidocaine and prilocaine).

Infiltration/Peripheral nerve block: 1–15 mL (0.5–2.0% solution) or 0.5–6.0 mg/kg.

Brachial plexus block: 300–750 mg (30–50 mL of 1.0–1.5% solution). (Children, 0.5–0.75 mL/kg.) With high doses add epinephrine 1:200,000 to decrease systemic toxicity (in the absence of any contraindications). Add tetracaine 0.5–1.0 mg/kg to prolong the block.

> *Epidural:* 10–25 mL (1–2% solution) or 100–500 mg. Maximum safe dose: 6 mg/kg without epinephrine; 9 mg/kg with epinephrine 1:200,000. Solutions containing preservatives should not be used for epidural block.

No more than 600 mg prilocaine should be administered within a 2-hour period in healthy adults. Except where contraindicated, vasoconstrictor drugs may be added to increase effect and prolong local or regional anesthesia. For dosage and route guidelines, see the "Dosing" section of Epinephrine. Do not use vasoconstrictor drugs for IV regional anesthesia or local anesthesia of end organs (digits, penis, ears).

Elimination: Hepatic, pulmonary.

Preparations

Prilocaine hydrochloride **(Citanest Plain):** Injection: 4%.

Prilocaine hydrochloride **(Citanest Forte):** Injection 4% with epinephrine bitartrate 1:200,000.

Pharmacology

This amide local anesthetic stabilizes the neuronal membrane and prevents the initiation and transmission of impulses. Equipotent to lidocaine but longer in duration, prilocaine is less toxic and undergoes rapid hepatic metabolism to *ortho*-toluidine, which oxidizes hemoglobin to methemoglobin. When the dose of prilocaine exceeds 600 mg there may be sufficient methemoglobin to cause the patient to appear cyanotic, and oxygen-carrying capacity is reduced. The unique ability to cause dose-related methemoglobinemia limits its clinical usefulness, with the exception of intravenous regional anesthesia.

Pharmacokinetics

Onset of Action: Infiltration, 1–2 minutes. Epidural, 5–15 minutes.
Peak Effect: Infiltration/Epidural, <30 minutes. IV, 15–20 minutes.
Duration of Action: Infiltration, 0.5–1.5 hours; with epinephrine, 2–6 hours. Epidural, 1–3 hours, prolonged with epinephrine.

Interactions

Methemoglobinemia at high doses (greater than 600 mg); reduced clearance with coadministration of β-blockers, cimetidine; benzodiazepines, barbiturates, and volatile anesthetics increase seizure threshold; duration of regional anesthesia prolonged by vasoconstrictor agents (e.g., epinephrine) and α_2-agonists (e.g., clonidine); alkalinization increases rate of onset and potency of local or regional anesthesia.

Toxicity

Toxic Range: >6 μg/mL.
Manifestations: Hypotension, confusion, slurred speech, perioral numbness, tinnitus, seizures, arrhythmias, respiratory depression, circulatory collapse, cardiac arrest.
Antidote: No specific antidote. Treat methemoglobinemia with oxygen and methylene blue (IV 1–2 mg/kg injected over 5 minutes).

Management: Discontinue or reduce medication. Support ventilation and circulation (patent airway, oxygen, IV fluids, vasopressors). Benzodiazepines (diazepam IV 0.05–0.2 mg/kg, midazolam IV/IM 0.025–0.1 mg/kg) or barbiturates (thiopental sodium IV 0.5–2.0 mg/kg) to control seizures. Prolonged cardiopulmonary resuscitation with cardiac arrest: Sodium bicarbonate IV 1–2 mEq/kg to treat cardiac toxicity (sodium channel blockade); bretylium IV 5 mg/kg; DC cardioversion/defibrillation for ventricular arrhythmias. Administer antidote for dose-related methemoglobinemia. Remove ingested drug by induced emesis followed by activated charcoal. Hypersensitivity reactions: Remove from further exposure and treat dermatitis.

Guidelines/Precautions

1. Treat methemoglobinemia with oxygen and methylene blue (1–2 mg/kg injected over 5 minutes).
2. Use with caution in patients with hypovolemia, severe congestive heart failure, shock, or any form of heart block.
3. Prilocaine is contraindicated in infants younger than 6 months (low dose may cause severe methemoglobinemia) and in patients with hypersensitivity to amide-type local anesthetics.
4. In intravenous regional blocks, deflate the cuff after 40 minutes and no less than 20 minutes. Between 20 and 40 minutes, the cuff can be deflated, reinflated immediately, and finally deflated after a minute to reduce the sudden absorption of anesthetic into the systemic circulation.
5. The level of sympathetic blockade (bradycardia with block above T5) determines the degree of hypotension (often heralded by nausea and vomit-

ing) following epidural or intrathecal prilocaine. Fluid hydration (10–20 mL/kg normal saline or lactated Ringer's solution), vasopressor agents (e.g., ephedrine), and left uterine displacement in pregnant patients may be used for prophylaxis and/or treatment. Administer atropine to treat bradycardia.

6. Epidural injections should be avoided when the patient has hypovolemic shock, septicemia, infection at the injection site, or coagulopathy.

Principal Adverse Reactions

Cardiovascular: Hypotension, arrhythmia, collapse.
Pulmonary: Respiratory depression, paralysis.
CNS: Seizures, tinnitus, blurred vision.
Hematologic: Methemoglobinemia.
Allergic: Urticaria, anaphylactoid reactions.
Epidural/Caudal: High spinal, urinary retention, lower extremity weakness and paralysis, loss of sphincter control, headache, backache, cranial nerve palsies, slowing of labor.

PROCAINE HYDROCHLORIDE

Class: Local Anesthetic

Use(s): Regional anesthesia, systemic analgesia for treatment of painful conditions (e.g., neuropathic pain, reflex sympathetic dystrophy, burn or sickle cell pain); pruritus.

Dosing: *Infiltration:* <500 mg of 0.5–2.0% solution.
Epidural: 10–25 mL (<500 mg) of 1–2% solution.

Spinal: 0.5–2.0 mL (50–200 mg) of 10% solution with glucose 5%.

Maximum safe dose: 10 mg/kg without epinephrine; 15 mg/kg with epinephrine. Solutions containing preservatives should not be used for epidural or spinal block. Except where contraindicated, vasoconstrictor drugs may be added to increase effect and prolong local or regional anesthesia. For dosage and route guidelines, see the "Dosing" section of Epinephrine (p. 204). Do not use vasoconstrictor drugs for IV regional anesthesia or local anesthesia of end organs (digits, penis, ears).

Systemic analgesia and pruritus: Slow IV 4–5 mg/kg (0.1% solution). Administer over 20 to 30 minutes. Observe for symptoms of toxicity (e.g., hypotension, slurred speech, drowsiness) and adjust rate accordingly.

Elimination: Plasma pseudocholinesterase.

Preparations

Procaine hydrochloride **(Novocain)**
  Injection: 1%, 2%.
  Spinal (hyperbaric solution): 10%.

Pharmacology

Procaine is a benzoic acid ester local anesthetic. It stabilizes the neuronal membrane and prevents the initiation and transmission of impulses. It possesses vasodilator activity and is ineffective as a surface anesthetic. When administered intravenously, procaine may produce central analgesia. This may be due to local anesthetic effects, inhibition of release of neurotransmitters (e.g., substance P, ATP from nociceptive afferent C fibers), modulation of information transfer along primary afferents, and central sympathetic blockade with decrease in pain-induced reflex vasoconstriction. Procaine has a rapid onset of action and a relatively short duration that depends on the anesthetic technique, the type of block, the concentration, and the individual patient. Vasoconstrictor drugs may be added to the procaine solution to delay systemic absorption and prolong the duration of action.

Pharmacokinetics

Onset of Action: Infiltration/Spinal, 2–5 minutes. Epidural, 5–25 minutes.
Peak Effect: Infiltration/Epidural/Spinal, <30 minutes.
Duration of Action: Infiltration, 0.25–0.5 hours; with epinephrine, 0.5–1.5 hours. Epidural/Spinal, 0.5–1.5 hours, prolonged with epinephrine.

Interactions

Prolongs the effect of succinylcholine; metabolite (PABA) inhibits action of sulfonamides and aminosalicylic acid; toxicity enhanced by anti-cholinesterases (which inhibit degradation); benzodiazepines, barbiturates, and volatile anesthetics increase seizure threshold; duration of regional anesthesia prolonged by vasoconstrictor agents (e.g., epinephrine) and α_2-agonists (e.g., clonidine); alkalinization increases rate of onset and potency of local or regional anesthesia.

Toxicity

Toxic Range: Not routinely monitored.

Manifestations: Hypotension, confusion, slurred speech, perioral numbness, tinnitus, seizures, arrhythmias, respiratory depression, circulatory collapse, cardiac arrest.

Antidote: No specific antidote.

Management: Discontinue or reduce medication. Support ventilation and circulation (patent airway, oxygen, IV fluids, vasopressors). Benzodiazepines (diazepam IV 0.05–0.2 mg/kg, midazolam IV/IM 0.025–0.1 mg/kg) or barbiturates (thiopental sodium IV 0.5–2.0 mg/kg) to control seizures. Prolonged cardiopulmonary resuscitation with cardiac arrest: Sodium bicarbonate IV 1–2 mEq/kg to treat cardiac toxicity (sodium channel blockade); bretylium IV 5 mg/kg; DC cardioversion/ defibrillation for ventricular arrhythmias. Remove ingested drug by induced emesis followed by activated charcoal. Hypersensitivity reactions: Remove from further exposure and treat dermatitis.

Guidelines/Precautions

1. Use with caution in patients with severe disturbances of cardiac rhythm, shock, or heart block.
2. Reduce doses in obstetric and in elderly patients.
3. Contraindicated in patients with hypersensitivity to procaine or ester-type local anesthetics and patients with allergy to suntan lotion (contains PABA derivatives).
4. Epidural, caudal, or intrathecal injections should be avoided when the patient has hypovolemic shock, septicemia, infection at the injection site, or coagulopathy.

Principal Adverse Reactions

Cardiovascular: Hypotension, bradycardia, arrhythmias, heart block.

Pulmonary: Respiratory depression, arrest.

CNS: Tinnitus, seizures, dizziness, restlessness, loss of hearing, euphoria, diplopia, postspinal headache, arachnoiditis, palsies.

Allergic: Urticaria, pruritus, angioneurotic edema.

Epidural/Caudal/Spinal: High spinal; loss of bladder and bowel control; permanent motor, sensory, and autonomic (sphincter control) deficit of lower segments.

PROCHLORPERAZINE

Class: Phenothiazine

Use(s): Antiemetic, antipsychotic, adjunct treatment of migraine and neuropathic pain (e.g., diabetic neuropathy, postherpetic neuralgia).

Dosing: *Antiemetic/Pain*

PO: 5–10 mg three to four times daily.

Rectal: 25 mg twice daily.

IV/IM: 5–10 mg (at 5 mg/mL/min).

Do not administer subcutaneously because of local irritation.

Antipsychotic

PO: 5–10 mg three to four times daily. Titrate doses upward every 2 or 3 days until symptoms are controlled or adverse effects become troublesome.

IM initial dose: 10–20 mg. Repeat every 1–4 hours to control symptoms if necessary.

Generally no more than three or four
doses are necessary.

IM prolonged therapy: 10–20 mg every 4–6
hours. After control of symptoms, replace with oral medication at the same
dosage level or higher.

Elimination: Hepatic.

Preparations

Prochlorperazine **(Compazine):** Rectal suppositories:
2.5 mg, 5 mg, 25 mg.
Prochlorperazine edisylate **(Compazine)**
Oral solution: 1 mg/mL.
Injection: 5 mg/mL.
Prochlorperazine maleate **(Compazine)**
Capsules, extended release: 10 mg, 15 mg, 30 mg.
Tablets, film coated: 5 mg, 10 mg, 25 mg.

Pharmacology

Prochlorperazine is a phenothiazine tranquilizer with
pharmacologic actions similar to those of chlorpromazine, and with strong antiemetic, antiadrenergic, anticholinergic, and sedative effects. It has weak
antiserotonergic, antihistaminic, and ganglion-blocking
activity. The neuroleptic actions are most likely due to
antagonism of dopamine as a synaptic neurotransmitter
in the basal ganglia and limbic portions of the forebrain.
Moderate extrapyramidal side effects are evidence of
interference with the normal actions of dopamine. The
strong antiemetic effects are mediated by dopamine
receptor blockade in the medullary chemoreceptor
trigger zone. Prochlorperazine may lower the seizure

threshold and cause EEG changes. Therapeutic doses have little effect on respiration, but the drug may enhance respiratory depression produced by other CNS depressants.

Prochlorperazine is commonly used to control the emetic effects of opioid analgesics. The drug may be useful in chronic pain syndromes by altering the perception of pain and, where applicable, relieving psychosis and/or anxiety. Prochlorperazine has been used in the abortive and antiemetic therapy of migraine, either as a sole agent or in combination with other drugs (e.g., narcotics, dexamethasone). Prochlorperazine may be useful in postherpetic neuralgia and other neuropathies in which burning dyesthetic pain and lancinating sensations are prominent features. Unlike the anticonvulsant drugs, prochlorperazine may be helpful in the management of both qualities of pain. Due to the risk of serious adverse effects (e.g., permanent tardive dyskinesia), prochlorperazine is not a drug of first choice for neuropathic pain. It should be used after initial therapy with antidepressants, narcotics, and/or nonsteroidal anti-inflammatory drugs. It is advisable to obtain informed consent before instituting prochlorperazine therapy for chronic pain management.

Pharmacokinetics

Onset of Action: Antiemetic effects: IV, few minutes; IM, 10–20 minutes; PO, 30–40 minutes; rectal, 60 minutes.

Peak Effect: Antiemetic effects: IV/IM/PO, 15–30 minutes.

Duration of Action: Antiemetic effects: IV/IM/PO/Rectal, 3–4 hours; PO extended release, 10–12 hours.

Interactions

Potentiates depressant effects of barbiturates, narcotics, anesthetics; additive anticholinergic effects with atropine, glycopyrrolate, and other anticholinergics; decreases hepatic metabolism and increases serum levels and pharmacologic/toxic effects of tricyclic antidepressants; inhibits neuronal uptake and antihypertensive effects of guanethidine; blocks α-adrenergic effects of epinephrine, leaving unopposed β activity; may potentiate neuromuscular blockade in conjunction with polypeptide antibiotics; interferes with metabolism of phenytoin and may precipitate toxicity; encephalopathic syndrome with coadministration of lithium; mephentermine, epinephrine, and thiazide diuretics potentiate prochlorperazine-induced hypotension; concomitant administration of propranolol increases plasma levels of both drugs.

Toxicity

Toxic Range: Not routinely monitored.
Manifestations: Hypotension, QT interval prolongation, respiratory depression, tardive dyskinesia (rhythmic involuntary movement of the tongue, face, mouth, or jaw), extrapyramidal symptoms (akathisia, cogwheel rigidity, oculogyric crisis), neuroleptic malignant syndrome (hyperpyrexia, muscle rigidity, altered mental status, autonomic instability).
Antidote: No specific antidote.
Management: Discontinue or reduce medication. Support ventilation and circulation (patent airway, oxygen, IV fluids, vasopressors). Phenylephrine or norepinephrine should be used to treat hypotension; epinephrine should not be used because it may paradoxically fur-

ther lower the blood pressure. Treat extrapyramidal symptoms with anticholinergic antiparkinsonian agents (e.g., benztropine IV/PO 1–2 mg two or three times daily, or trihexyphenidyl PO 5–15 mg daily) or with H_1 receptor antagonists such as diphenhydramine (IV/PO 25 mg). Treat neuroleptic malignant syndrome symptomatically and with dantrolene (IV 1.0–2.5 mg/kg every 6 hours for up to 2 days) or bromocriptine (PO 2.5–10.0 mg three times daily). Symptomatic treatment.

Guidelines/Precautions

1. Extrapyramidal reactions may consist of dystonic reactions, feelings of motor restlessness (akathisia), and parkinsonian signs and symptoms. Dystonic reactions occur more frequently in children, especially those with acute infections, whereas parkinsonian symptoms predominate in geriatric patients.
2. Use cautiously in geriatric patients; in patients with glaucoma, prostatic hypertrophy, or seizure disorders; and in children with acute illnesses (e.g., chickenpox, measles).
3. Neuroleptic malignant syndrome (hyperpyrexia, tachycardia, muscle rigidity) should be managed by immediate discontinuation of prochlorperazine and symptomatic and supportive treatment, including correction of fluid and electrolyte imbalances, administration of dantrolene or bromocriptine, cooling of the patient, maintenance of renal function, management of cardiovascular instability, and prevention of respiratory complications.
4. Prochlorperazine possesses little or no anti-motion-sickness activity.
5. Do not crush or chew sustained-release capsules.

6. Do not use epinephrine to treat prochlorperazine-induced hypotension. Phenothiazines cause a reversal of epinephrine's vasopressor effects and a further lowering of blood pressure. Treat the drug-induced hypotension with norepinephrine or phenylephrine.

Principal Adverse Reactions

Cardiovascular: Hypotension, hypertension.
Pulmonary: Bronchospasm, laryngeal edema.
CNS: Drowsiness, dizziness, extrapyramidal reactions, tardive dyskinesia.
Gastrointestinal/Hepatic: Cholestatic jaundice, nausea, vomiting.
Endocrinologic: Gynecomastia, amenorrhea, hyperglycemia.
Allergic: Angioneurotic edema, anaphylactoid reactions.

PROMETHAZINE HYDROCHLORIDE

Class: Phenothiazine

Use(s): Antiemetic; sedative; adjunct to analgesics for treatment of migraine, acute, chronic, and cancer pain.

Dosing: *Antiemetic, sedative, analgesic adjunct:* IV/ Deep IM/PO/Rectal: 12.5–50.0 mg. (Do not administer subcutaneously.)

Elimination: Hepatic.

Preparations

Promethazine hydrochloride **(Phenergan):** Tablets: 12.5 mg, 25 mg, 50 mg.

Promethazine hydrochloride **(Phenergan Syrup, Pherazine Syrup):** Oral solution: 6.25 mg/5 mL, 25 mg/5 mL.

Promethazine hydrochloride **(Phenergan, Promethazine Hydrochloride Suppositories, Promethegan):** Rectal suppositories: 12.5 mg, 25 mg, 50 mg.

Promethazine hydrochloride **(Phenergan, Anergan 25, Phenazine 25, Prorex, V-Gan-25):** Injection: 25 mg/mL.

Promethazine hydrochloride **(Phenergan, Anergan 50, Phenazine 50, Phencen-50, Phenoject-50, Prorex, V-Gan-50):** Injection, for IM use only: 50 mg/mL.

Promethazine hydrochloride and meperidine hydrochloride **(Mepergan Fortis):** Oral capsules: Promethazine hydrochloride 25 mg and meperidine hydrochloride 50 mg.

Promethazine hydrochloride and phenylephrine hydrochloride **(Phenergan VC, Promethazine Hydrochloride VC):** Oral solution: Promethazine hydrochloride 6.25 mg/5 mL and phenylephrine hydrochloride 5 mg/5 mL.

Promethazine hydrochloride and meperidine hydrochloride **(Mepergan):** Injection: Promethazine hydrochloride 25 mg/mL and meperidine hydrochloride 25 mg/mL.

Pharmacology

This phenothiazine derivative does not possess neuroleptic or antipsychotic activity in typical standard doses. It is a good histamine H_1 receptor antagonist with sedative, antiemetic, anticholinergic, and anti-motion-sickness effects. Promethazine is commonly used to

control the emetic effects of opioid analgesics. Promethazine lacks analgesic activity but may potentiate other
analgesic agents (e.g., in the treatment of migraine
attacks). The drug competitively antagonizes in varying
degrees most but not all of the pharmacologic effects
of histamine mediated at H_1 receptors. The drug is
not effective in the treatment of bronchial asthma, allergic reactions, or angioedema in which chemical mediators other than histamine are responsible for the
symptoms.

Pharmacokinetics

Onset of Action: IV, 2–5 minutes. IM/PO/Rectal, 15–30
minutes.
Peak Effect: IV/IM/PO/Rectal, <2 hours.
Duration of Action: IV/IM/PO/Rectal, 2–8 hours.

Interactions

Potentiates CNS and circulatory depressant effect of
alcohol, opioid analgesics, volatile anesthetics, and
sedative-hypnotics, including barbiturates, tranquilizers;
intra-arterial or subcutaneous injection may result in
necrosis and gangrene; may reverse vasopressor effect
of epinephrine; extrapyramidal reactions at high doses
and with concomitant use of monoamine oxidase
(MAO) inhibitors.

Toxicity

Toxic Range: Not routinely monitored.
Manifestations: Hypotension, QT interval prolongation, respiratory depression, tardive dyskinesia (rhythmic involuntary movement of the tongue, face, mouth,
or jaw), extrapyramidal symptoms (akathisia, cogwheel

rigidity, oculogyric crisis), neuroleptic malignant syndrome (hyperpyrexia, muscle rigidity, altered mental status, autonomic instability).

Antidote: No specific antidote.

Management: Discontinue or reduce medication. Support ventilation and circulation (patent airway, oxygen, IV fluids, vasopressors). Phenylephrine or norepinephrine should be used to treat hypotension; epinephrine should not be used because it may paradoxically further lower the blood pressure. Treat extrapyramidal symptoms with anticholinergic antiparkinsonian agents (e.g., benztropine IV/PO 1–2 mg two or three times daily, or trihexyphenidyl PO 5–15 mg daily) or with H_1 receptor antagonists such as diphenhydramine (IV/PO 25 mg). Treat neuroleptic malignant syndrome symptomatically and with dantrolene (IV 1.0–2.5 mg/kg every 6 hours for up to 2 days) or bromocriptine (PO 2.5–10.0 mg three times daily). Symptomatic treatment.

Guidelines/Precautions

1. Extrapyramidal reactions may consist of dystonic reactions, feelings of motor restlessness (akathisia), and parkinsonian signs and symptoms. Dystonic reactions occur more frequently in children, especially those with acute infections, whereas parkinsonian symptoms predominate in geriatric patients.
2. Use with caution in patients with cardiovascular disease, liver dysfunction, asthmatic attack, narrow-angle glaucoma, bone marrow depression, prostatic hypertrophy, stenosing peptic ulcer, or pyloroduodenal and bladder neck obstruction.
3. Use with caution, if at all, in children.

4. Produces a high degree of drowsiness and sedation at clinically effective doses. Doses of opioid analgesics should be reduced when used in combination with promethazine.
5. Do not use epinephrine to treat promethazine-induced hypotension. Phenothiazines cause a reversal of epinephrine's vasopressor effects and a further lowering of blood pressure. Treat the drug-induced hypotension with norepinephrine or phenylephrine.

Principal Adverse Reactions

Cardiovascular: Hypotension, bradycardia, tachycardia, extrasystoles.
Pulmonary: Bronchospasm, nasal stuffiness.
CNS: Drowsiness, sedation, dizziness, confusion, tremors.
Gastrointestinal: Nausea, vomiting.
Hematologic: Leukopenia, agranulocytosis, thrombocytopenia.

PROPOXYPHENE HYDROCHLORIDE

Class: Narcotic Agonist

Use(s): Treatment of acute, chronic, and cancer pain.

Dosing: *Analgesia:* PO 65 mg every 4 hours. Maximum daily dose 390 mg. Each 65 mg of propoxyphene hydrochloride is equivalent to 100 mg of propoxyphene napsylate. Administer analgesic regularly (not as needed). Due to impaired elimination, accumulation and excess sedation may occur in patients with renal or hepatic dysfunction. Analgesia may be enhanced by addition of adjuvant drugs such as non-steroidal anti-inflammatory drugs (NSAIDs) and antidepressant agents (see pages xxvi–xliv for drug combinations) and use of nondrug therapies such as transcutaneous electrical nerve stimulation (TENS).

Elimination: Hepatic, renal.

Preparations

Propoxyphene hydrochloride **(Darvon):** Tablets/Capsules: 65 mg.

Propoxyphene hydrochloride and acetaminophen **(Genagesic, E-Lor, Wygesic):** Tablets/Capsules: Propoxyphene 65 mg and acetaminophen 650 mg.

Propoxyphene hydrochloride, aspirin, and caffeine **(Darvon Compound):** Capsules: Propoxyphene 65 mg, aspirin 389 mg, and caffeine 32.4 mg.

Propoxyphene napsylate **(Darvon-N):** Tablets: 100 mg.

Propoxyphene napsylate combinations **(Darvocet-N 50, Darvocet-N 100)**

Tablets: Propoxyphene 50 mg and acetaminophen 325 mg; propoxyphene 100 mg and acetaminophen 325 mg.

Tablets/Capsules: Propoxyphene 65 mg and acetaminophen 650 mg.

Pharmacology

A synthetic narcotic analgesic, propoxyphene is structurally related to methadone and exerts its analgesic actions on the central nervous system. Its analgesic effects are mild. Propoxyphene is 1/50 to 1/25 as potent as morphine, and 32–65 mg of the hydrochloride or 50–100 mg of the napsylate salt is as potent as or less potent than 30–60 mg codeine or 600 mg aspirin or acetaminophen. Propoxyphene is more effective when combined with other analgesics (e.g., codeine, aspirin, acetaminophen). The drug has no antitussive or antipyretic effects. Norpropoxyphene, the active metabolite, has local anesthetic effects and, like lidocaine, may cause cardiac conduction delay (increased PR interval and QRS prolongation). Over long periods of time, psychological dependence, physical dependence, and tolerance may accompany propoxyphene's use. The abuse liability is similar to that of codeine. Propoxyphene will only partially suppress the withdrawal syndrome in patients physically dependent on other narcotics. Propoxyphene crosses the placenta, and low levels may be detected in breast milk; however, no adverse effects have been noted in nursing infants.

Pharmacokinetics

Onset of Action: PO, 15–60 minutes.
Peak Effect: PO, 2–3 hours.
Duration of Action: PO, 4–6 hours.

Interactions

Potentiates CNS and circulatory depressant effects of other narcotic analgesics, volatile anesthetics, phenothiazines, sedative-hypnotics, alcohol, tricyclic antidepressants; analgesia enhanced and prolonged by narcotic and non-narcotic analgesics (e.g., aspirin, acetaminophen), α_2-agonists (e.g., clonidine); increases serum levels and toxic effects of carbamazepine; hepatic metabolism increased and efficacy of propoxyphene decreased in cigarette smokers; hypoprothrombinemic effects of warfarin increased by propoxyphene-acetaminophen combination.

Toxicity

Toxic Range: Not routinely monitored.

Manifestations: Somnolence, coma, respiratory arrest, apnea, cardiac arrhythmias, combined respiratory and metabolic acidosis, circulatory collapse, cardiac arrest, death.

Antidote: Naloxone IV/IM/SC 0.4–2.0 mg. Repeat dose every 2 to 3 minutes to a maximum of 10–20 mg.

Management: Discontinue or reduce medication. Support ventilation and circulation (patent airway, oxygen, IV fluids, vasopressors). Administer antidote. Monitor blood gases, pH, and electrolytes. Correct acidosis and electrolyte disturbance (lactic acidosis may require sodium bicarbonate IV 1–2 mEq/kg). Symptomatic treatment. Airway-protected, ipecac syrup–induced emesis (30 mL or 0.5 mL/kg ipecac syrup followed by 200 mL or 4 mL/kg of water or clear fluid) or gastric lavage (with drug ingestion) followed by administration of activated charcoal (PO 50–100 g or 1–2 g/kg).

Guidelines/Precautions

1. Inadvertent brachial artery injection, as may occur in abuse, may result in digital gangrene and amputation.
2. Reduce dosage in elderly patients and with concomitant use of narcotics and sedative-hypnotics.

3. Prescribe or supply an antiemetic (e.g., metoclopramide) for use in the event of nausea and/or vomiting.

4. Constipation may be more difficult to control than pain. Prevent and/or treat by daily administration of stool softeners or laxatives, for example, Colace (docusate sodium) 100–300 mg/day. Do not administer bulk-forming agents that contain methylcellulose, psyllium, or polycarbophil. Temporary arrest in the passage through the gastrointestinal tract may lead to fecal impaction or bowel obstruction.

5. Tolerance is manifested by decreased duration of effect and increasing need for the drug. In these cases, add adjuvant drugs (e.g., NSAIDs, antidepressant agents) or switch to alternative opioids (starting at one-half the equianalgesic dose) or supplement with nondrug therapies (e.g., TENS).

6. Abrupt discontinuation of opioids in patients with physical dependence may manifest with withdrawal symptoms. To avoid withdrawal, doses should be reduced slowly (e.g., dose reduction of 75% every 2 days). Withdrawal should be treated symptomatically.

7. Addiction occurs rarely (frequency of <1:3000) and should not be considered in deciding the proper dose and schedule of propoxyphene.

8. Drug combinations with adjuvant drugs enhance analgesia (see pages xxvi–xliv).

9. Adjuvant drug therapies also include regional blockade, trigger-point injections (with local anesthetics and steroids), and intravenous regional anesthesia.

10. Adjuvant nondrug therapies include TENS and modalities such as ice or heat application, ultrasound, and soft tissue mobilization.
11. Patients should be warned that propoxyphene may impair their ability to perform hazardous tasks requiring mental alertness or physical coordination (e.g., driving a motor vehicle, operating heavy machinery).
12. Propoxyphene is subject to control under the Federal Controlled Substances Act of 1970 as a Schedule V (C-V) drug.

Principal Adverse Reactions

Cardiovascular: Hypotension, circulatory depression, bradycardia, syncope.
Pulmonary: Respiratory depression.
CNS: Sedation, somnolence, euphoria, dysphoria, disorientation.
Genitourinary: Urinary retention.
Gastrointestinal: Nausea, vomiting, abdominal pain, biliary tract spasm, constipation, anorexia, hepatic dysfunction.
Ocular: Miosis.
Allergic: Rash, pruritus, urticaria.

PROPRANOLOL HYDROCHLORIDE

Class: β-Blocker, Antihypertensive, Antianginal, Antiarrhythmic

Use(s): Antihypertensive; antianginal; antiarrhythmic (supraventricular and ventricular arrhythmias); treat-

ment of acute myocardial infarction; migraine prophylaxis; treatment of phantom limb pain; symptomatic
treatment of thyrotoxicosis, pheochromocytoma, and
tremors.

Dosing: *Hypertension*

IV: 0.5–3.0 mg (10–30 μg/kg) every 2 minutes to maximum of 6–10 mg.

PO: 20–40 mg twice daily.

PO, long-acting preparation: 60–80 mg once
daily.

Titrate doses upward at 3- to 7-day intervals until optimal response is obtained.
Usual maintenance range: 120–160 mg
daily. Therapeutic concentration: 50–
100 ng/mL.

Arrhythmia

PO: 10–30 mg three or four times daily.

IV: 0.5–3.0 mg (10–30 μg/kg) every 2 minutes to maximum of 6–10 mg.

Angina

PO: 10–20 mg three or four times daily.

PO, long-acting preparation: 80 mg once
daily.

Titrate doses upward at 3- to 7-day intervals until optimal response is obtained.
Usual maintenance range: 160 mg daily.

Acute myocardial infarction: IV 1–3 mg. Do
not exceed 1 mg/min to avoid lowering the
blood pressure and causing cardiac stand-
still. If necessary, give a second dose after
2 minutes. Then PO 180–240 mg/day in
three or four divided doses.

Migraine prophylaxis
Initial: PO 20 mg one to four times daily. (PO, long-acting preparation: 80 mg once daily.)
Maintenance: PO 20–80 mg one to four times daily. (PO, long-acting preparation: 80–240 mg once daily.)
Titrate doses upward at 3- to 7-day intervals until optimal response is obtained. Effective dose range: 160–240 mg daily. A trial of at least 2 months is indicated.
Phantom limb pain: PO 80 mg one to three times daily.

Elimination: Hepatic, pulmonary.

Preparations

Propranolol hydrochloride **(Inderal):** Tablets: 10 mg, 20 mg, 40 mg, 60 mg, 80 mg, 90 mg.

Propranolol hydrochloride **(Inderal LA):** Capsules, extended release: 60 mg, 80 mg, 120 mg, 160 mg.

Propranolol hydrochloride **(Inderal, Propranolol Hydrochloride):** Injection: 1 mg/mL.

Propranolol hydrochloride and hydrochlorothiazide **(Inderide):** Tablets: Propranolol hydrochloride 40 mg and hydrochlorothiazide 25 mg; propranolol hydrochloride 80 mg and hydrochlorothiazide 25 mg.

Propranolol hydrochloride and hydrochlorothiazide **(Inderide LA):** Capsules, extended release: Propranolol hydrochloride 80 mg and hydrochlorothiazide 50 mg; propranolol hydrochloride 120 mg and hydrochlorothiazide 50 mg; propranolol hydrochloride 160 mg and hydrochlorothiazide 50 mg.

Pharmacology

Propranolol is a nonselective β-adrenergic receptor antagonist without intrinsic sympathomimetic activity. The degree of β blockade depends on the ongoing β activity at the time of administration. Thus, decreases in heart rate and cardiac output (β_1-receptor blockade) are greater in the presence of increased sympathetic nervous system activity. Blockade of β_2-receptors increases peripheral and coronary vascular resistance. Reduced cardiac work is the basis for use of the drug after myocardial infarction and in the treatment of angina. Propranolol depresses automaticity and conduction velocity in cardiac muscle. Propranolol may prevent common migraine and reduce the number of attacks in some patients. It is not effective for a migraine attack that has already started. The antimigraine effect may be partly due to inhibition of vasodilatation. The drug may also inhibit arteriolar spasm of the pial vessels in the brain. Propranolol prophylaxis may result in increased effectiveness of abortive migraine agents when these are required.

Pharmacokinetics

Onset of Action: Antihypertensive effects: IV, <2 minutes; PO, <30 minutes.
Peak Effect: Antihypertensive effects: IV, within 1 minute; PO, variable. Antimigraine effects: PO, 4–6 weeks.
Duration of Action: Antihypertensive effects: IV, 1–6 hours; PO, 6–12 hours.

Interactions

Potentiates myocardial depression of inhaled and injected anesthetics; additive effects with catecholamine-depleting drugs (e.g., reserpine), calcium channel blockers; antagonizes cardiac-stimulating and bronchodilating effects of sympathomimetics; potentiates vasoconstrictive effect of epinephrine; increased serum levels with concomitant use of chlorpromazine, cimetidine, halothane; decreased serum levels with enzyme inducers (e.g., phenytoin, phenobarbital, rifampin); potentiates effects of digoxin, succinylcholine, nondepolarizing muscle relaxants (e.g., tubocurarine); produces hypoglycemia, prolongs the hypoglycemic effect of insulin, and may mask symptoms of hypoglycemia (e.g., tachycardia); may unmask direct negative inotropic effects of ketamine.

Toxicity

Toxic Range: Not routinely monitored.

Manifestations: Bradycardia, hypotension, atrioventricular block, cardiogenic shock, asystole, convulsions, hypoglycemia, hyperkalemia.

Antidote: No specific antidote, but glucagon (diluted in preservative-free saline) IV 5–10 mg followed by 1–5 mg/hr infusion may be used to treat bradycardia and hypotension. Sodium bicarbonate IV 0.5–1.0 mEq/kg bolus repeated as needed may be used to treat wide complex conduction defects.

Management: Discontinue or reduce medication. Support ventilation and circulation (patent airway, oxygen, IV fluids, vasopressors). Bradycardia may be treated with IV atropine (1–2 mg), IV isoproterenol (0.02–0.15 μg/kg/min), or a transvenous cardiac pacemaker. Administer antidote. Symptomatic treatment. Airway-protected, ipecac syrup–induced emesis (30 mL or 0.5 mL/kg ipecac syrup followed by 200 mL or 4 mL/

kg of water or clear fluid) or gastric lavage (with drug ingestion) followed by administration of activated charcoal (PO 50–100 g or 1–2 g/kg) and cathartics.

Guidelines/Precautions

1. Propranolol is contraindicated in cardiogenic shock, sinus bradycardia, greater than first-degree block, bronchial asthma, and congestive heart failure unless the failure is secondary to a tachyarrhythmia treatable with propranolol.
2. Use with caution in patients with diabetes and nonallergic bronchospastic disease (e.g., bronchitis).
3. There is increased risk of ischemia or infarction in patients with coronary artery disease if drug is withdrawn abruptly.
4. Epinephrine use in patients receiving propranolol may result in rapid blood pressure increase and decreased pulse rate with first- or second-degree heart block. The β-adrenergic activity of epinephrine is blocked, while α-adrenergic effects are unopposed.

Principal Adverse Reactions

Cardiovascular: Bradycardia, hypotension, congestive heart failure, atrioventricular block.
Pulmonary: Bronchospasm.
CNS: Depression, disorientation, dizziness, memory loss.
Gastrointestinal: Nausea, vomiting, mesenteric thrombosis.
Hematologic: Agranulocytosis, thrombocytopenic purpura, nonthrombocytopenic purpura.

PROTRIPTYLINE HYDROCHLORIDE

Class: Tricyclic Antidepressant

Use(s): Treatment of neurotic and endogenous depression; adjunct treatment of neuropathic pain syndromes, including diabetic neuropathy, postherpetic neuralgia, tic douloureux, and cancer pain; anxiety disorders; migraine; phobias; panic disorders; enuresis; eating disorders.

Dosing: *Pain syndromes*

Initial: PO 5 mg (0.1 mg/kg) three times daily.

Maintenance: PO 5–10 mg (0.1–0.2 mg/kg) three times daily. Doses should be decreased if unacceptable side effects occur. Serum levels should be determined if there are signs of toxicity. The higher end of the dose range may be required in the management of painful diabetic neuropathy.

Depression

Initial: PO 5 mg (0.1 mg/kg) three times daily.

Maintenance: PO 5–20 mg (0.1–0.2 mg/kg) three times daily. Maximum dose 60 mg daily.

Use lower doses for adolescent and geriatric patients.

Doses for pain are generally smaller than those used for treatment of affective disorders. Medication should be administered on a fixed schedule and not as needed. Administration of the entire daily dose at bedtime may reduce daytime sedation. After symptoms are controlled, dosage should be gradually reduced to the lowest level that will maintain relief of symptoms. Analgesia may be enhanced by addition of opioid analgesics (see pages xxvi–xliv for drug combinations), nonsteroidal anti-inflammatory drugs (NSAIDs), and use of nondrug therapies such as transcutaneous electrical nerve stimulation (TENS). In geriatric patients and patients with decreased renal or hepatic function, decrease doses by one-third to one-half. The possibility for suicide is inherent in depression and may persist until significant remission occurs. The quantity of drug dispensed should reflect this consideration.

Elimination: Hepatic, renal.

Preparations

Protriptyline hydrochloride **(Vivactil):** Tablets, film coated: 5mg, 10mg.

Pharmacology

Protriptyline hydrochloride is a dibenzocycloheptene derivative and a secondary amine tricyclic antidepressant. Antidepressant activity may be partly due to inhibition of the amine-pump uptake of neurotransmitters (e.g., norepinephrine and serotonin) at the presynaptic neuron and down-regulation of β-receptor sensitivity.

The drug has mild sedative, antihistaminic, and anti-cholinergic effects. Protriptyline may have a more rapid onset of action than imipramine or amitriptyline. Although blockade of neurotransmitter uptake may occur immediately, the initial antidepressant response may take a week. Patients with low norepinephrine levels may respond better to protriptyline compared with serotonin-deficient patients. Protriptyline does not inhibit the monoamine oxidase (MAO) system.

The analgesic effects of protriptyline may occur partly through the alleviation of depression, which may be responsible for increased pain suffering, but also by mechanisms that are independent of mood effects. Serotonin and norepinephrine activity may be increased in descending pain-inhibitory pathways. Activation of these pathways decreases the transmission of nociceptive impulses from primary afferent neurons to first-order cells in laminae I and V of the spinal cord dorsal horn. Protriptyline may also potentiate the analgesic effect of opioids by increasing their binding efficacy to opioid receptors. Protriptyline has varying degrees of efficacy in different pain syndromes and may be better at relieving the burning, aching, and dyesthetic component of neuropathic pain. The drug is seldom useful in the management of lancinating, shooting paroxysmal pain.

Protriptyline may produce abnormal EEG patterns and lower the seizure threshold. Therapeutic doses do not affect respiration, but toxic doses may lead to respiratory depression. The direct quinidine-like effects may manifest at toxic doses and produce cardiovascular disturbances (e.g., conduction blockade). Protriptyline does not have addiction liability and its use is not associated with drug-seeking behavior. Withdrawal symptoms may be precipitated by acute withdrawal. Tolerance develops to the sedative and anticholinergic effects, but there are no reports of tolerance to the analgesic effects. Protriptyline crosses the placenta and is excreted in breast milk. Usage in pregnant or nursing mothers should occur only if the potential benefit justifies the potential risk.

Pharmacokinetics

Onset of Action: Analgesic effect: PO, <5 days. Antidepressant effect: PO, <7 days.
Peak Effect: Antidepressant effect: PO, 2–4 weeks.
Duration of Action: Antidepressant effect: PO, variable.

Interactions

Increased risk of hyperthermia with concomitant administration of anticholinergics (e.g., atropine), phenothiazines, thyroid medications; serum levels and toxic effects of protriptyline increased by concomitant methylphenidate, fluoxetine, cimetidine, quinidine, phenothiazines, and haloperidol; ventilatory and circulatory depressant effects of CNS depressant drugs and alcohol potentiated by protriptyline; antihypertensive response to guanethidine antagonized by protriptyline; increases the pressor and cardiac effects of sympathomimetics (e.g., isoproterenol, phenylephrine, norepinephrine, epinephrine, amphetamine); decreases serum levels and pharmacologic effects of levodopa and phenylbutazone; increases serum levels and toxic effects of dicumarol; onset of therapeutic effects shortened and adverse cardiac effects of protriptyline increased with concomitant administration of levothyroxine and liothyronine; fatal hyperpyretic crisis or seizures with concomitant use of MAO inhibitors; uptake-dependent efficacy of IV regional bretylium decreased by protriptyline.

Toxicity

Toxic Range: >50 ng/mL.

Manifestations: *Chronic:* Dream and sleep disturbances, akathisia, anxiety, chills, coryza, malaise, myalgia, headache, dizziness, nausea and vomiting. *Acute:* In addition to the previously listed symptoms, CNS stimulation with excitement, delirium, hallucinations, hyperreflexia, myoclonus, choreiform movements, parkinsonian symptoms, seizures, hyperpyrexia, then CNS depression with drowsiness, areflexia, hypothermia, respiratory depression, cyanosis, hypotension, coma; peripheral anticholinergic symptoms, including urinary retention, dry mucous membranes, mydriasis, constipation, adynamic ileus; cardiac irregularities, including tachycardia, QRS prolongation; metabolic and/or respiratory acidosis; polyradiculoneuropathy; renal failure; vomiting; ataxia; dysarthria; bullous cutaneous lesions; pulmonary consolidation.

Antidote: None.

Management: Discontinue or reduce medication. Correct fluid, electrolyte, and acid-base disturbances. Airway-protected, ipecac syrup–induced emesis (30 mL or 0.5 mL/kg ipecac syrup) or gastric lavage (with drug ingestion) followed by administration of activated charcoal (PO 50–100 g or 1–2 g/kg). These purging actions should be performed even if several hours have elapsed after ingestion because the anticholinergic effects may delay gastric emptying, and the drug may also be secreted into the stomach. Control seizures: Intravenous benzodiazepines are the first choice because IV barbiturates may enhance respiratory depression; however, IV barbiturates may be useful in refractory seizures. Control hyperpyrexia with ice packs and cooling sponge baths. Support ventilation and circulation (patent airway, oxygen, IV fluids, vasopressors). Continuous EKG monitoring. Treat cardiac arrhythmias with IV lidocaine or propranolol. Digoxin, quinidine, procainamide, and diisopyramide should be avoided because they may further depress myocardial conduction and/or contractility. Temporary pacemakers may be necessary in patients with advanced atrioventricular block, severe bradycardia, and/or life-threatening ventricular arrhythmias unresponsive to drug therapy. Physostigmine (slow IV 1–3 mg) may be used in the treatment of life-threatening anticholinergic toxicity. Routine use of physostigmine is not advisable due to its serious adverse effects (e.g., seizures, bronchospasm, and severe bradyarrhythmias). Hemodialysis or peritoneal dialysis is ineffective because the drug is highly protein bound. Symptomatic treatment. Consider the possibility of multiple drug involvement. Counseling prior to and after discharge for patients who attempted suicide.

Guidelines/Precautions

1. To avoid withdrawal symptoms, the medication should be tapered down over a couple of weeks and not discontinued abruptly.
2. Use with caution in patients with cardiovascular disease, thyroid disease, or seizure disorders and in those in whom excessive anticholinergic activity

may be harmful (e.g., patients with benign prostatic hypertrophy, a history of urinary retention, or increased intraocular pressure). The drug should be used in close-angle glaucoma only when the glaucoma is adequately controlled by drugs and closely monitored.

3. Protriptyline is contraindicated in patients receiving MAO inhibitors (concurrently or within the past 2 weeks), patients in the acute recovery phase following myocardial infarction, and those with demonstrated hypersensitivity to protriptyline.
   Cross-sensitivity with other tricyclic antidepressants may occur.

4. Patients should be warned of the possibility of drowsiness that may impair performance of potentially hazardous tasks such as driving an automobile or operating machinery. Persisting daytime drowsiness may be decreased by administering a lower dose, administering the dose earlier in the evening, or substituting a less sedating alternative.

Principal Adverse Reactions

Cardiovascular: Postural hypotension, arrhythmias, conduction disturbances, hypertension, sudden death.

Pulmonary: Respiratory depression.

CNS: Confusion, disorientation, extrapyramidal symptoms.

Gastrointestinal: Hepatic dysfunction, jaundice, nausea, vomiting, constipation, decrease in lower esophageal sphincter tone.

Genitourinary: Urinary retention, paradoxical nocturia, urinary frequency.

Ocular: Blurred vision, mydriasis, increased intraocular pressure.

Dermatologic: Pruritus, urticaria, petechiae, photosensitivity.

Hematologic: Leukopenia, thrombocytopenia, eosinophilia, agranulocytosis, purpura.

Endocrinologic: Increased or decreased libido, impotence, gynecomastia, SIADH.

Other: Hyperthermia.

RANITIDINE

Class: Histamine H_2 Antagonist

Use(s): Treatment of duodenal ulcer, gastroesophageal reflux, pathologic hypersecretory conditions; prophylaxis against acid pulmonary aspiration, stress ulcers, upper GI bleeding in critically ill patients.

Dosing: PO: 150 mg twice daily; alternately, 150–300 mg at bedtime.

IV/IM: 50 mg every 6–8 hours (dilute IV dose in 20 mL normal saline and give over 5–15 minutes).

Infusion: 6.25 mg/hr (10.7 mL/hr of 0.6 mg/mL solution).

Elimination: Hepatic.

Preparations

Ranitidine **(Zantac)**
   Tablet: 150 mg, 300 mg.
   Oral solution: 15 mg/mL.
   Injection: 25 mg/mL.

Dilution for Infusion: 150 mg (6 mL) in 250 mL D5W or normal saline (0.6 mg/mL).

Pharmacology

This histamine H_2-receptor antagonist blocks histamine-, pentagastrin-, and acetylcholine-induced secretion of hydrogen ions by gastric parietal cells. Nocturnal and food-induced gastric secretion are also inhibited. Ranitidine has no significant effect on gastric emptying time, volume, or pancreatic secretions. A single oral dose of 150 mg will provide acid inhibition for a period of 8 to 12 hours. Ranitidine also suppresses histamine-induced peripheral vasodilatation and inotropic effects. There is minimal entrance into the central nervous system; thus, in contrast with cimetidine, ranitidine produces fewer side effects such as CNS dysfunction in elderly patients. Ranitidine produces less inhibition of microsomal drug-metabolizing enzymes and less antiandrogenic effects than cimetidine.

Pharmacokinetics

Onset of Action: IV/IM, <15 min; PO, <30 min.
Peak Effect: IV/IM, 1–2 hours; PO, 2–3 hours.
Duration of Action: IV/IM, 6–8 hours; PO, 8–12 hours.

Interactions

Absorption decreased by concurrent antacids; may decrease absorption of diazepam; may increase hypoglycemic effect of glipizide; may interfere with warfarin clearance; may antagonize neuromuscular blockade of nondepolarizing muscle relaxants (by an intrinsic anticholinesterase effect); may potentiate succinylcholine depolarizing blockade.

Toxicity

Toxic Range: Not routinely monitored.
Manifestations: Tachycardia, respiratory failure, headache, delirium, psychosis.
Antidote: No specific antidote.
Management: Discontinue or reduce medication. Support ventilation and circulation (patent airway, oxygen, IV fluids, vasoactive drugs). Treat tachycardia with a β-blocker (e.g., esmolol IV 10–40 mg or propranolol IV 0.5–3.0 mg). Remove ingested drug by induced emesis. Symptomatic treatment.

Guidelines/Precautions

1. Use with caution in elderly patients.
2. Full daily dose may be given once a day.

Principal Adverse Reactions

Cardiovascular: Tachycardia, bradycardia, premature ventricular beats with rapid IV injection.
Pulmonary: Bronchospasm.
CNS: Headache, depression, dizziness, confusion.
Gastrointestinal/Hepatic: Nausea, vomiting, hepatitis, diarrhea.
Hematologic: Leukopenia, granulocytopenia, thrombocytopenia.
Dermatologic: Erythema multiforme, alopecia.

ROPIVACAINE HYDROCHLORIDE

Class: Local Anesthetic

Use(s): Local and regional anesthesia, sympathetic blockade.

Dosing: *Infiltration/Peripheral nerve block:* <200 mg
(0.2–0.5% solution).

Caudal: 30–150 mg (15–30 mL of 0.2–0.5%
solution). Children, 0.4–0.7–1.0 mL/kg (L2-
T10-T7 level of anesthesia). At higher
volumes (>0.6 mL/kg), utilize lower concentrations of ropivacaine (0.1–0.2% solutions). Maximum safe dose: 2.5 mg/kg.

Brachial plexus block: 175–250 mg (35–50 mL
of 0.35–0.5% solution). Children, 0.5–
0.75 mL/kg. Regional blockade may be
potentiated by the addition of tetracaine
0.5–1.0 mg/kg or fentanyl 1–2 μg/kg or
preservative-free morphine 0.05–0.1 mg/kg.

Stellate ganglion block: 10–20 mL of 0.2%
(25–50 mg) solution.

Paravertebral block: 3–4 mL of 0.5% solution
per segment.

Epidural

Bolus: 20–200 mg (0.1–0.75% solution).
Children, 0.5–2.5 mg/kg or 0.3–0.5 mL/kg
(0.1–0.5% solution).

Infusion: 4–15 mL/hr (0.1–0.2% solution
with or without epidural narcotics). Children, 0.1–0.35 mL/kg/hr.

Rate of onset and potency of local anesthetic action may be enhanced by carbonation. (Add 0.1 mL of 7.5% or 8.4%
sodium bicarbonate with 20 mL of 0.2%
ropivacaine. Do not use if there is precipitation.)

Spinal bolus: 15–22 mg (0.5–0.75% solution
without glucose).

Note: Intrathecal use of ropivacaine is not approved by the FDA.

Intrapleural: Bolus, <100 mg (0.4 mL/kg) (20 mL of 0.2–0.5% solution). Infusion, 5–7 mL/hr (0.125 mL/kg/hr) (0.1–0.2% solution).

Intra-articular (knee joint block for arthroscopy): <150 mg (30 mL of 0.5% solution). If desired, add morphine 0.5–1.0 mg.

Maximum safe dose: 2.5 mg/kg with or without epinephrine. Ropivacaine single-dose vials, ampules, and infusion bottles are preservative free and may be used for epidural or caudal block.

Elimination: Hepatic, renal.

Preparations

Ropivacaine hydrochloride **(Naropin):** Injection: 0.2%, 0.5%, 0.75%, 1%. Store at room temperature (20°C to 25°C). Continuous-infusion bottles should not be left in place for longer than 24 hours.

Dilution for Infusion: Epidural use only: Use undiluted 0.2% solution (2 mg/mL) or dilute 40 mL of 0.2% in 40 mL preservative-free normal saline (0.1% solution). Discard after use or within 24 hours after ampules or vials have been opened.

Pharmacology

This amino amide local anesthetic stabilizes neuronal membranes by blocking the generation and conduction of nerve impulses. The progression of anesthesia is related to the diameter, myelination, and conduction velocity of affected nerve fibers, with the order of loss of function being as follows: 1) autonomic, 2) pain,

3) temperature, 4) touch, 5) proprioception, and 6) skeletal muscle tone. The onset, depth, and duration of sensory block with ropivacaine are similar to those of bupivacaine. However, ropivacaine produces a less intense and shorter-lasting motor block compared with bupivacaine. Addition of epinephrine improves the quality of analgesia, but has no major effect on the time of onset, duration of action, or systemic absorption of ropivacaine. Hypotension results from loss of sympathetic tone, as in spinal or epidural anesthesia. At recommended doses, ropivacaine has decreased arrhythmogenic and cardiodepressant effects compared with bupivacaine, although both are considerably more toxic than lidocaine. Higher than recommended doses of ropivacaine may negate these advantages. The incidence of successful resuscitation is not significantly different with ropivacaine or bupivacaine. At high plasma levels, ropivacaine produces uterine vasoconstriction and decrease in uterine blood flow. Such plasma levels are seen in paracervical blocks but not with epidural or spinal blocks.

Pharmacokinetics

Onset of Action: Infiltration, 1–15 minutes. Epidural, 10–20 minutes. Spinal, <2 minutes.
Peak Effect: Infiltration/Epidural, 20–45 minutes. Spinal, 10–13 minutes.
Duration of Action: Infiltration/Epidural, 120–400 minutes. Spinal, 120 minutes.

Interactions

Seizures and respiratory and circulatory depression at high plasma levels; reduced clearance with concomitant

use of theophylline, imipramine, verapamil, and fluvoxamine; additive toxic effects with concomitant use
of other amide-type local anesthetics; benzodiazepines,
barbiturates, and volatile anesthetics increase seizure
threshold; reduced dose requirements in pregnant
patients.

Toxicity

Toxic Range: Not routinely monitored.
Manifestations: Seizures, arrhythmias, circulatory collapse, respiratory depression, cardiac arrest.
Antidote: No specific antidote.
Management: Discontinue or reduce medication. Support ventilation and circulation (patent airway, oxygen,
IV fluids, vasopressors). Benzodiazepines (diazepam
IV 0.05–0.2 mg/kg, midazolam IV/IM 0.025–0.1 mg/kg)
or barbiturates (thiopental sodium IV 0.5–2.0 mg/kg)
to control seizures. Prolonged cardiopulmonary resuscitation with cardiac arrest: Sodium bicarbonate IV 1–
2 mEq/kg to treat cardiac toxicity (sodium channel
blockade); bretylium IV 5 mg/kg; DC cardioversion/
defibrillation for ventricular arrhythmias. Remove ingested drug by induced emesis followed by activated
charcoal. Hypersensitivity reactions: Remove from
further exposure and treat dermatitis. Exchange transfusions in newborns with toxicity.

Guidelines/Precautions

1. Ropivacaine is not recommended for obstetrical
   paracervical block. The drug may cause fetal
   bradycardia or death.
2. Ropivacaine is not recommended for IV regional
   anesthesia. High plasma concentrations may occur

following tourniquet release and result in refractory cardiac arrest and death.

3. Intravenous access is essential during major regional block.

4. Use with caution in patients with hypovolemia, severe congestive heart failure, shock, or any form of heart block.

5. Ropivacaine is contraindicated in patients with hypersensitivity to amide-type local anesthetics.

6. Toxic plasma levels (e.g., from accidental intravascular injection) may cause cardiopulmonary collapse and seizures. Premonitory signs and symptoms manifest as numbness of the tongue and circumoral tissues, metallic taste, restlessness, tinnitus, and tremors. Support of circulation (IV fluids, vasopressors), sodium bicarbonate IV 1–2 mEq/kg to treat cardiac toxicity (sodium channel blockade), bretylium IV 5 mg/kg, DC cardioversion/defibrillation for ventricular arrhythmias, and securing a patent airway (ventilate with 100% oxygen) are paramount. Thiopental (IV 0.5–2.0 mg/kg), midazolam (IV 0.02–0.04 mg/kg), or diazepam (IV 0.1 mg/kg) may be used for prophylaxis and/or treatment of seizures.

7. The level of sympathetic blockade (bradycardia with block above T5) determines the degree of hypotension (often heralded by nausea and vomiting) following epidural or intrathecal ropivacaine (or other local anesthetic). Fluid hydration (10–20 mL/kg normal saline or lactated Ringer's solution), vasopressor agents (e.g., ephedrine), and left uterine displacement in pregnant patients may be used for prophylaxis and/or treatment. Administer atropine to treat bradycardia.

8. Unintentional subarachnoid administration during epidural anesthesia may result in persistent anesthesia, paresthesia, weakness, paralysis of the lower extremities, and loss of sphincter control, all of which may have slow, incomplete, or no recovery.

9. Epidural, caudal, or intrathecal injections should be avoided when the patient has hypovolemic shock, septicemia, infection at the injection site, or coagulopathy.

10. Epidural motor blockade may be reversed by the epidural injection of 20 mL of 0.9% saline.

Principal Adverse Reactions

Cardiovascular: Hypotension, arrhythmias, cardiac arrest.

Pulmonary: Respiratory impairment, arrest.

CNS: Seizures, tinnitus, blurred vision.

Allergic: Urticaria, angioneurotic edema, anaphylactoid symptoms.

Epidural/Caudal/Spinal: High spinal, hypotension, urinary retention, lower extremity weakness and paralysis, loss of sphincter control, headache, back pain, cranial nerve palsies, slowing of labor.

SALSALATE

Class: Nonsteroidal Anti-inflammatory Drug

Use(s): Symptomatic treatment of mild to moderate pain, inflammatory conditions (e.g., rheumatic fever, rheumatoid arthritis, osteoarthritis), chronic pain, cancer pain (especially with bone metastasis).

Dosing: *Pain or inflammatory disease:* PO 2–4 g (40–80 mg/kg) daily in two or three divided doses.

Dosage should be adjusted according to the patient's response, tolerance, and serum salicylate levels. Administer analgesic regularly (not as needed). Analgesia may be enhanced by addition of opioid analgesics (see pages xxvi–xliv for drug combinations), antidepressant agents, and use of nondrug therapies such as transcutaneous electrical nerve stimulation (TENS). In rheumatoid arthritis or juvenile rheumatoid arthritis, second-line rheumatoid agents may include leflunomide (Arava), entanercept (Enbrel), antimalarials, or methotrexate. In geriatric patients and patients with decreased renal or hepatic function, decrease doses by one-third to one-half. The incidence of salsalate-induced gastropathy may be decreased by concomitant administration of antacids or sucralfate (PO 1 g four times daily). Misoprostol (PO 100–200 μg four times daily) may be used to prevent gastric ulcers in high-risk patients.

Elimination: Hepatic, renal.

Preparations

Salsalate **(Disalcid)**
   Oral Capsules: 500 mg.
   Tablets, film coated: 500 mg, 750 mg.
Salsalate **(Argesic):** Tablets: 500 mg.
Salsalate **(Arthra-G):** Tablets: 750 mg.

Pharmacology

Salsalate, a nonsteroidal anti-inflammatory drug (NSAID), is the salicylate ester of salicylic acid. Salsalate is hydrolyzed to salicylic acid in the intestinal lumen and plasma. The analgesic and anti-inflammatory activity of salsalate may be mediated by inhibition of the biosynthesis and release of prostaglandins that sensitize C fibers' nociceptors to mechanical stimuli and chemical mediators (e.g., bradykinin, histamine) and that may interfere with the endogenous descending pathways that inhibit pain transmission. Salsalate irreversibly acetylates and inactivates cyclooxygenase (prostaglandin synthetase), an enzyme that catalyzes the formation of prostaglandin precursors (endoperoxides) from arachidonic acid. The analgesic and anti-inflammatory effects of salsalate are comparable with those of aspirin. In contrast to aspirin, salsalate (and other salicylate salts) does not inhibit platelet aggregation and should not be substituted for aspirin in the prophylaxis of thrombosis. Salsalate is better tolerated than aspirin and is associated with less gastric mucosal abnormalities. The drug is particularly useful in patients with GI intolerance to aspirin or in patients in whom interference with normal platelet function by aspirin or other NSAIDs is undesirable. Salsalate (like other NSAIDs) exhibits a ceiling effect for analgesia. Exceeding recommended doses results in increased toxicity without improvement in analgesia. Inhibition of prostaglandin synthesis may result in decreased uterine tone and contractility and prolonged gestation in the parturient and premature closure of the ductus arteriosus in the fetus.

Pharmacokinetics

Onset of Action: PO, analgesic effect 5–30 minutes.
Peak Effect: PO, analgesic effect 0.5–2.0 hours.
Duration of Action: PO, analgesic effect 3–7 hours.

Interactions

Incidence of GI side effects increased with concomitant NSAID therapy, alcohol ingestion; enhances toxicity of lithium, methotrexate, valproic acid; serum levels of salsalate increased by carbonic anhydrous inhibitors; decreases diuretic effects of spirinolactone; decreased serum concentration of salsalate with concomitant corticosteroids; enhances hypoglycemic effects of sulfonylureas; decreases antihypertensive effects of β-adrenergic blockers, angiotensin-converting enzyme (ACE) inhibitors; enhances hypotensive effects of nitroglycerin; urinary excretion of salsalate increased by antacids and urinary alkalinizers; absorption delayed by food, milk, and concomitant administration of activated charcoal; prostaglandin-mediated natriuretic effects of spirinolactone and furosemide antagonized by salsalate.

Toxicity

Toxic Range: Salicylic acid >250 μg/mL (mild salicylism); salicylic acid >400–500 μg/mL (severe toxicity).
Manifestations: *Chronic:* Tinnitus, hearing loss, dimness of vision, headache, hyperventilation, GI ulceration, dyspepsia, dizziness, mental confusion, drowsiness, sweating, thirst, nausea and vomiting, diarrhea, tachycardia. *Acute:* In addition to the previously listed symptoms, acid-base and electrolyte disturbances, dehydration, hyperpyrexia, oliguria, acute renal failure, hyperthermia, restlessness, irritability, vertigo, asterixis,

tremor, diplopia, delirium, mania, hallucinations, EEG abnormalities, seizures, lethargy, coma.

Antidote: None.

Management: Discontinue or reduce medication. Correct fluid, electrolyte, and acid-base disturbances. Support ventilation and circulation (patent airway, oxygen, IV fluids, vasopressors). Airway-protected, ipecac syrup–induced emesis (30 mL or 0.5 mL/kg ipecac syrup followed by 200 mL or 4 mL/kg of water or clear fluid) or gastric lavage (with drug ingestion) followed by administration of activated charcoal (PO 50–100 g or 1–2 g/kg). Forced alkaline diuresis with IV sodium bicarbonate (IV furosemide if necessary) after correction of dehydration. Hemodialysis or hemoperfusion. Symptomatic treatment.

Guidelines/Precautions

1. Avoid the use of salsalate in children or teenagers with influenza or chickenpox. There is an increased risk of developing Reye's syndrome, an acute life-threatening condition characterized by vomiting, lethargy, delirium, and coma.
2. Discontinue use of the drug if dizziness, tinnitus, or hearing loss occurs. Tinnitus may herald the approach of salicylate levels to the upper limit of the therapeutic range. The temporary hearing loss remits gradually upon discontinuation of salsalate.
3. Salicylate salts should not be used for self-medication of fever for longer than 3 days in adults or children or for self-medication of pain for longer than 10 days in adults or 5 days in children unless directed by a physician.
4. Use with caution in patients with active GI lesions

(e.g., erosive gastritis, peptic ulcer), a history of recurrent GI lesions, hepatic or renal dysfunction, preexisting hypoprothrombinemia, or vitamin K deficiency. Salsalate may precipitate renal failure in patients with impaired renal function, heart failure, and liver dysfunction.

5. Electrolyte-containing salicylate salts (e.g., sodium salicylate or magnesium salicylate) should be used with caution in patients in whom a high sodium or magnesium intake would be harmful (e.g., patients with congestive heart and acute renal failure, respectively).

6. Patient response to NSAIDs is variable. Patients who do not respond to or cannot tolerate salsalate may be successfully treated with another NSAID.

7. Contraindicated in patients with previously demonstrated hypersensitivity to salsalate or with the complete or partial syndrome of nasal polyps, angioedema, or bronchospastic reactivity to aspirin or other NSAIDs.

8. Signs and symptoms of infection or other diseases may be masked by the antipyretic and anti-inflammatory effects of salsalate.

9. Monitor stool for blood every 14 days, and monitor BUN, serum creatinine, and urinalysis every 1 to 2 months when administering salsalate at chronic high doses.

Principal Adverse Reactions

Cardiovascular: Vasodilatation, pallor, angina.
Pulmonary: Dyspnea, asthma.
CNS: Drowsiness, dizziness, headache, sweating, depression, euphoria.

Gastrointestinal: Ulceration, bleeding, dyspepsia, nausea, vomiting, diarrhea, hepatic dysfunction.

Genitourinary: Dysuria, interstitial nephritis, renal papillary necrosis.

Dermatologic: Pruritus, urticaria.

Hematologic: Leukopenia, thrombocytopenia, purpura, decreased plasma iron concentration, shortened erythrocyte survival time.

SERTRALINE HYDROCHLORIDE

Class: Selective Serotonin Reuptake Inhibitor—Antidepressant

Use(s): Treatment of neurotic and endogenous depression; adjunct treatment of neuropathic pain syndromes, including diabetic neuropathy, postherpetic neuralgia, tic douloureux, and cancer pain; anxiety disorders; phobias; panic disorders; alcohol dependency; enuresis; eating disorders.

Dosing: *Pain syndrome*

Initial: PO 25–50 mg daily, preferably in the morning or evening.

Maintenance: PO 50–200 mg daily in the morning or evening. Doses may be titrated upward in increments of 50 mg per day at 1-week intervals. Doses should be decreased if unacceptable side effects occur. Serum levels should be determined if there are signs of toxicity. The higher end of the dose range may be required in the management of painful diabetic neuropathy.

Depression:

Initial: PO 25–50 mg daily, preferably in one dose in the morning or evening.

Maintenance: PO 50–200 mg daily in one dose in the morning or evening. Doses may be titrated upward in increments of 50 mg per day at 1-week intervals.

Doses for pain are generally smaller than those used for treatment of affective disorders. Medication should be administered on a fixed schedule and not as needed. After symptoms are controlled, dosage should be gradually reduced to the lowest level that will maintain relief of symptoms. Analgesia may be enhanced by addition of opioid analgesics (see pages xxvi–xliv for drug combinations) and nonsteroidal anti-inflammatory drugs (NSAIDs) and use of nondrug therapies such as transcutaneous electrical nerve stimulation (TENS). In geriatric patients and patients with decreased renal or hepatic function, decrease doses by one-third to one-half. The possibility for suicide is inherent in depression and may persist until significant remission occurs. The quantity of drug dispensed should reflect this consideration.

Elimination: Hepatic, renal.

Preparations

Sertraline hydrochloride **(Zoloft):** Tablets: 25 mg, 50 mg, 100 mg.

Pharmacology

A naphthalenamine-derivative antidepressant agent, sertraline differs structurally and pharmacologically from currently available antidepressant agents, including other selective serotonin reuptake inhibitors (SSRIs) (e.g., fluoxetine, paroxetine) and tricyclic/tetracyclic agents. Antidepressant activity is comparable to fluoxetine, amitriptyline, or nefazodone, with fewer adverse effects, and may be partly due to highly selective reuptake inhibition of serotonin. Sertraline is more potent than fluoxetine, fluvoxamine, or clomipramine as a serotonin-reuptake inhibitor. Sertraline has little or no effect on norepinephrine and dopamine neuronal uptake. Synaptic concentrations of serotonin are increased, with enhanced serotonergic neurotransmission and numerous CNS effects (e.g., appetite suppression, decreased alcohol intake). Sertraline and other SSRI agents correct the dysregulation of serotonin that is responsible for obsessive-compulsive disorders.

Sertraline may be associated with some anxiety and activation of mania/hypomania. Unlike with the tricyclics, sedating and cardiovascular effects are minimal due to the lack of substantial antihistaminic, anticholinergic, α_1-adrenergic-blocking, catecholamine-potentiating, and quinidine-like cardiotoxic effects. Sertraline undergoes hepatic metabolism to inactive metabolites. Sertraline does not appear to affect cardiac conduction and is not arrhythmogenic. Sertraline does not inhibit the reuptake of tyramine and has no effect on the pressor response to tyramine. Sertraline does not inhibit the monoamine oxidase (MAO) system. Onset of action and relief of associated anxiety symptoms occur earlier compared with fluoxetine and the tricyclic anti-depressants. Although blockade of neurotransmitter uptake may occur immediately, antidepressant response may take days to weeks.

The analgesic effects of sertraline may occur partly through the alleviation of depression, which may be responsible for increased pain suffering, but also by mechanisms that are independent of mood effects. Sertraline may potentiate the analgesic effect of opiate agonists, possibly by enhancing serotonergic transmission. The drug may produce abnormal EEG patterns and lower the seizure threshold. Therapeutic doses do not affect respiration, but the effects of higher doses remain to be established. Sertraline does not appear to have addiction liability. Sertraline crosses the placenta and is excreted in breast milk. It should be used with caution in pregnant and nursing mothers.

Pharmacokinetics

Onset of Action: Analgesic effect: PO, <5 days. Antidepressant effect: PO, 1–2 weeks.
Peak Effect: Antidepressant effect: PO, 3–4 weeks.
Duration of Action: Antidepressant effect: PO, variable (up to 44 weeks following 8 weeks of acute treatment).

Interactions

Increased risk of serotonin syndrome (myoclonus, rigidity, hyperreflexia, seizures, hyperthermia, hypertension, restlessness, diaphoresis, shivering, diarrhea, and tremor) with concomitant administration of serotonergics (e.g., clomipramine, tryptophan, pseudoephedrine, tricyclic antidepressant agents, cocaine, lithium, and MAO inhibitors); serum levels and toxic effects of sertraline increased by cimetidine; serum levels of sertraline decreased by enzyme inducers (e.g., phenytoin, phenobarbital, rifampin); extrapyramidal effects of antipsychotic drugs may be potentiated by sertraline; sertraline may increase the risks of bleeding in patients receiving warfarin.

Toxicity

Toxic Range: Not routinely monitored.

Manifestations: Serotonin syndrome (myoclonus, rigidity, hyperreflexia, seizures, hyperthermia, hypertension, restlessness, diaphoresis, shivering, diarrhea, and tremor), nausea and vomiting, drowsiness, sinus tachycardia, dilated pupils.

Antidote: Serotonin antagonists: Cyproheptadine PO 4–12 mg stat *or* methysergide PO 2 mg twice daily (three doses may be sufficient).

Management: Discontinue medication. Administer antidote. Correct fluid, electrolyte, and acid-base disturbances. Airway-protected, ipecac syrup–induced emesis (30 mL or 0.5 mL/kg ipecac syrup) or gastric lavage (with drug ingestion) followed by administration of activated charcoal (PO 50–100 g or 1–2 g/kg). Activated charcoal may be administered every 4 to 6 hours during the first 24 to 48 hours after ingestion. Control seizures: Intravenous benzodiazepines are the first choice; however, IV barbiturates or phenytoin may be useful in refractory seizures. Support ventilation and circulation (patent airway, oxygen, IV fluids, vasopressors). Control hyperpyrexia with ice packs and cooling sponge baths. Hemodialysis or peritoneal dialysis is ineffective because the drug is highly protein bound. Symptomatic treatment. Consider the possibility of multiple drug involvement. Counseling is recommended prior to and after discharge for patients who attempted suicide.

Guidelines/Precautions

1. To avoid withdrawal symptoms, the medication should be tapered down over a couple of weeks and not discontinued abruptly.
2. Use with caution in patients with cardiovascular disease, diabetes mellitus, anorexia nervosa, thyroid disease, or seizure disorders.
3. Sertraline is contraindicated in patients receiving MAO inhibitors (concurrently or within the past 2 weeks), in patients in the acute recovery phase following myocardial infarction, and in those with demonstrated hypersensitivity to sertraline. The combination of sertraline and MAO inhibitors may result in the serotonin syndrome (see "Interactions").
4. Loss of libido and significant sexual dysfunction may occur in patients on sertraline (and other SSRI antidepressants). In late stages of chronic regional pain syndrome and in patients treated with morphine or hydromorphone pumps, serum levels of estrogen and testosterone are at or below the lower limits of normal. The low sex hormone levels in these patients are often accompanied by edema, fatigue, hot flashes in females, and tendency for inactivity. SSRI antidepressants may aggravate these symptoms and preclude their use. Supplemental estrogen or testosterone may counteract the chronic fatigue and cold extremities and improve the level of analgesia.

5. Patients should be warned of the possibility of drowsiness that may impair performance of potentially hazardous tasks such as driving an automobile or operating machinery. Persisting daytime drowsiness may be decreased by administering a lower dose, administering the dose earlier in the evening, or substituting a less sedating alternative.

Principal Adverse Reactions

Cardiovascular: Tachycardia, bradycardia, hypertension.

Pulmonary: Respiratory depression.

CNS: Amnesia, CNS stimulation, emotional lability, vertigo, ataxia, seizures, extrapyramidal symptoms, activation of mania/hypomania.

Gastrointestinal: Hepatic dysfunction, jaundice, nausea, vomiting, diarrhea.

Genitourinary: Amenorrhea, dysmenorrhea, dysuria, urinary urgency, urinary retention.

Ocular: Blurred vision, mydriasis, increased intraocular pressure.

Dermatologic: Pruritus, urticaria, petechiae, photosensitivity.

Hematologic: Anemia, thrombocytopenia, eosinophilia, agranulocytosis.

Endocrinologic: Increased or decreased libido, impotence, gynecomastia, SIADH.

Other: Hyperthermia.

SODIUM HYALURONATE

Class: Elasto-Viscous Fluid

Use(s): Treatment of pain in osteoarthritis of the knee.

Dosing: *Intra-articular:* 20 mg/2 mL per painful knee joint; one injection per affected joint once a week, for a total of three to five injections. Use an 18- to 20-G needle. Strict aseptic technique must be followed. Remove joint effusion if present before injecting hyaluronate. Do not use the same syringe for removing joint effusion and for injecting hyaluronate. Prior subcutaneous infiltration with local anesthetic should be done to make injection comfortable. Do not inject anesthetic intra-articularly. This may dilute hyaluronate and affect its safety and effectiveness. Do not use skin disinfectants containing quarternary ammonium salts because hyaluronate can precipitate in their presence. Do not inject hyaluronate extra-articularly or into the synovial tissues and capsule. This has been reported to cause a systemic adverse event.

Elimination: Renal.

Preparations

Sodium hyaluronate **(Hyalgan, Synvisc):** Vial/Prefilled syringe: 20 mg/2 mL.

Pharmacology

Hyalgan is a sterile elasto-viscous mixture that is made up mostly of a natural, highly purified sodium hyaluronate that comes from rooster combs. Sodium hyaluronate is a natural chemical found in the body; it is present in a particularly high amount in joint tissues and in the fluids that fill the joint. It acts like a lubricant and a shock absorber in the joint and is needed for the joint to work properly. In osteoarthritis, there may not be enough hyaluronate and there may be a change in the quality of the hyaluronate found in joint tissue. Intra-articular hyaluronate provides pain relief comparable with that of oral naproxen.

Pharmacokinetics

Onset of Action: Intra-articular, 3–4 weeks.
Peak Effect: Intra-articular, 5 weeks.
Duration of Action: Intra-articular, >26 weeks.

Interactions

Hyaluronate is precipitated by skin disinfectants containing quartenary ammonium salts.

Toxicity

Toxic Range: Not routinely monitored.
Manifestations: Hypotension, tachycardia, diaphoresis.
Antidote: No specific antidote.
Management: Discontinue or reduce medication. Support ventilation and circulation (patent airway, oxygen, IV fluids). Symptomatic treatment.

Guidelines/Precautions

1. The patient should avoid any strenuous activities or prolonged (i.e., more than 1 hour) weight-bearing activities, such as jogging or tennis, within 48 hours following the intra-articular injection.
2. Do not administer to patients with known hyper-sensitivity to hyaluronate preparations.

3. Intra-articular injections are contraindicated in cases of infection or skin diseases in the area of injection.

Principal Adverse Reactions

Musculoskeletal: Transient pain and/or swelling and effusion of the joint, rash, itching or bruising around the joint, joint infection, fever.
CNS: Hypotension, anaphylactoid reaction.
Dermatologic: Rash, pruritus.

SUCRALFATE

Class: Disaccharide Antiulcer Agent

Use(s): Prophylaxis and treatment of peptic ulcer and gastric erosions

Dosing: *Prophylaxis/Treatment:* PO 1 g two to four times daily.

Elimination: Gastrointestinal.

Preparations

Sucralfate **(Carafate)**
   Tablets: 1 g.
   Oral suspension: 1 g/10 mL.

Pharmacology

This anionic sulfated disaccharide is an inhibitor of pepsin and an antiulcer agent. Sucralfate is a basic aluminum complex of sucrose sulfate. Sucralfate is structurally related to heparin, but lacks anticoagulant activity. Although structurally related to sucrose, sucralfate is not utilized as a sugar in vivo in humans. Sucralfate binds to normal gastric mucosa, with a greater affinity for gastric and duodenal erosions and ulcer sites. Sucralfate reacts with hydrochloric acid in the stomach and gradually dissociates to release aluminum ions. It binds electrostatically to positively charged protein molecules in the damaged mucosa of the GI tract to form insoluble stable complexes. These complexes form an adherent protective barrier at the ulcer site. Sucralfate may be administered concomitantly with nonsteroidal anti-inflammatory drugs (NSAIDs) to minimize gastric irritation from the latter.

Pharmacokinetics

Onset of Action: PO, variable.
Peak Effect: PO, variable.
Duration of Action: PO, 6 hours.

Interactions

May decrease GI absorption of ciprofloxacin, norfloxacin, cimetidine, digoxin, phenytoin, ranitidine, tetracycline, or theophylline; increases serum aluminum with concomitant administration of aluminum-containing antacids.

Toxicity

Toxic Range: Not routinely monitored.
Manifestations: Diarrhea, constipation, nausea, vomiting, headache, sleepiness, vertigo.
Antidote: No specific antidote.
Management: Discontinue or reduce medication. Support ventilation and circulation (patent airway, oxygen, IV fluids). Symptomatic treatment.

Guidelines/Precautions

1. Antacids may be used as adjuncts to sucralfate therapy but should not be taken within 30 minutes before or after administration of sucralfate.
2. Patients with chronic renal failure may be at risk for aluminum intoxication. Use sucralfate with caution.

Principal Adverse Reactions

CNS: Sleepiness, vertigo, dizziness.
Gastrointestinal: Diarrhea, constipation, nausea, vomiting, indigestion, flatulence.
Dermatologic: Rash, pruritus.
Musculoskeletal: Back pain.
Other: Dry mouth.

SUFENTANIL CITRATE

Class: Narcotic Agonist

Use(s): Treatment of acute, chronic, and cancer pain.

Dosing: *Pain*

       IV/IM: 10–30µg (0.2–0.6µg/kg).

       Intranasal: 1.5–3.0µg/kg. Use undiluted injectate solution for the intranasal route.

       Epidural

          Bolus: 10–50µg (0.2–1.0µg/kg).

          Infusion: 5–30µg/hr (0.1–0.6µg/kg/hr).

       Spinal: 1–10µg (0.01–0.02µg/kg).

       Patient-controlled analgesia IV

       Bolus: 2–10µg (0.04–0.2µg/kg).

       Infusion: 2–20µg/hr (0.04–0.4µg/kg/hr).

       Lockout interval: 3–10 minutes.

Patient-controlled analgesia epidural:
> Bolus: 4–8 µg (0.08–0.16 µg/kg).
> Infusion: 4–8 µg/hr (0.08–0.16 µg/kg/hr).
> Lockout interval: 10–20 minutes.

Due to impaired elimination, accumulation and excess sedation may occur in patients with hepatic dysfunction. Analgesia may be enhanced by addition of adjuvant drugs such as nonsteroidal anti-inflammatory drugs (NSAIDs) and antidepressant agents (see pages xxvi–xliv for drug combinations) and use of nondrug therapies such as transcutaneous electrical nerve stimulation (TENS).

Elimination: Hepatic.

Preparations

Sufentanil citrate **(Sufenta):** Injection: 50 µg/mL.

Dilution for Infusion

IV: 500 µg in 100 mL normal saline (5 µg/mL).
Epidural
> Bolus: 10–30 µg in 15–20 mL local anesthetic or preservative-free normal saline.
> Infusion: 100 µg in 100 mL local anesthetic or preservative-free normal saline (1 µg/mL).

Pharmacology

A potent narcotic, sufentanil is a thiamyl analogue of fentanyl with five to seven times the parenteral analgesic potency and two to five times the epidural/intrathecal analgesic potency. Compared with fentanyl, sufentanil has a shorter duration of action. The cardiovascular effects of both drugs are generally similar. Sufentanil may produce a dose-dependent bradycardia, probably by stimulation of the vagal nucleus in the medulla. Depression of ventilation is due to a decrease in response of the respiratory centers in the brain stem to increases in carbon dioxide. Sufentanil (and fentanyl) is more lipophilic than morphine, and segmentation of epidural analgesia reflects rapid vascular uptake as well as incorporation in the lipid structures of the spinal space (epidural fat and white matter). The segmental limitation of analgesia requires placement of the epidural catheter at sites adjacent to the dermatomes to be covered. Large volumes of diluent may enable more dermatomes to be included. Sufentanil crosses the placental barrier and may produce depression in the neonate. The drug may appear in breast milk and should be used with caution in nursing mothers.

Pharmacokinetics

Onset of Action: IV, 1–3 minutes. Intranasal, <5 minutes. Epidural/Spinal, 4–10 minutes.
Peak Effect: IV, 3–5 minutes. Intranasal, 10 minutes. Epidural/Spinal, <30 minutes.
Duration of Action: IV, 20–45 minutes. IM, 2–4 hours. Epidural/Spinal, 2–4 hours.

Interactions

Circulatory and ventilatory depressant effects potentiated by other narcotics, sedatives, nitrous oxide, volatile anesthetics; ventilatory depressant effects potentiated by monoamine oxidase (MAO) inhibitors, phenothiazines, and tricyclic antidepressants; analgesia enhanced and prolonged by α_2-agonists (e.g., clonidine, epinephrine); addition of epinephrine to intrathecal/epidural sufentanil results in increased side effects (e.g., nausea) and prolonged motor block; in higher dosages, skeletal muscle rigidity sufficient to interfere with ventilation occurs; increased incidences of bradycardia with use of vecuronium.

Toxicity

Toxic Range: Not routinely monitored.

Manifestations: Somnolence, coma, respiratory arrest, apnea, cardiac arrhythmias, combined respiratory and metabolic acidosis, circulatory collapse, cardiac arrest, death.

Antidote: Naloxone IV/IM/SC 0.4–2.0 mg. Repeat dose every 2 to 3 minutes to a maximum of 10–20 mg.

Management: Discontinue or reduce medication. Support ventilation and circulation (patent airway, oxygen, IV fluids, vasopressors). Administer antidote. Monitor blood gases, pH, and electrolytes. Correct acidosis and electrolyte disturbance (lactic acidosis may require sodium bicarbonate IV 1–2 mEq/kg). Symptomatic treatment. Airway-protected, ipecac syrup–induced emesis (30 mL or 0.5 mL/kg ipecac syrup followed by 200 mL or 4 mL/kg of water or clear fluid) or gastric lavage (with drug ingestion) followed by administration of activated charcoal (PO 50–100 g or 1–2 g/kg).

Guidelines/Precautions

1. Reduce doses in elderly patients and with concomitant use of sedatives and other narcotics. Incremental doses should be determined from effect of initial dose.
2. Narcotic effect reversed with naloxone (IV 0.2–0.4 mg or higher). Duration of reversal may be shorter than duration of narcotic effect.

3. Sufentanil may produce a dose-related rigidity of skeletal muscles.

4. The drug crosses the placental barrier, and usage in labor may produce depression of respiration in the neonate. Resuscitation may be required; have naloxone available.

5. Undesirable side effects of epidural, caudal, or intrathecal sufentanil include delayed respiratory depression (up to 8 hours), pruritus, nausea and vomiting, and urinary retention. Naloxone (IV/IM/SC 0.2–0.4 mg as needed or infusion 5–10 μg/kg/hr) is effective for prophylaxis and/or treatment. Ventilatory support for respiratory depression must be readily available. Antihistamines, such as diphenhydramine (IV/IM 12.5–25.0 mg every 6 hours as needed), may be used in treating pruritus. Metoclopramide (IV 10 mg every 6 hours as needed) may be used in treating nausea and vomiting. Urinary retention that does not respond to naloxone may require straight bladder catheterization. Bethanechol (Urecholine) PO 15–30 mg three times daily or SC 2.5–5.0 mg three or four times daily as required may be used as an alternative to naloxone. (Bethanechol increases the tone of the detrusor urinae muscle. It should not be given IV or IM, which may result in cholinergic overstimulation. Have atropine available [IV/SC 0.5 mg].)

6. Epidural, caudal, or intrathecal injections should be avoided when the patient has septicemia, infection at the injection site, or coagulopathy.

7. Patients should be warned that sufentanil may impair their ability to perform hazardous tasks requiring mental alertness or physical coordination

(e.g., driving a motor vehicle, operating heavy machinery).
8. Sufentanil is subject to control under the Federal Controlled Substances Act of 1970 as a Schedule II (C-II) drug.

Principal Adverse Reactions

Cardiovascular: Hypotension, bradycardia.
Pulmonary: Respiratory depression, apnea.
CNS: Dizziness, sedation, euphoria, dysphoria, anxiety.
Gastrointestinal: Nausea, vomiting, delayed gastric emptying, biliary tract spasm.
Ocular: Miosis.
Musculoskeletal: Muscle rigidity.

SULINDAC

Class: Nonsteroidal Anti-inflammatory Drug

Use(s): Symptomatic treatment of moderate to severe inflammatory and degenerative arthritis, primary dysmenorrhea, migraine, ankylosing spondylitis, gouty arthritis, Reiter's syndrome, posttraumatic pain, chronic pain, cancer pain (especially with bone metastasis).

Dosing: *Pain or inflammatory diseases:* PO 150–200 mg (3–4 mg/kg) twice daily. Maximum dose 400 mg daily. After initial therapy, dosage may be reduced according to patient response.

Administer analgesic regularly (not as needed). Addition of opioid analgesics, antidepressant agents, and nondrug therapies such as transcutaneous electrical nerve stimulation (TENS) may enhance analgesia (see pages xxvi–xliv for drug combinations). In rheumatoid arthritis or juvenile rheumatoid arthritis, second-line rheumatoid agents may include leflunomide (Arava), entanercept (Enbrel), antimalarials, or methotrexate. In geriatric patients and patients with decreased renal or hepatic function, decrease doses by one-third to one-half. The incidence of sulindac-induced gastropathy may be decreased by administration with meals, milk, antacids, or sucralfate (PO 1g four times daily). Misoprostol (PO 100–200μg four times daily) may be used to prevent gastric ulcers in high-risk patients.

Elimination: Hepatic, renal.

Preparations

Sulindac **(Clinoril):** Tablets: 150mg, 200mg.

Pharmacology

A pyrroleacetic acid derivative and nonsteroidal anti-inflammatory drug (NSAID), sulindac is structurally and pharmacologically related to indomethacin. The analgesic and anti-inflammatory activities of sulindac are similar to those of indomethacin and are partly due to the inhibition of prostaglandin synthesis and/or release secondary to the inhibition of cyclooxygenase. Cyclooxygenase enzyme catalyzes the formation of prostaglandin precursors (endoperoxides) from arachidonic acid. Sulindac may cause gastric mucosal damage that may result in ulceration or bleeding. However, sulindac is better tolerated than indomethacin, and equipotent doses are associated with less gastric mucosal abnormalities. This may be attributable to the fact that sulindac is an inactive prodrug that is converted by hepatic microsomal enzymes to an active metabolite, sulindac disulfide. The antipyretic activity of sulindac may occur secondary to inhibition of pyrogen-induced release of prostaglandins in the central nervous system (including the hypothalamus) and possibly to centrally mediated peripheral vasodilatation.

Sulindac (like other NSAIDs) exhibits a ceiling effect for analgesia. Exceeding recommended doses results in increased toxicity without improvement in analgesia. Inhibition of prostaglandin synthesis may result in decreased uterine tone and contractility and prolonged gestation in the parturient and premature closure of the ductus arteriosus in the fetus. Sulindac inhibits platelet aggregation and prolongs bleeding time. However, unlike the irreversible effects of aspirin, these effects are transient and platelet function and aggregation return to normal within 24 hours. The drug has no uricosuric activity.

Pharmacokinetics

Onset of Action: PO, analgesic effect 15–30 minutes; anti-inflammatory effect <7 days.
Peak Effect: PO, analgesic effect 1–2 hours; anti-inflammatory effect 2–3 weeks.
Duration of Action: PO, analgesic effect 3–4 hours.

Interactions

Risks of bleeding increased with concomitant NSAIDs, anticoagulant or heparin therapy, alcohol ingestion;

decreases antihypertensive effects of β-adrenergic blocking agents; serum levels of sulindac's active sulfide metabolite are decreased slightly by concomitant aspirin; serum levels of sulindac increased by concomitant probenecid; renal elimination decreased and serum levels and toxic effects of methotrexate and lithium increased by concomitant sulindac; GI absorption of sulindac delayed by food and milk; antihypertensive effects of thiazide diuretics and β-adrenergic blocking agents antagonized by sulindac; prostaglandin-mediated natriuretic effects of loop diuretics antagonized by sulindac.

Toxicity

Toxic Range: Not routinely monitored.

Manifestations: *Acute:* Drowsiness, nausea, vomiting, lethargy, paresthesia, disorientation, seizures, abdominal pain, GI bleeding.

Antidote: None.

Management: Discontinue or reduce medication. Correct fluid, electrolyte, and acid-base disturbances. Support ventilation and circulation (patent airway, oxygen, IV fluids, vasopressors). Airway-protected, ipecac syrup–induced emesis (30 mL or 0.5 mL/kg ipecac syrup followed by 200 mL or 4 mL/kg of water or clear fluid) or gastric lavage (with drug ingestion) followed by administration of activated charcoal (PO 50–100 g or 1–2 g/kg). Forced alkaline diuresis with IV sodium bicarbonate (IV furosemide if necessary) after correction of dehydration. Symptomatic treatment. Monitor for several days due to the risk of delayed GI ulceration.

Guidelines/Precautions

1. Use with caution in patients with active GI lesions (e.g., erosive gastritis, peptic ulcer), a history of recurrent GI lesions, hepatic or renal dysfunction, preexisting hypoprothrombinemia, or vitamin K deficiency. Sulindac should be used cautiously in patients with heart failure, hypertension, or other conditions associated with fluid retention.
2. Renal prostaglandins may have a supportive role in maintaining renal perfusion in patients with prerenal conditions. Sulindac should be avoided in such patients because it may cause a dose-dependent decrease in prostaglandin formation and thus precipitate renal decompensation.
3. Carefully observe patients with coagulation disorders and those receiving drug therapy that interferes with hemostasis.
4. Avoid the use of sulindac during pregnancy. In the third trimester, the drug may produce adverse fetal effects, including constriction of the ductus arteriosus, neonatal primary pulmonary hypertension, and fetal death.
5. Patient response to NSAIDs is variable. Patients who do not respond to or cannot tolerate sulindac may be successfully treated with another NSAID.
6. Sulindac and salicylates should not be administered concomitantly because there may not be any therapeutic advantage and incidences of adverse GI side effects may be increased.
7. Contraindicated in patients with previously demonstrated hypersensitivity to sulindac or with the

complete or partial syndrome of nasal polyps, angioedema, or bronchospastic reactivity to aspirin or other NSAIDs.
8. Signs and symptoms of infection or other diseases may be masked by the antipyretic and anti-inflammatory effects of sulindac.
9. Monitor stool for blood every 14 days, and monitor BUN, serum creatinine, and urinalysis every 1 to 2 months when administering sulindac at chronic high doses.

Principal Adverse Reactions

Cardiovascular: Congestive heart failure, peripheral edema, fluid retention, hypertension, tachycardia, arrhythmias.

Pulmonary: Dyspnea, bronchospasm.

CNS: Drowsiness, dizziness, headache, anxiety, confusion.

Gastrointestinal: Ulceration, bleeding, dyspepsia, nausea, vomiting, diarrhea, hepatic dysfunction, jaundice.

Genitourinary: Renal dysfunction, acute renal failure, azotemia, cystitis, hematuria.

Dermatologic: Pruritus, urticaria.

Hematologic: Prolongation of bleeding time, leukopenia, thrombocytopenia, aplastic anemia, hemolytic anemia.

Other: Tinnitus, blurred vision.

SUMATRIPTAN SUCCINATE

Class: Serotonin Agonist

Use(s): Acute treatment of migraine attacks with or without auras.

Dosing: SC: 3–6 mg. Dose may be repeated after 1 hour if needed, or oral medication may be utilized. Maximum daily SC dosage: 12 mg.

PO: 25–100 mg. Dose may be repeated every 2 hours. Maximum 24-hour PO dosage: 300 mg. Maximum 24-hour PO dosage after initial SC dose: 200 mg.

Intranasal: 20 mg per 0.1 mL insufflation. Administer two insufflations of 20 mg 15 minutes apart.

Slow IV: 1–2 mg (20–30 μg/kg). Dilute in normal saline and infuse over 10 minutes.

Sumatriptan is approved for only subcutaneous, intranasal, and oral administration in the United States. Intravenous administration may be associated with coronary vasospasm.

Elimination: Hepatic.

Preparations

Sumatriptan succinate **(Imitrex)**
Tablets: 25 mg, 50 mg.
Injection: 12 mg/mL.
Nasal spray: 5 mg/0.1 mL and 20 mg/0.1 mL.
Sumatriptan succinate **(Imitrex SELFdose System kit):**
Injection: 12 mg/mL.

Pharmacology

Sumatriptan is a selective serotonin 5-hydroxytryptamine (5-HT$_1$) receptor agonist. It produces brief and selective vasoconstriction of the arteriovenous anastomosis of the carotid distribution and prevents neurogenic dural plasma extravasation. Sumatriptan is a stronger vasoconstrictor of the dural arteries than cerebral and temporal arteries. The drug has no effect on α-, β-, dopamine, and other serotonin (5-HT$_2$, 5-HT$_3$) receptors. There is no effect on cerebral blood flow, peripheral arteries, or perfusion of peripheral organs. Sumatriptan reduces the incidence of nausea, vomiting, photophobia, and phonophobia. It appears to be more effective than Cafergot (ergotamine and caffeine) in the acute treatment of migraine. The efficacy of sumatriptan for migraine is unaffected by the absence or presence of aura, the duration of attack, the gender of the patient, or concomitant use of common migraine prophylactic drugs (e.g., β-blockers).

Pharmacokinetics

Onset of Action: SC/Intranasal, <10 minutes.
Peak Effect: SC/Intranasal, 20 minutes.
Duration of Action: 2 hours.

Interactions

Additive adverse cardiovascular effects may occur with concomitant use of ergot compounds.

Toxicity

Toxic Range: Not routinely monitored.
Manifestations: Hypertension, coronary vasospasm, palpitations, arrhythmias, seizures, respiratory depression, cyanosis, ataxia.
Antidote: No specific antidote.

Management: Discontinue or reduce medication. Support ventilation and circulation (patent airway, oxygen, IV fluids, vasodilators). Monitoring should continue while symptoms and signs persist and for at least 10 hours afterward. Symptomatic treatment.

Guidelines/Precautions

1. Patients who will self-administer sumatriptan injections should receive instructions on the proper use of the product prior to doing so for the first time. Parenteral administration should be avoided in patients with ischemic heart disease or Prinzmetal's angina. In patients with identifiable cardiac risk factors, the initial dose should be given in the physician's office to determine if there is any unrecognized cardiovascular disease. Do not administer intravenously due to the risk of inducing coronary vasospasm.

2. Use with caution in patients with impaired renal or hepatic function.

3. Sumatriptan should not be used within 24 hours of administration of an ergot compound or other 5-HT_1 receptor agonists (e.g., zolmitriptan).

4. Sumatriptan should not be administered in patients with basilar or hemiplegic migraine.

5. Chest, jaw, or neck tightness is relatively common after administration of sumatriptan injection, but has only rarely been associated with ischemic EKG changes. However, because sumatriptan may cause coronary artery vasospasm, patients who experience signs and symptoms suggestive of angina following sumatriptan should be evaluated

for the presence of coronary artery disease or a predisposition to variant angina before receiving additional doses of sumatriptan. Similarly, patients who experience other symptoms or signs suggestive of decreasing arterial flow (such as ischemic abdominal syndromes or Raynaud's syndrome) following sumatriptan administration should be evaluated for arteriosclerosis or predisposition to vasospasm.

6. Do not administer sumatriptan to patients with cerebral vascular disease. Cerebral hemorrhage, subarachnoid hemorrhage, stroke, and other cerebrovascular events have occurred in patients treated with 5-HT$_1$ agonist drugs. It is believed that the severe headaches were secondary to an evolving neurologic lesion. Patients with migraine may be at increased risk of certain cerebrovascular events (e.g., hemorrhage, stroke, transient ischemic attacks). For a given attack, if a patient does not respond to the first dose of sumatriptan, the diagnosis of migraine or cluster headache should be reconsidered before administration of a second dose.

Principal Adverse Reactions

Cardiovascular: Hypertension, angina, arrhythmias, peripheral vasoconstriction, palpitations.
Pulmonary: Dyspnea, bronchospasm.
CNS: Dizziness, malaise, drowsiness, weakness, seizures, paresthesias.
Gastrointestinal: Bad taste.
Other: Visual disturbances; neck, throat, jaw, and/or chest pain, tightness, or pressure.

TETRACAINE

Class: Local Anesthetic

Use(s): Regional and topical anesthesia.

Dosing: *Spinal:* Bolus/Infusion, 5–20 mg (1% solution). (Children, 0.4 mg/kg, with a minimum of 1 mg.) Dilute dose with equal volume of supplied dextrose solution (hyperbaric) or cerebrospinal fluid (isobaric) or sterile water (hypobaric).

Brachial plexus block: Combine 0.5–1.0 mg/kg tetracaine with 30–50 mL (0.5–0.75 mL/kg) of bupivacaine (0.25–0.375%) or lidocaine (1%) or mepivacaine (1%).

Topical (spray): Apply 2% solution for 1 second (never more than 2 seconds). Average expulsion rate of residue from spray is 200 mg per second.

Maximum safe dose: 1.0–1.5 mg/kg without epinephrine; 2.5 mg/kg with epinephrine. Solutions containing preservatives should not be used for spinal block. Except where contraindicated, vasoconstrictor drugs may be added to increase effect and prolong local or regional anesthesia. For dosage and route guidelines, see the "Dosing" section of Epinephrine (p. 204). Do not use vasoconstrictor drugs for IV regional anesthesia or local anesthesia of end organs (digits, penis, ears).

Elimination: Plasma cholinesterase.

Preparations

Tetracaine hydrochloride **(Pontocaine)**
  Injection: 1% with 10% dextrose, 0.2% in 6% dextrose,
    0.3% in 6% dextrose.
  Powder for reconstitution: 20 mg.
Tetracaine hydrochloride, benzocaine, and butyl ami-
  nobenzoate **(Cetacaine Topical):** Topical solution:
  Tetracaine 2%, benzocaine 14%, butyl aminobenzoate
  2%.

Pharmacology

This ester of *para*-aminobenzoic acid is a potent,
long-acting local anesthetic. Tetracaine stabilizes the
neuronal membrane and prevents initiation and transmission of nerve impulses. It has a prolonged duration
of action compared with procaine and chloroprocaine
due to a much slower rate of hydrolysis by plasma
cholinesterase. The duration of action may be further
prolonged by the addition of vasoconstrictor drugs to
delay systemic absorption. High plasma levels may
produce seizures and cardiovascular collapse secondary
to a decrease in peripheral vascular resistance and direct
myocardial depression.

Pharmacokinetics

Onset of Action: Topical, <30 seconds; infiltration, 15
minutes; spinal, <10 minutes.
Peak Effect: Infiltration/Spinal, 0.25–1.0 hours.
Duration of Action: Infiltration, 2–3 hours; spinal,
1.25–3.0 hours.

Interactions

Prolongs the effect of succinylcholine; metabolite
(PABA) inhibits the action of sulfonamides and ami-

nosalicylic acid; toxicity enhanced by cimetidine, anticholinesterases (which inhibit degradation); benzodiazepines, barbiturates, and volatile anesthetics increase seizure threshold; duration of regional anesthesia prolonged by vasoconstrictor agents (e.g., epinephrine) and α_2-agonists (e.g., clonidine); alkalinization increases rate of onset and potency of local or regional anesthesia.

Toxicity

Toxic Range: Serum levels >8µg/mL.

Manifestations: Hypotension, confusion, slurred speech, perioral numbness, tinnitus, seizures, arrhythmias, circulatory collapse, respiratory depression, cardiac arrest.

Antidote: No specific antidote.

Management: Discontinue or reduce medication. Support ventilation and circulation (patent airway, oxygen, IV fluids, vasopressors). Benzodiazepines (diazepam IV 0.05–0.2 mg/kg, midazolam IV/IM 0.025–0.1 mg/kg) or barbiturates (thiopental sodium IV 0.5–2.0 mg/kg) to control seizures. Prolonged cardiopulmonary resuscitation with cardiac arrest: Sodium bicarbonate IV 1–2 mEq/kg to treat cardiac toxicity (sodium channel blockade), bretylium IV 5 mg/kg, DC cardioversion/defibrillation for ventricular arrhythmias. Remove ingested drug by induced emesis followed by activated charcoal. Hypersensitivity reactions: Remove from further exposure and treat dermatitis.

Guidelines/Precautions

1. Do not use on eyes.
2. To minimize systemic absorption, do not apply topically to large areas of denuded or inflamed tissue.

3. Use with caution in patients with severe disturbances of cardiac rhythm, shock, or heart block.
4. Reduce doses in obstetric and elderly patients.
5. Cauda equina syndrome with permanent neurologic deficit has occurred in patients receiving more than 20 mg of a 1% tetracaine solution with a continuous spinal technique.
6. There is potential for allergic reaction with repeated use.
7. Contraindicated in patients with hypersensitivity to tetracaine or ester-type local anesthetics and in patients with allergy to suntan lotion (contains PABA derivatives).
8. The level of sympathetic blockade determines the degree of hypotension following intrathecal administration of tetracaine. Blocks above T5 affect cardiac sympathetic nerves and are associated with bradycardia and decreased cardiac output. Fluid hydration (10–20 mL/kg normal saline or lactated Ringer's solution), vasopressor agents (e.g., ephedrine), and left uterine displacement in pregnant patients may be used for prophylaxis and/or treatment. Administer atropine to treat bradycardia.
9. Caudal or intrathecal injections should be avoided when the patient has hypovolemic shock, septicemia, infection at the injection site, or coagulopathy.

Principal Adverse Reactions

Cardiovascular: Hypotension, bradycardia, heart block, arrhythmias, peripheral vasodilatation.
Pulmonary: Respiratory impairment or paralysis.

CNS: Postspinal headache, tinnitus, seizures, blurred vision, restlessness.
Allergic: Urticaria, erythema, angioneurotic edema.
Spinal: High spinal, loss of perineal sensation and sexual function, backache, weakness and paralysis of the lower extremities, loss of sphincter control, slowing of labor, cranial nerve palsies, meningitis.

TIZANIDINE

Class: Skeletal Muscle Relaxant

Use(s): Treatment of spasticity related to spinal cord pathology and multiple sclerosis; adjunct treatment of acute compression radiculopathy, chronic regional pain syndrome (CRPS/RSD), multiple sclerosis, trigeminal neuralgia, pretrigeminal neuralgia, glossopharyngeal neuralgia, vagoglossopharyngeal neuralgia, organic (nontraction) headache, neuropathic pain, postherpetic neuralgia, fibromyalgia; perioperative sedation.

Dosing: *Spasticity, trigeminal neuralgia, organic headache, neuropathic pain, fibromyalgia, CRPS/RSD*

Initial: PO 2 mg (half tablet) in the morning and afternoon, 4 mg (one tablet) at bedtime.
Maintenance: PO 4–12 mg three times daily.
For increased muscle relaxation, tizanidine doses may be supplemented with baclofen.
Monitoring of aminotransferase levels is recommended during the first 6 months of treatment (e.g., baseline and 1, 3, and 6

months) and periodically thereafter based on clinical status. Because of the potential toxic hepatic effect of tizanidine, the drug should be used only with extreme caution in patients with impaired hepatic function.

Perioperative sedation: PO 4 mg (one tablet). Administer 90 minutes prior to induction.

Elimination: Renal.

Preparations

Tizanidine **(Zanaflex):** Tablets: 4 mg, 8 mg, 12 mg.

Pharmacology

A short-acting α_2-adrenergic receptor agonist, tizanidine is structurally and pharmacologically similar to clonidine and other α_2-adrenergic receptor agonists. However, tizanidine has one-tenth to one-fiftieth the antihypertensive potency of these drugs. In sedative and sympatholytic activity, 12 mg of tizanidine is equipotent with 150 µg of clonidine. The antispasmodic activity of tizanidine results from agonism at central presynaptic α_2-receptors. The response to agonism at these receptors is a decrease in the release of excitatory neurotransmitters (such as glutamic acid), which in turn leads to the inhibition of spinal motor neurons. Both tizanidine and baclofen inhibit spinal interneuron firing; however, tizanidine's effects are mediated by α_2-receptors, whereas baclofen may exert a direct effect on the polarization state of the neuron membrane. Tizanidine and baclofen are equally effective in antispastic activity; however, tizanidine may be associated with fewer side effects such as severe muscle weakness.

Tizanidine or baclofen is the drug of choice for muscle spasm in patients with multiple sclerosis and other spinal cord lesions, where the decrease in the number and severity of muscle spasms (especially flexor spasms) alleviates associated pain, clonus, and muscle rigidity and improves mobility. Either tizanidine or intrathecal baclofen is preferable to intrathecal injections of sclerosing agents (e.g., phenol), rhizotomy, or cordotomy. Tizanidine (like clonidine) mediates gastric mucosal protection and may reduce the incidence of gastric irritation induced by nonsteroidal anti-inflammatory drugs (NSAIDs). Tizanidine may have antinociceptive properties. It has been reported to relieve neuropathic (lancinating, shooting) and causalgic (hot, burning, cramping) components of phantom limb pain. Oral tizanidine may be effective in the adjunctive treatment of reflex sympathetic dystrophy, trigeminal neuralgia, fibromyalgia, and nonvascular headache. Tizanidine may relieve the episodic and allodynic pain in postherpetic neuralgia. In large doses, tizanidine may produce excess sedation and hypotension.

Pharmacokinetics

Onset of Action: Antispastic effects: PO, hours to weeks.
Peak Effect: Antispastic effects: PO, variable; intrathecal bolus, 4 hours.
Duration of Action: Antispastic effects: PO, variable.

Interactions

Potentiates CNS depressant effects of alcohol, barbiturates, narcotics, volatile anesthetics; additive muscle relaxant effects when coadministered with baclofen.

Toxicity

Toxic Range: Not routinely monitored.

Manifestations: Vomiting, muscle hypotonia, salivation, drowsiness, confusion, blurred vision, respiratory depression, coma, seizures, elevated serum lactate dehydrogenase and AST (SGOT) concentrations.

Antidote: No specific antidote.

Management: Discontinue or reduce medication. Support ventilation and circulation (patent airway, oxygen, IV fluids, vasopressors). Airway-protected, ipecac syrup–induced emesis (30 mL or 0.5 mL/kg ipecac syrup followed by 200 mL or 4 mL/kg of water or clear fluid) or gastric lavage (with drug ingestion) followed by administration of activated charcoal (PO 50–100 g or 1–2 g/kg). Symptomatic treatment.

Guidelines/Precautions

1. Tizanidine occasionally causes liver injury, most often hepatocellular in type. In controlled clinical studies, approximately 5% of patients treated with tizanidine had elevations of liver function tests (>3 times normal). Most cases resolved rapidly on drug withdrawal.
2. Deterioration in seizure control may occur in epileptic patients receiving tizanidine. The EEG should be monitored periodically.
3. Use with caution in patients who must use spasticity to maintain an upright posture or balance in locomotion or whenever spasticity is utilized to obtain increased function.
4. Abrupt withdrawal may lead to hallucinations, seizures, and acute exacerbation of spasticity.

Dosage should be reduced gradually if the drug is to be discontinued.
5. Patients should be warned that tizanidine may impair their ability to perform activities requiring mental alertness or physical coordination (e.g., operating heavy machinery, driving a motor vehicle).

Principal Adverse Reactions

Cardiovascular: Tachycardia, hypotension, palpitations, angina, syncope.
Pulmonary: Dyspnea, respiratory depression.
CNS: Drowsiness, fatigue, vertigo, dizziness, hypotonia, mental depression, excitation, headache, hallucinations, euphoria, anxiety, dysarthria, strabismus.
Gastrointestinal: Nausea and vomiting, constipation, diarrhea, taste disorders, abdominal pain.
Musculoskeletal: Muscle pain.
Other: Rash, pruritus.

TOLMETIN SODIUM

Class: High-Potency Anti-inflammatory Agent

Use(s): Symptomatic treatment of moderate to severe inflammatory and degenerative arthritis, primary dysmenorrhea, migraine, ankylosing spondylitis, posttraumatic pain, chronic pain, and cancer pain (especially with bone metastasis).

Dosing: *Pain or inflammatory diseases:* PO 400–600 mg (8–12 mg/kg) three times daily (preferably including a dose on arising and at bedtime). Maximum dose 2000 mg/day.

Administer analgesic regularly (not as needed). Addition of opioid analgesics and antidepressant agents and use of nondrug therapies such as transcutaneous electrical nerve stimulation (TENS) may enhance analgesia (see pages xxvi–xliv for drug combinations). In rheumatoid arthritis or juvenile rheumatoid arthritis, second-line rheumatoid agents may include leflunomide (Arava), etanercept (Enbrel), antimalarials, or methotrexate. In geriatric patients and patients with decreased renal or hepatic function, decrease doses by one-third to one-half. The incidence of tolmetin-induced gastropathy may be decreased by administration with meals, milk, antacids, or sucralfate (PO 1 g four times daily). Misoprostol (PO 100–200 μg four times daily) may be used to prevent gastric ulcers in high-risk patients.

Elimination: Hepatic, renal.

Preparations

Tolmetin sodium **(Tolectin)**
    Tablets: 200 mg.
    Tablets, film coated: 600 mg.
Tolmetin sodium **(Tolectin DS):** Capsules: 400 mg.

Pharmacology

A pyrroleacetic acid derivative and nonsteroidal anti-inflammatory drug (NSAID), tolmetin is structurally and pharmacologically related to zomepirac. The analgesic and anti-inflammatory activities of tolmetin are similar to those of indomethacin and are partly due to the inhibition of prostaglandin synthesis and/or release secondary to the inhibition of cyclooxygenase. Cyclooxygenase enzyme catalyzes the formation of prostaglandin precursors (endoperoxides) from arachidonic acid. Tolmetin may cause gastric mucosal damage that may result in ulceration or bleeding. However, tolmetin is better tolerated than aspirin, and equipotent doses are associated with less gastric mucosal abnormalities. The antipyretic activity of tolmetin may occur secondary to inhibition of pyrogen-induced release of prostaglandins in the central nervous system (including the hypothalamus) and possibly to centrally mediated peripheral vasodilatation.

Tolmetin (like other NSAIDs) exhibits a ceiling effect for analgesia. Exceeding recommended doses results in increased toxicity without improvement in analgesia. Inhibition of prostaglandin synthesis may result in decreased uterine tone and contractility and prolonged gestation in the parturient and premature closure of the ductus arteriosus in the fetus. Tolmetin inhibits platelet aggregation and prolongs bleeding time. The drug has no uricosuric activity.

Pharmacokinetics

Onset of Action: PO, analgesic effect 15–30 minutes; anti-inflammatory effect <7 days.
Peak Effect: PO, analgesic effect 1–2 hours; anti-inflammatory effect 2–3 weeks.
Duration of Action: PO, analgesic effect 3–4 hours.

Interactions

Risks of bleeding increased with concomitant NSAIDs, anticoagulant or heparin therapy, alcohol ingestion; decreases antihypertensive effects of β-adrenergic blocking agents; serum levels of tolmetin decreased slightly by concomitant aspirin; serum levels of tolmetin increased by concomitant probenecid; serum levels and toxic effects of phenytoin, oral anticoagulants, salicylates, sulfonamides, sulfonylureas (e.g., tolbutamide), methotrexate, and lithium increased by concomitant tolmetin; GI absorption of tolmetin delayed by food and milk.

Toxicity

Toxic Range: Not routinely monitored.
Manifestations: *Acute:* Drowsiness, nausea, vomiting, lethargy, paresthesia, disorientation, abdominal pain, GI bleeding, thrombocytopenia.
Antidote: None.
Management: Discontinue or reduce medication. Correct fluid, electrolyte, and acid-base disturbances. Support ventilation and circulation (patent airway, oxygen, IV fluids, vasopressors). Airway-protected, ipecac syrup–induced emesis (30 mL or 0.5 mL/kg ipecac syrup followed by 200 mL or 4 mL/kg of water or clear fluid) or gastric lavage (with drug ingestion) followed by administration of activated charcoal (PO 50–100 g or 1–2 g/kg). Forced alkaline diuresis with IV sodium bicarbonate (IV furosemide if necessary) after correction of dehydration. Symptomatic treatment.

Guidelines/Precautions

1. Use with caution in patients with active GI lesions (e.g., erosive gastritis, peptic ulcer), a history of

recurrent GI lesions, hepatic or renal dysfunction, preexisting hypoprothrombinemia, or vitamin K deficiency. Tolmetin may cause peripheral edema and should be used cautiously in patients with heart failure, hypertension, or conditions associated with fluid retention.

2. Renal prostaglandins may have a supportive role in maintaining renal perfusion in patients with prerenal conditions. Tolmetin should be avoided in such patients because it may cause a dose-dependent decrease in prostaglandin formation and thus precipitate renal decompensation.

3. Carefully observe patients with coagulation disorders and those receiving drug therapy that interferes with hemostasis.

4. Avoid the use of tolmetin during pregnancy. In the third trimester, the drug may produce adverse fetal effects, including constriction of the ductus arteriosus, neonatal primary pulmonary hypertension, and fetal death.

5. Tolmetin and salicylates should not be administered concomitantly because there may not be any therapeutic advantage and incidences of adverse GI side effects may be increased.

6. Patient response to NSAIDs is variable. Patients who do not respond to or cannot tolerate tolmetin may be successfully treated with another NSAID.

7. Contraindicated in patients with previously demonstrated hypersensitivity to tolmetin or with the complete or partial syndrome of nasal polyps, angioedema, or bronchospastic reactivity to aspirin or other NSAIDs.

8. Signs and symptoms of infection or other diseases may be masked by the antipyretic and anti-
inflammatory effects of tolmetin.
9. Monitor stool for blood every 14 days, and
monitor BUN, serum creatinine, and urinalysis
every 1 to 2 months when administering tolmetin
at chronic high doses.
10. Use of tolmetin and other NSAIDs is not recommended during pregnancy (especially during the
last trimester) or during labor and delivery. Tolmetin and other NSAIDs inhibit prostaglandin synthesis, which may cause dystocia, interfere with
labor, and delay parturition. Prostaglandin synthesis inhibitors may also have adverse effects on the
fetal cardiovascular system (e.g., premature
closure of ductus arteriosus).

Principal Adverse Reactions

Cardiovascular: Congestive heart failure, peripheral
edema, fluid retention, hypertension, tachycardia, arrhythmias.
Pulmonary: Dyspnea, bronchospasm.
CNS: Drowsiness, dizziness, headache, anxiety, confusion.
Gastrointestinal: Ulceration, bleeding, dyspepsia, nausea, vomiting, diarrhea, hepatic dysfunction, jaundice.
Genitourinary: Renal dysfunction, acute renal failure,
azotemia, cystitis, hematuria.
Dermatologic: Pruritus, urticaria.
Hematologic: Prolongation of bleeding time, leukopenia, thrombocytopenia, aplastic anemia, hemolytic
anemia.
Other: Tinnitus, blurred vision, optic neuropathy.

TRAMADOL HYDROCHLORIDE

Class: Central-Acting Analgesic

Use(s): Treatment of acute, chronic, and cancer pain.

Dosing: *Analgesia:* PO 50–100 mg (1–2 mg/kg) every 4 to 6 hours. Maximum daily dose 400 mg (300 mg for patients >75 years). Reduce dose for patients with renal or hepatic impairment.

Renal impairment:

Creatine clearance ≥30 mL/min: No dosage adjustment needed.

Creatine clearance <30 mL/min: PO 50 mg every 12 hours. Maximum daily dose 200 mg.

Hepatic impairment (cirrhosis): PO 50 mg every 12 hours.

Administer analgesic regularly (not as needed). Analgesia may be enhanced by addition of adjuvant drugs such as nonsteroidal anti-inflammatory drugs (NSAIDs) and antidepressant agents (see pages xxvi–xliv for drug combinations) and use of nondrug therapies such as transcutaneous electrical nerve stimulation (TENS).

Elimination: Hepatic, renal.

Preparations

Tramadol hydrochloride **(Ultram):** Tablets: 50 mg.

Pharmacology

Tramadol is a centrally acting synthetic analgesic with moderate analgesic efficacy comparable with that of codeine or pentazocine. For analgesia, 50 mg of tramadol is equal to 60 mg of codeine. The analgesic activity is mediated by binding of the drug to opioid receptors and antidepressant-like inhibition of reuptake of serotonin and norepinephrine. This unique mechanism of action may allow tramadol to be utilized in place of combination therapy (analgesic and antidepressant) for the treatment of neuropathic pain syndromes. Unlike typical opioid analgesics, tramadol is associated with fewer incidences of analgesic tolerance or side effects such as respiratory depression or constipation. Tramadol crosses the placental barrier and may produce depression in the neonate. The drug may appear in breast milk, but at usual doses the effects on the infant may not be clinically significant.

Pharmacokinetics

Onset of Action: PO, <1 hour.
Peak Effect: PO, 2–3 hours.
Duration of Action: PO, 3–6 hours.

Interactions

Increased seizure risk in patients with epilepsy, history of seizures, or decreased seizure threshold (e.g., with head trauma), metabolic disorders, alcohol and drug withdrawal, or CNS infections, and in patients receiving tricyclic antidepressants, selective serotonin reuptake inhibitors, monoamine oxidase (MAO) inhibitors, neuroleptics, or other drugs that reduce the seizure threshold; increased metabolism and dosage requirements of tramadol in patients receiving carbamazepine; potentiates CNS and circulatory depressant effects of other narcotic analgesics, volatile anesthetics, phenothiazines, sedative-hypnotics, alcohol, tricyclic antidepressants; analgesia enhanced and prolonged by narcotic and non-narcotic analgesics (e.g., aspirin, acetaminophen), α_2-agonists (e.g., clonidine).

Toxicity

Toxic Range: Not routinely monitored.

Manifestations: Seizures, respiratory depression, apnea, death.

Antidote: Treat seizures with barbiturates or benzodiazepines. Risk of seizures may be increased with naloxone.

Management: Discontinue or reduce medication. Support ventilation and circulation (patent airway, oxygen, IV fluids, vasopressors). Administer antidote. Monitor blood gases, pH, and electrolytes. Correct acidosis and electrolyte disturbance (lactic acidosis may require sodium bicarbonate IV 1–2 mEq/kg). Symptomatic treatment. Hemodialysis is not expected to be helpful because it removes less than 7% of the administered drug in a 4-hour dialysis period.

Guidelines/Precautions

1. Tramadol should not be used in opioid-dependent patients. The drug can reinitiate physical dependence in patients who have been previously dependent or chronically using other opioids.
2. Constipation may be more difficult to control than pain. Prevent and/or treat by daily administration of laxatives and stool softeners, for example, Colace (docusate sodium) 100–300 mg/day. Do not administer bulk-forming agents that contain methylcellulose, psyllium, or polycarbophil. Temporary arrest

in the passage through the gastrointestinal tract may lead to fecal impaction or bowel obstruction.

3. Tolerance may develop in patients taking tramadol for more than a couple of weeks. The first sign is a decrease in duration of effective analgesia. To delay the development of tolerance, add adjuvant drugs (e.g., NSAIDs, antidepressant agents, dextromethorphan) or switch to alternative opioids (starting at one-half the equianalgesic dose) or supplement with nondrug therapies (e.g., TENS).

4. Physical dependence may be revealed with abrupt discontinuation of chronically administered tramadol (longer than 2 weeks). Withdrawal symptoms may manifest by anxiety, nervousness, irritability, chills alternating with hot flashes, diaphoresis, insomnia, abdominal cramps, nausea, vomiting, and myoclonus. To avoid withdrawal, doses should be reduced slowly (e.g., dose reduction of 75% every 2 days). Withdrawal should be treated symptomatically.

5. Addiction (psychological dependence) is characterized by a continued craving for a narcotic and the need to use tramadol for effects other than for pain relief. The patient exhibits drug-seeking behavior. Most patients with psychological dependence are also physically dependent, but the reverse is rare in patients using opioid agonists for the management of pain.

6. Drug combinations with adjuvant drugs enhance analgesia (see pages xxvi–xliv).

7. Adjuvant drug therapies also include regional blockade, trigger-point injections (with local anesthetics and steroids), and intravenous regional anesthesia.

8. Adjuvant nondrug therapies include TENS and modalities such as ice or heat application, ultrasound, and soft tissue mobilization.
9. Patients should be warned that tramadol may impair their ability to perform hazardous tasks requiring mental alertness or physical coordination (e.g., driving a motor vehicle, operating heavy machinery).
10. Tramadol is contraindicated in patients who have previously demonstrated hypersensitivity to tramadol or opioids.
11. Large doses of tramadol may cause seizures. Caution is advised in concomitant administration of tramadol with MAO inhibitors, phenothiazines, antidepressants, antipsychotics, naloxone, and other drugs that reduce the seizure threshold.

Principal Adverse Reactions

Cardiovascular: Orthostatic hypotension, vasodilatation, syncope.
Pulmonary: Respiratory depression.
CNS: Sedation, somnolence, euphoria, dysphoria, disorientation.
Genitourinary: Urinary retention, urinary frequency.
Gastrointestinal: Nausea, vomiting, dyspepsia, constipation, abdominal pain, anorexia, flatulence.
Dermatologic: Rash, urticaria.

TRAZODONE HYDROCHLORIDE

Class: Antidepressant

Use(s): Treatment of neurotic and endogenous depression; adjunct treatment of neuropathic pain syndromes, including diabetic neuropathy, postherpetic neuralgia, tic douloureux, and cancer pain; anxiety disorders; phobias; panic disorders; alcohol dependency; enuresis; eating disorders.

Dosing: *Pain syndromes*

Initial: PO 150 mg daily in divided doses, with a major portion of the daily dose preferably at bedtime.

Maintenance: PO 150–400 mg daily in divided doses, with a major portion of the daily dose preferably at bedtime. Doses may be titrated upward in increments of 50 mg/day every 3 to 4 days. Doses should be decreased if unacceptable side effects occur. Serum levels should be determined if there are signs of toxicity. The higher end of the dose range may be required in the management of painful diabetic neuropathy.

Depression

Initial: PO 150 mg daily in divided doses, with a major portion of the daily dose preferably at bedtime.

Maintenance: PO 150–600 mg daily in divided doses, with a major portion of the daily dose preferably at bedtime. The higher end of the dose range (400–600 mg/day) may be required for inpatients with severe depression.

Doses for pain are generally smaller than those used for treatment of affective disorders. Medication should be administered on a fixed schedule and not as needed. After symptoms are controlled, dosage should be gradually reduced to the lowest level that will maintain relief of symptoms. Analgesia may be enhanced by addition of opioid analgesics (see pages xxvi–xliv for drug combinations), nonsteroidal anti-inflammatory drugs (NSAIDs), and use of nondrug therapies such as transcutaneous electrical nerve stimulation (TENS). In geriatric patients and patients with decreased renal or hepatic function, decrease doses by one-third to one-half. The possibility for suicide is inherent in depression and may persist until significant remission occurs. The quantity of drug dispensed should reflect this consideration.

Elimination: Hepatic, renal.

Preparations

Trazodone hydrochloride **(Desyrel):** Tablets: 50 mg, 100 mg, 150 mg, 300 mg.

Pharmacology

A triazolopyridine-derivative antidepressant agent, trazodone is chemically unrelated to other currently available antidepressant agents, including tricyclics, tetracyclics, or selective serotonin reuptake inhibitors (SSRIs). Antidepressant activity occurs earlier and is comparable with amitriptyline, imipramine, or doxepin, with fewer adverse effects. Trazodone selectively inhibits serotonin uptake at the presynaptic neuronal membrane. Synaptic concentrations of serotonin are increased, with enhanced serotonergic neurotransmission and numerous CNS effects (e.g., appetite suppression, decreased alcohol intake). Unlike other antidepressant agents, trazodone may have a dual effect on the central serotonergic system. At high doses (6–8 mg/kg) trazodone may act as a serotonin agonist, whereas at low doses (0.05–1.0 mg/kg) the drug antagonizes the actions of serotonin. Trazodone does not appear to influence the reuptake of dopamine or norepinephrine within the CNS but may enhance the release of norepinephrine from neuronal tissue. Trazodone does not inhibit the monoamine oxidase (MAO) system. Trazodone does not inhibit the reuptake of tyramine and has no effect on the pressor response to tyramine. Unlike the tricyclic antidepressants, trazodone exhibits little if any anticholinergic activity and thus has a lower incidence of anticholinergic side effects (e.g., dry mouth, blurred vision, urinary retention, constipation). The drug has also not been associated with activation of hypomanic or manic attacks in patients with bipolar disorders. Unlike with the tricyclics, sedating and cardiovascular effects are less pronounced due to the lack of substantial antihistaminic, α_1-adrenergic-blocking, catecholamine-potentiating, and quinidine-like cardiotoxic effects. Trazodone has anxiolytic and weak skeletal muscle relaxant activity. Although trazodone does not affect cardiac conduction or appear to have substantial arrhythmogenic activity, arrhythmias have occurred in some patients with preexisting cardiac disease during trazodone therapy. Blockade of neurotransmitter uptake may occur immediately, but antidepressant response may take days to weeks.

The analgesic effects of trazodone may occur partly

through the alleviation of depression, which may be responsible for increased pain suffering, but also by mechanisms that are independent of mood effects. Trazodone may potentiate the analgesic effect of opiate agonists, possibly by enhancing serotonergic transmission. The analgesic effects of trazodone occur early (< 24 hours) compared to the delayed effects of tricyclic antidepressants (5–7 days). The drug may produce abnormal EEG patterns and lower the seizure threshold. Therapeutic doses do not affect respiration, but the effects of higher doses remain to be established. Trazodone does not appear to have addiction liability. Trazodone crosses the placenta and is excreted in breast milk. It should be used with caution in pregnant and nursing mothers.

Pharmacokinetics

Onset of Action: Analgesic effect: PO, < 24 hours. Antidepressant effect: PO, 1 week.
Peak Effect: Antidepressant effect: PO, 2–4 weeks.
Duration of Action: Antidepressant effect: PO, variable.

Interactions

Increased risk of serotonin syndrome (myoclonus, rigidity, hyperreflexia, seizures, hyperthermia, hypertension, restlessness, diaphoresis, shivering, diarrhea, and tremor) with concomitant administration of serotonergics (e.g., clomipramine, tryptophan, pseudoephedrine, tricyclic antidepressant agents, cocaine, lithium, and MAO inhibitors); serum levels and toxic effects of trazodone increased by cimetidine; serum levels of trazodone decreased by enzyme inducers (e.g., phenytoin, phenobarbital, rifampin); trazodone may increase serum levels of digoxin or phenytoin with concomitant administration.

Toxicity

Toxic Range: Not routinely monitored.

Manifestations: Serotonin syndrome (myoclonus, rigidity, hyperreflexia, seizures, hyperthermia, hypertension, restlessness, diaphoresis, shivering, diarrhea, and tremor), priapism, nausea and vomiting, drowsiness, sinus tachycardia, dilated pupils.

Antidote: Serotonin antagonists: Cyproheptadine PO 4–12 mg stat *or* methysergide PO 2 mg twice daily (three doses may be sufficient).

Management: Discontinue medication. Administer antidote. Correct fluid, electrolyte, and acid-base disturbances. Airway-protected, ipecac syrup–induced emesis (30 mL or 0.5 mL/kg ipecac syrup) or gastric lavage (with drug ingestion) followed by administration of activated charcoal (PO 50–100 g or 1–2 g/kg). Activated charcoal may be administered every 4 to 6 hours during the first 24 to 48 hours after ingestion. Control seizures: Intravenous benzodiazepines are the first choice; however, IV barbiturates or phenytoin may be useful in refractory seizures. Support ventilation and circulation (patent airway, oxygen, IV fluids, vasopressors). Control hyperpyrexia with ice packs and cooling sponge baths. Hemodialysis or peritoneal dialysis is ineffective because the drug is highly protein bound. Symptomatic treatment. Consider the possibility of multiple drug involvement. Counseling prior to and after discharge for patients who attempted suicide.

Guidelines/Precautions

1. Trazodone has been associated with the occurrence of priapism. In many of the cases reported, surgical intervention has been required, and in some of these cases permanent impairment of erectile function or impotence resulted. Male patients with prolonged or inappropriate erections should immediately discontinue the drug and consult their physician. The detumescence of priapism and drug-induced penile erections has been accomplished by pharmacologic (e.g., the intracavernosal injection of α-adrenergic stimulants such as epinephrine and norepinephrine) as well as surgical procedures. Any pharmacologic or surgical procedure utilized in the treatment of priapism should be performed under the supervision of a urologist or physician familiar with the procedure and should not be initiated without urologic consultation if the priapism has persisted for more than 24 hours.

2. Trazodone is not recommended for use during the initial recovery phase of myocardial infarction. Use with caution and monitor closely in patients with cardiac disease. Trazodone has been associated with the occurrence of cardiac arrhythmias (e.g., isolated premature ventricular contractions) in these populations.

3. Use with caution in patients with diabetes mellitus, anorexia nervosa, thyroid disease, or seizure disorders.

4. Occasional decreases in leukocyte and neutrophil

counts have occurred in some patients receiving trazodone. The changes were not clinically significant and did not require discontinuation of the drug. Leukocyte and differential counts should be monitored if patients develop fever, sore throat, or other signs of infection while receiving trazodone. The drug should be discontinued if the counts decrease to less than normal levels.

5. Trazodone is contraindicated in patients receiving MAO inhibitors (concurrently or within the past 2 weeks), patients in the acute recovery phase following myocardial infarction, and those with demonstrated hypersensitivity to trazodone. The combination of trazodone and MAO inhibitors may result in the serotonin syndrome (see "Interactions").

6. Patients should be warned of the possibility of drowsiness that may impair performance of potentially hazardous tasks such as driving an automobile or operating machinery. Persisting daytime drowsiness may be decreased by administering a lower dose, administering the dose earlier in the evening, or substituting a less sedating alternative.

Principal Adverse Reactions

Cardiovascular: Tachycardia, bradycardia, hypertension.

Pulmonary: Shortness of breath.

CNS: Drowsiness, dizziness, light headedness, impaired memory.

Gastrointestinal: Abdominal and gastric disorders, nausea, vomiting, diarrhea.

Genitourinary: Priapism, impotence, decreased libido, inhibited female orgasm, increased urinary frequency.

Ocular: Blurred vision, mydriasis, increased intraocular pressure.
Dermatologic: Pruritus, dermatitis.
Hematologic: Anemia, decreases in leukocyte and neutrophil counts.
Other: Weight gain, weight loss.

TRIMIPRAMINE MALEATE

Class: Tricyclic Antidepressant

Use(s): Treatment of neurotic and endogenous depression; migraine prophylaxis; adjunct treatment of neuropathic pain syndromes, including diabetic neuropathy, postherpetic neuralgia, tic douloureux, and cancer pain; anxiety disorders; phobias; panic disorders; enuresis; eating disorders.

Dosing: *Pain syndromes*

Initial: PO 25–100 mg (0.5–2.0 mg/kg) daily at bedtime. Titrate dose upward every 3 to 4 weeks by increments of 25–50 mg as necessary.

Maintenance: PO 25–200 mg (0.5–4.0 mg/kg) daily at bedtime. Doses should be decreased if unacceptable side effects occur. Serum levels should be determined if there are signs of toxicity. The higher end of the dose range may be required in the management of painful diabetic neuropathy.

Depression

Initial PO: 75–100 mg daily in one to four divided doses.

Maintenance PO: 50–300 mg daily in one to four divided doses. Doses greater than 200 mg daily are not recommended for outpatients.

IM: 100 mg daily in divided doses. Replace with oral medication as soon as possible. Do not administer intravenously.

Doses for pain are generally smaller than those used for treatment of affective disorders. Medication should be administered on a fixed schedule and not as needed. Administration of the entire daily dose at bedtime may reduce daytime sedation. After symptoms are controlled, dosage should be gradually reduced to the lowest level that will maintain relief of symptoms. Analgesia may be enhanced by addition of opioid analgesics (see pages xxvi–xliv for drug combinations), nonsteroidal anti-inflammatory drugs (NSAIDs), and use of nondrug therapies such as transcutaneous electrical nerve stimulation (TENS). In geriatric patients and patients with decreased renal or hepatic function, decrease doses by one-third to one-half. The possibility for suicide is inherent in depression and may persist until significant remission occurs. The quantity of drug dispensed should reflect this consideration.

Elimination: Hepatic, renal.

Preparations

Trimipramine hydrochloride **(Surmontil):** Capsules: 25 mg, 50 mg, 100 mg.

Pharmacology

A dibenzazepine derivative and a tertiary amine tricyclic antidepressant, trimipramine differs structurally from imipramine by the addition of a methyl group to the side chain. Antidepressant activity may be partly due to inhibition of the amine-pump uptake of neurotransmitters (e.g., norepinephrine and serotonin) at the presynaptic neuron and down-regulation of β-receptor sensitivity. Trimipramine has anxiolytic, sedative, antihistaminic, and anticholinergic effects. Trimipramine enhances ulcer healing and may be as effective as cimetidine. Trimipramine produces orthostatic hypotension secondary to peripheral α_1-adrenergic blockade. Antidepressant response may take days to weeks even though blockade of neurotransmitter uptake may occur immediately. Trimipramine does not inhibit the monoamine oxidase (MAO) system.

The analgesic effects of trimipramine may occur partly through the alleviation of depression, which may be responsible for increased pain suffering, but also by mechanisms that are independent of mood effects. Serotonin and norepinephrine activity may be increased in descending pain-inhibitory pathways. Activation of these pathways decreases the transmission of nociceptive impulses from primary afferent neurons to first-order cells in laminae I and V of the spinal cord dorsal horn. Trimipramine may also potentiate the analgesic effect of opioids by increasing their binding efficacy to opioid receptors. Trimipramine has varying degrees of efficacy in different pain syndromes and may be better at relieving the burning, aching, and dyesthetic component of neuropathic pain. The drug is seldom useful in the management of lancinating, shooting paroxysmal pain. Trimipramine may produce abnormal EEG patterns and lower the seizure threshold. Therapeutic doses do not affect respiration, but toxic doses may lead to respiratory depression. The direct quinidine-like effects may manifest at toxic doses and produce cardiovascular disturbances (e.g., conduction blockade). Trimipramine does not have addiction liability and its use is not associated with drug-seeking behavior. Withdrawal symptoms, including sleep disruption with vivid dreams, may be precipitated by acute withdrawal. Tolerance develops to the sedative and anticholinergic effects, but there are no reports of tolerance to the analgesic effects. Trimipramine crosses the placenta, and use in pregnancy may be associated with fetal malformations. The drug is excreted in breast milk and has a potential for serious adverse effects in nursing infants.

Pharmacokinetics

Onset of Action: Analgesic effect: PO, <5 days. Antidepressant effect: PO, 1–2 weeks.
Peak Effect: Antidepressant effect: PO, 2–4 weeks.
Duration of Action: Antidepressant effect: PO, variable.

Interactions

Increased risk of hyperthermia with concomitant administration of anticholinergics (e.g., atropine), phenothiazines, thyroid medications; serum levels and toxic effects of trimipramine increased by concomitant methylphenidate, fluoxetine, cimetidine, phenothi-azines, and haloperidol; ventilatory and circulatory depressant effects of CNS depressant drugs and alcohol potentiated by trimipramine; increases the pressor and cardiac effects of sympathomimetics (e.g., isopro-terenol, phenylephrine, norepinephrine, epinephrine, amphetamine); decreases serum levels and pharmaco-logic effects of levodopa and phenylbutazone; increases serum levels and toxic effects of dicumarol; onset of therapeutic effects shortened and adverse cardiac effects of trimipramine increased with concomitant administration of levothyroxine and liothyronine; fatal hyperpyretic crisis or seizures with concomitant use of MAO inhibitors; uptake-dependent efficacy of IV re-gional bretylium decreased by trimipramine.

Toxicity

Toxic Range: Not routinely monitored. Blood and urine levels may not correlate with the degree of intox-ication and are not reliable guides for clinical manage-ment.

Manifestations: *Chronic:* Dream and sleep distur-bances, akathisia, anxiety, chills, coryza, malaise, myalgia, headache, dizziness, nausea and vomiting. *Acute:* In addition to the previously listed symptoms, CNS stimulation with excitement, delirium, hallucina-tions, hyperreflexia, myoclonus, choreiform move-ments, parkinsonian symptoms, seizures, hyperpyrexia, then CNS depression with drowsiness, areflexia, hypo-thermia, respiratory depression, cyanosis, hypotension, coma; peripheral anticholinergic symptoms, including urinary retention, dry mucous membranes, mydriasis, constipation, adynamic ileus; cardiac irregularities, including tachycardia, QRS prolongation; metabolic and/or respiratory acidosis; polyradiculoneuropathy; renal failure; vomiting; ataxia; dysarthria; bullous cutaneous lesions; pulmonary consolidation.

Antidote: None.

Management: Discontinue or reduce medication. Correct fluid, electrolyte, and acid-base disturbances. Airway-protected, ipecac syrup–induced emesis (30 mL or 0.5 mL/kg ipecac syrup) or gastric lavage (with drug ingestion) followed by administration of activated charcoal (PO 50–100 g or 1–2 g/kg). These purging actions should be performed even if several hours have elapsed after ingestion because the anticholinergic effects may delay gastric emptying, and the drug may also be secreted into the stomach. Control seizures: Intravenous benzodiazepines are the first choice because IV barbiturates may enhance respiratory depression; however, IV barbiturates or phenytoin may be useful in refractory seizures. Support ventilation and circulation (patent airway, oxygen, IV fluids, vasopressors). Continuous EKG monitoring. Treat cardiac arrhythmias with IV lidocaine or propranolol. Digoxin, quinidine, procainamide, and diisopyramide should be avoided because they may further depress myocardial conduction and/or contractility. Temporary pacemakers may be necessary in patients with advanced atrioventricular block, severe bradycardia, and/or life-threatening ventricular arrhythmias unresponsive to drug therapy. Control hyperpyrexia with ice packs and cooling sponge baths. Physostigmine (slow IV 1–3 mg) may be used in the treatment of life-threatening anticholinergic toxicity. Routine use of physostigmine is not advisable due to its serious adverse effects (e.g., seizures, bronchospasm, and severe bradyarrhythmias). Hemodialysis or peritoneal dialysis is ineffective because the drug is highly protein bound. Symptomatic treatment. Consider the possibility of multiple drug involvement. Counseling prior to and after discharge for patients who attempted suicide.

Guidelines/Precautions

1. To avoid withdrawal symptoms, the medication should be tapered down over a couple of weeks and not discontinued abruptly.

2. Use with caution in patients with cardiovascular disease, thyroid disease, or seizure disorders and in those in whom excessive anticholinergic activity may be harmful (e.g., patients with benign prostatic hypertrophy, a history of urinary retention, or increased intraocular pressure). The drug should be used in close-angle glaucoma only when the glaucoma is adequately controlled by drugs and closely monitored.

3. Trimipramine is contraindicated in patients receiving MAO inhibitors (concurrently or within the past 2 weeks), patients in the acute recovery phase following myocardial infarction, and those with demonstrated hypersensitivity to trimipramine. Cross-sensitivity with other tricyclic antidepressants may occur.

4. Patients should be warned of the possibility of drowsiness that may impair performance of potentially hazardous tasks such as driving an automobile or operating machinery. Persisting daytime drowsiness may be decreased by administering a lower dose, administering the dose earlier in the evening, or substituting a less sedating alternative.

Principal Adverse Reactions

Cardiovascular: Postural hypotension, arrhythmias, conduction disturbances, hypertension, sudden death.

Pulmonary: Respiratory depression.

CNS: Confusion, disorientation, extrapyramidal symptoms.

Gastrointestinal: Hepatic dysfunction, jaundice, nausea, vomiting, constipation, decrease in lower esophageal sphincter tone.

Genitourinary: Urinary retention, paradoxical nocturia, urinary frequency.

Ocular: Blurred vision, mydriasis, increased intraocular pressure.

Dermatologic: Pruritus, urticaria, petechiae, photosensitivity.

Hematologic: Leukopenia, thrombocytopenia, eosinophilia, agranulocytosis, purpura.

Endocrinologic: Increased or decreased libido, impotence, gynecomastia, SIADH.

Other: Hyperthermia.

VALPROIC ACID

Class: Anticonvulsant

Use(s): Anticonvulsant; treatment of lancinating neuropathic pain, such as trigeminal neuralgia (tic douloureux) and other cranial neuralgias, postsympathectomy neuralgia, postherpetic neuralgia, diabetic neuropathy, phantom limb pain, the thalamic syndrome, or lightning tabetic pain; migraine prophylaxis; prevention of recurrent febrile seizures in children.

Dosing: *Pain:* PO 250–2000 mg (5–15 mg/kg) daily at bedtime or in three divided doses. Titrate dose upward by 5–10 mg/kg/day at weekly intervals. Maximum dose 40 mg/kg/day. It is advisable to obtain informed consent before institution of valproic acid for chronic pain management, given the potential for side effects. Analgesia may be enhanced by combination with other anti-convulsants (e.g., phenytoin), benzodi-azepines (e.g., diazepam), antidepressant agents (e.g., paroxetine), and use of nondrug therapies such as transcutaneous electrical nerve stimulation (TENS).

Migraine prophylaxis: PO 250 mg twice daily. Some patients may benefit from doses up to PO 500 mg twice daily. Higher doses do not appear to improve efficacy.

Anticonvulsant

PO: 15 mg/kg/day in two or three divided doses.

IV infusion: 15 mg/kg/day. Administer over 60 minutes. Rapid infusion (>20 mg/min) may be associated with an increase in adverse reactions. Dilute IV dose in at least 50 mL of normal saline, D5W or LR solution.

Oral or intravenous doses may be in-creased by 5–10 mg/kg/day at weekly intervals until seizures are controlled or side effects preclude further increases. Maximum dose 60 mg/kg/day. Adminis-tration at bedtime may minimize sedative

> effects. Doses that exceed 250 mg/ day should be given in two or more divided doses. Therapeutic range: 50–100 μg/mL.
>
> Hepatic function tests, platelet counts, bleeding times, and coagulation studies should be determined prior to and at regular intervals during pain or anticonvulsant therapy.

Elimination: Hepatic, renal.

Preparations

Valproic acid **(Depakene):** Capsules: 250 mg.

Valproate sodium **(Depakene, Depa, Valproic Acid):** Oral solution: 50 mg/mL.

Valproate sodium **(Depacon):** Injection: 100 mg/mL.

Divalproex sodium **(Depakote Sprinkle):** Capsules: 125 mg (equivalent to valproic acid).

Divalproex sodium **(Depakote):** Tablets, sustained release: 125 mg, 250 mg, 500 mg (equivalent to valproic acid).

Dilution for Infusion: Dilute prescribed dose in 50 mL normal saline, D5W, or LR.

Pharmacology

A carboxylic acid–derivative anticonvulsant, valproic acid is structurally unrelated to the other anticonvulsants. Derivatives of valproic acid include valproate sodium (the sodium salt) and divalproex sodium, a stable coordination compound containing equal proportions of valproic acid and valproate sodium. The anticonvulsant activity of valproic acid may be partly related to inhibition of catabolism [by γ-aminobutyric acid (GABA) transferase and succinic acid dehydrogenase enzymes] and increased brain concentrations of the inhibitory neurotransmitter GABA. Neuronal activity may also be inhibited by increase in potassium conductance. Valproic acid, alone or in conjunction with other anticonvulsants, is used in the management of simple and complex absence (petit mal) seizures. Valproic acid use in chronic pain syndromes is primarily for suppression of the sharp lancinating and paroxysmal electrical shooting qualities common in neuropathic pain, such as in idiopathic trigeminal neuralgia. It is less effective than carbamazepine. Valproic acid is not as useful for the more chronic aching pains (e.g., in posttraumatic trigeminal pain). The drug is also effective for migraine prophylaxis but because of the potential side effects is reserved for patients who have failed to respond to first-line agents (e.g., β-blockers, antidepressants). Valproic acid crosses the placenta and is distributed in breast milk. It should be avoided in pregnant and nursing mothers except in situations when discontinuation of therapy may pose a serious threat to the mother.

Pharmacokinetics

Onset of Action: Anticonvulsant effects: PO, <15 minutes. Analgesic effects: 3–5 days.
Peak Effect: Anticonvulsant effects: PO, 1–4 hours.
Duration of Action: Anticonvulsant effects: 5–20 hours (half-life).

Interactions

May potentiate the CNS depressant effects of alcohol, other anticonvulsants, sedatives; increases serum levels and toxicity of phenobarbital, primidone; alters serum levels of phenytoin; potentiates the effects of MAO inhibitors, other antidepressants, coumarin anticoagulants; potentiates antiplatelet effects of salicylates; serum levels and toxicity of valproic acid increased by salicylates; increased risk of absence seizures with concomitant administration of clonazepam.

Toxicity

Toxic Range: Not routinely monitored.

Manifestations: Coma, visual hallucinations, asterixis, death.

Antidote: No specific antidote. Naloxone may reverse the CNS depressant effects; however, use with caution because it may reverse the anticonvulsant effects as well.

Management: Discontinue or reduce medication. Support ventilation and circulation (patent airway, oxygen, IV fluids, vasopressors). Symptomatic treatment. Airway-protected, ipecac syrup–induced emesis (30 mL or 0.5 mL/kg ipecac syrup followed by 200 mL or 4 mL/kg of water or clear fluid) or gastric lavage (with drug ingestion) followed by administration of activated charcoal (PO 50–100 g or 0.5–1.0 g/kg). Efficacy may depend on time since ingestion. Hemodialysis and hemoperfusion may be useful.

Guidelines/Precautions

1. A trial of withdrawal of valproic acid therapy in chronic pain may be attempted after 4 to 6 months of therapy. Patients occasionally may maintain pain relief once they are off the medication.
2. Valproic acid may be associated with exfoliative dermatitis and the Stevens-Johnson syndrome as a

non–dose-related hypersensitivity reaction. Discontinue the drug if a rash occurs.

3. Patients should be warned that valproic acid may impair their ability to perform activities requiring mental alertness or physical coordination (e.g., operating heavy machinery, driving a motor vehicle).

4. Abrupt withdrawal in epileptic patients may precipitate status epilepticus. Reduce dosage, discontinue, or substitute other anticonvulsant medications gradually.

Principal Adverse Reactions

Cardiovascular: Hypotension, cardiovascular collapse, atrial and ventricular conduction depression, ventricular fibrillation.

CNS: Ataxia, confusion, dizziness, tremors, headaches, peripheral neuropathy.

Gastrointestinal: Nausea, vomiting, indigestion, diarrhea, constipation, hypersalivation, abdominal cramps, hepatic dysfunction.

Dermatologic: Stevens-Johnson syndrome, lupus erythematosus, rash, pruritus, alopecia.

Hematologic: Thrombocytopenia, petechiae, prolonged bleeding time, leukopenia.

Other: Enuresis, muscular weakness, fatigue.

VERAPAMIL HYDROCHLORIDE

Class: Calcium Channel Blocker

Use(s): Treatment of supraventricular tachyarrhythmias [e.g., paroxysmal supraventricular tachycardia (PSVT)], temporary control of rapid ventricular rate in atrial flutter or fibrillation not associated with accessory bypass tracts; treatment of angina and hypertension; migraine prophylaxis.

Dosing: *PSVT/Atrial flutter or fibrillation:* IV: 5–10 mg (0.075–0.25 mg/kg). Administer over 2 minutes. Dose may be repeated 30 minutes later if necessary.

Chronic atrial fibrillation (digitalized patients): PO, regular release: 240–320 mg/day in three or four divided doses.

PSVT (nondigitalized patients): PO, regular release: 240–480 mg/day in three or four divided doses.

Angina: PO, regular release: 40–120 mg three times a day.

Antihypertensive

PO, regular release: 40–80 mg three times a day.

PO, sustained release (Calan SR/Isoptin SR): 120–480 mg daily in one or two divided doses.

PO, sustained release (Verelan): 120–480 mg once daily.

IV: 2.5–10.0 mg (0.05–0.2 mg/kg). Titrate to patient response.

Migraine prophylaxis: PO, regular release, 80–120 mg three times a day.

Elimination: Renal.

Preparations

Verapamil hydrochloride **(Calan, Isoptin, Verapamil):** Tablets, film coated: 40 mg, 80 mg, 120 mg.

Verapamil hydrochloride **(Calan SR, Isoptin SR):** Tablets, sustained release: 120 mg, 180 mg, 240 mg.

Verapamil hydrochloride **(Covera-HS):** Tablets, sustained release: 180 mg, 240 mg.

Verapamil hydrochloride **(Verelan):** Capsules, sustained release: 120 mg, 180 mg, 240 mg, 360 mg.

Verapamil hydrochloride **(Isoptin Injection):** Injection: 2.5 mg/mL.

Pharmacology

Verapamil is a calcium channel blocker that selectively inhibits the transmembrane influx of calcium ions into cardiac muscle and smooth muscle. The antiarrhythmic effect is due to inhibition of calcium influx through the slow channel in cells of the cardiac conduction system. It slows atrioventricular (AV) conduction and prolongs the effective refractory period within the AV node in a rate-related manner. It reduces ventricular rate in atrial flutter or fibrillation, and interrupts reentry at the AV node and restores normal sinus rhythm in patients with paroxysmal supraventricular tachycardia. Verapamil increases antegrade conduction across accessory bypass tracts, which may result in an increase in the ventricular response rate. It decreases myocardial contractility, systemic vascular resistance, and arterial pressure. Decreased myocardial demand accounts for the effectiveness in the treatment of angina pectoris. Verapamil may alter excessive vasomotor reactivity and thus is useful for the prophylaxis of migraine and symptomatic relief of ischemic pain. Verapamil may increase the pain threshold and enhance analgesia when combined with opiates. This may be a central effect resulting from modulation of opiate effects and pain transmission secondary to calcium channel blockade.

Pharmacokinetics

Onset of Action: IV, 2–5 minutes; PO, 30 minutes.
Peak Effect: IV, within 10 minutes; PO, 1.2–2.0 hours.
Duration of Action: IV, 30–60 minutes; PO, 3–7 hours (half-life).

Interactions

Potentiates effects of depolarizing and nondepolarizing muscle relaxants; additive cardiovascular depressant effects with use of volatile anesthetics, other antihypertensives (e.g., diuretics, angiotensin-converting enzyme inhibitors, vasodilators); increases toxicity of digoxin, benzodiazepines, carbamazepine, oral hypoglycemics, and possibly quinidine and theophylline; cardiac failure, AV conduction disturbances, and sinus bradycardia with concurrent use of β-blockers; potentiates myocardial depressant effects (hypotension and bradycardia) of bupivacaine and local anesthetics; concomitant use of IV verapamil and IV dantrolene may result in cardiovascular collapse; decreases lithium effect and neurotoxicity; decreased clearance with cimetidine; chemically incompatible with solutions of bicarbonate or nafcillin; may displace other highly protein-bound drugs (e.g., oral anticoagulants, hydantoins, salicylates, sulfonamides, and sulfonylureas) from binding sites or may be displaced by such drugs.

Toxicity

Toxic Range: Not routinely monitored.
Manifestations: Nausea and vomiting, metabolic acidosis, hyperglycemia, hypotension, bradycardia, second- or third-degree atrioventricular block.

Antidote: Calcium chloride 10%, IV 500–1000 mg (5–10 mL) or calcium gluconate 10%, IV 500–2000 mg (5–20 mL). Calcium chloride or calcium gluconate reverses the depression of cardiac contractility but does not affect sinus node depression or peripheral vasodilatation. Calcium has variable effects on AV nodal conduction.

Management: Discontinue or reduce medication. Support ventilation and circulation (patent airway, oxygen, IV fluids, vasopressors). Excessive bradycardia or AV block may be treated with isoproterenol, calcium chloride, norepinephrine, atropine, or cardiac pacing. Rapid ventricular rate due to antegrade conduction in flutter/fibrillation with Wolff-Parkinson-White syndrome may be treated with procainamide, lidocaine, or DC cardioversion. Symptomatic treatment. Airway-protected gastric lavage (with drug ingestion); administer activated charcoal and cathartics.

Guidelines/Precautions

1. Verapamil may worsen heart failure in patients with poor left ventricular function.
2. Use with caution in patients receiving any highly protein-bound drug, such as oral anticoagulants, hydantoins, salicylates, sulfonamides, and sulfonylureas.
3. Do not chew or divide sustained-release tablets.

Principal Adverse Reactions

Cardiovascular: Hypotension, bradycardia, tachycardia.

Pulmonary: Bronchospasm, laryngospasm.

CNS: Dizziness, headache, seizures.
Gastrointestinal: Nausea, abdominal discomfort.
Allergic: Urticaria, pruritus.

ZOLMITRIPTAN

Class: Serotonin Agonist

Use(s): Acute treatment of migraine attacks with or without auras.

Dosing: PO: 2.5 mg (dose range 1–5 mg). Dose may be repeated every 2 hours. Maximum 24-hour PO dosage: 10 mg. Lower doses should be utilized and combined with blood pressure monitoring in patients with hepatic impairment.

Elimination: Hepatic.

Preparations

Zolmitriptan **(Zomig):** Tablets: 2.5 mg, 5 mg.

Pharmacology

Zolmitriptan is a selective serotonin agonist at 5-hydroxytryptamine (5-HT) type 1B and 1D receptors. Zolmitriptan has actions similar to those of sumatriptan, but, unlike sumatriptan, zolmitriptan can penetrate the blood-brain barrier to act centrally within the trigeminovascular system. The drug appears to have both peripheral and central sites of action. Migraine is believed to be caused by serotonin-induced local cranial vasodilatation and/or release of sensory neuropeptides (calcitonin gene-related peptide, substance P, and vasoactive intestinal peptide). 5-HT$_1$ type 1B and 1D receptors are present on intracranial blood vessels, including the arteriovenous anastomosis of the carotid distribution, and on sensory neurons of the trigemino-vascular system, which consist of bipolar nerves that innervate pain-sensitive intracranial structures. By binding to these receptors, zolmitriptan stimulates negative feedback, thereby shutting down further release of serotonin and leading to lower synaptic concentrations of serotonin. Peripherally, zolmitriptan causes selective vasoconstriction of inflamed and dilated cranial blood vessels in the carotid circulation. Centrally, zolmitriptan ultimately inhibits the production of pro-inflammatory neuropeptides in the trigeminovascular system. Zolmitriptan has no effect on α-, β-, dopamine, and other serotonin (5-HT$_2$, 5-HT$_3$) receptors. There is no effect on cerebral blood flow, peripheral arteries, or perfusion of peripheral organs. Zolmitriptan reduces the incidence of nausea, vomiting, photophobia, and phonophobia. The efficacy of zolmitriptan for migraine treatment is unaffected by the presence or absence of aura, the duration of attack, the gender of the patient, or the concomitant use of common migraine prophylactic drugs (e.g., β-blockers).

Pharmacokinetics

Onset of Action: PO, variable.
Peak Effect: PO, <2 hours.
Duration of Action: Half-life 3 hours.

Interactions

Additive adverse cardiovascular effects may occur with concomitant use of ergot compounds; type A

monoamine oxidase (MAO) inhibitors (e.g., moclobe-
mide), cimetidine, oral contraceptives, or propranolol
may potentiate the effects of zolmitriptan; type B MAO
inhibitors (e.g., selegeline) do not alter the pharmacokinetics of zolmitriptan; serotonin excess (weakness,
hyperreflexia, incoordination) may occur if zolmitriptan
is coadministered with selective serotonin reuptake
inhibitors such as paroxetine.

Toxicity

Toxic Range: Not routinely monitored.
Manifestations: Hypertension, coronary vasospasm,
palpitations, arrhythmias, seizures, respiratory depression, cyanosis, ataxia.
Antidote: No specific antidote.
Management: Discontinue or reduce medication. Support ventilation and circulation (patent airway, oxygen,
IV fluids, vasodilators). Monitoring should continue
while symptoms and signs persist and for at least 10
hours afterward. Symptomatic treatment.

Guidelines/Precautions

1. Use with caution in patients with impaired renal or
   hepatic function.
2. Zolmitriptan should not be administered in patients
   with basilar or hemiplegic migraine.
3. Other 5-HT$_1$ receptor agonists (e.g., sumatriptan)
   should not be administered within 24 hours of
   treatment with zolmitriptan.
4. Zolmitriptan should not be used in patients with
   peripheral vascular disease, cerebral vascular
   disease, ischemic heart disease, Prinzmetal's

angina, sepsis, a history of myocardial infarction, or uncontrolled hypertension. Zolmitriptan should not be given to patients in whom unrecognized coronary heart disease is predicted by the presence of risk factors (e.g., hypertension, hypercholesterolemia, current tobacco smoking, obesity, diabetes mellitus, strong family history of ischemic heart disease, postmenopausal females, or males older than 40) unless a cardiovascular evaluation provides sufficient evidence that the patient is reasonably free of ischemic heart disease.

5. Do not administer zolmitriptan to patients with symptomatic Wolff-Parkinson-White syndrome or cardiac arrhythmias associated with other cardiac accessory conduction pathway disorders. Serious cardiac events have occurred within a few hours of receiving other 5-HT$_1$ drugs.

6. Do not administer zolmitriptan to patients with cerebral vascular disease. Cerebral hemorrhage, subarachnoid hemorrhage, stroke, and other cerebrovascular events have occurred in patients treated with 5-HT$_1$ agonist drugs. It is believed that the severe headaches were secondary to an evolving neurologic lesion. Patients with migraine may be at increased risk of certain cerebrovascular events (e.g., hemorrhage, stroke, transient ischemic attacks).

Principal Adverse Reactions

Cardiovascular: Hypertension, angina, arrhythmias, peripheral vasoconstriction, palpitations.

Pulmonary: Dyspnea, bronchospasm.
CNS: Dizziness, malaise, drowsiness, weakness, seizures, paresthesias.
Gastrointestinal: Bad taste.
Other: Visual disturbances; xerostomia; neck, throat, jaw, and/or chest pain, tightness, or pressure.

Topical Agents //

Transdermal Drug Transport

Absorption through the skin is currently regarded as an important alternative to traditional methods of drug delivery. A definite advantage of topical therapy is area-specific targeting to obtain high tissue levels of the active ingredient. Topical absorption means a lack of systemic side effects. Also, low or undetectable blood levels avoid the need for dosage adjustment and the potential for problems with hepatic and renal impairment. Pluronic Lecithin Organogel (PLO) gels are microemulsion-based gels that originate from water-in-oil microemulsions. These gels are isotropic, thermoreversible, and optically transparent and reside in a cross-linked network lacking covalent bonds. At temperatures greater than 40°C, the gels become liquids with much lower viscosity; high-viscosity gels are re-formed by cooling and stirring.

PLO gels are stable compounds, show no harmful effect when applied to the skin for prolonged periods, and can solubilize sizable amounts of quite different chemicals. Lyophilic, hydrophilic, and amphoteric molecules, including enzymes, can be solubilized in the gels. The proposed mechanism of transport is an interaction between the layers of lipids in the stratum corneum and the phospholipids of the gel. Various pharmacologic substances, such as estradiol, amino acids, and peptides, can be transported transdermally via lecithin gels. Studies suggest that there are no great restrictions on the chemical structure of the drugs that can be incorporated into a properly compounded PLO gel. Proper preparation of this gel involves significant physical agitation to increase micelle formation and ensure efficacy. Micelles are spaghetti-like structures that produce a macroscopic viscosity, increasing the transdermal penetration of the gel. Appropriate agitation requires the use of an ointment mill or other homogenization process. Vanishing cream is sometimes added to the PLO gel to provide a better texture. Transdermal therapy has been shown to be effective without the side effects or concerns of systemic administration (e.g., gastrointestinal irritation or first-pass metabolism).

Compounding Medications for Pain Management

Compounding medications increases the therapeutic options available in the treatment of pain syndromes. Compounding pharmacies are able to provide custom formulations of commercially available medications.* These formulations may be modified in various ways, for example, minimizing acetaminophen toxicity by providing acetaminophen-free hydrocodone capsules. Preservative-free, dye-free, lactose-free formulations of commercially available medications may be compounded for improved patient tolerance, for example,

---

* Compounded topical medications are available (by prescription only) from L.A. Pain Clinic, 4019 W. Rosecrans Ave., Hawthorne, CA. Call 310-675-9121 or 1-800-9-MEDIC-9.

when a patient is allergic to the commercially available form. Providing customized dosages, such as higher dose strengths or slow-release formulations, enables the patient to reduce the quantity and/or frequency of medication required to achieve pain control. Most oral medications can be reformulated for alternate modes of administration, for example, as rectal suppositories or sublingual, topical, or nasal sprays. Custom-formulated topical gels, creams, and solutions of such drugs as anti-inflammatory agents, local anesthetics, muscle relaxants, anticonvulsants, antidepressants, and free radical scavengers offer site-specific treatment while decreasing or eliminating systemic side effects. Higher concentrations of preservative-free baclofen, clonidine, and narcotics may be compounded (with sterile techniques) for implantable pump infusions to enable delivery of smaller volumes.

AMITRIPTYLINE OINTMENT

Indication(s): Relief of diabetic and other peripheral neuropathies, arthritis pain.

Concentration: 2–5% (20–50 mg/mL), with or without 2% baclofen, in PLO gel placed in calibrated applicators.

Dosing: Apply 1 cc to the affected area three times daily. Titrate dosage to patient response. Gently rub gel into the skin until absorbed.

Pharmacology

A tricyclic antidepressant agent, amitriptyline increases serotonin and norepinephrine activity in descending pain-inhibitory pathways. Activation of these pathways decreases the transmission of nociceptive impulses from primary afferent neurons to first-order cells in laminae I and V of the spinal cord dorsal horn. Amitriptyline may also potentiate the analgesic effect of opioids by increasing their binding efficacy to opioid receptors. The topical route minimizes the dose-limiting side effects seen with systemic administration (e.g., sedation).

Onset of Action: 30–60 minutes.

Adverse Reactions: Drowsiness, sedation.

Comments

May be compounded in combination with nonsteroidal anti-inflammatory drugs (NSAIDs), dimethyl sulfoxide (DMSO), dextromethorphan, capsaicin, clonidine, or gabapentin.

BACLOFEN OINTMENT

Indication(s): Relief of neuropathic pain, flexor spasms, and concomitant clonus and muscular rigidity.

Concentration: 0.5–1.0% in a PLO ointment.

Dosing: Apply every 3 to 4 hours as needed. Gently rub ointment into the skin until absorbed. After obtaining pain relief, titrate dose downward to the minimum required for maintenance of pain control.

Pharmacology

Baclofen, a skeletal muscle relaxant, is a *p*-chlorophenyl derivative of γ-aminobutyric acid (GABA). Baclofen inhibits monosynaptic and polysynaptic reflexes at the spinal level, possibly by acting as an inhibitory neuro-transmitter and/or by hyperpolarization at afferent terminals.

Onset of Action: 30–60 minutes.

Comments

May be compounded in combination with nonsteroidal anti-inflammatory drugs (NSAIDs), dimethyl sulfoxide (DMSO), dextromethorphan, capsaicin, clonidine, or gabapentin.

CLONIDINE OINTMENT

Indication(s): Relief of neuropathic pain, musculoskeletal pain, treatment of hypertension.

Concentration: 0.1–0.15% in a PLO ointment. Available commercially as Catapres TTS (transdermal therapeutic system), which releases 0.1 mg, 0.2 mg, or 0.3 mg per 24 hours.

Dosing: *Compounded ointment:* Apply two to four times daily in the affected area. Gently rub ointment into the skin until absorbed. After initial response, titrate dose downward to the minimum required for maintenance of pain control.

Commercial transdermal system: Apply once a week. Dosage adjustments may be made at weekly intervals.

Pharmacology

Clonidine inhibits pain transmission by stimulating the presynaptic and postjunctional α_2-adrenoceptors located in the dorsal horn neurons of the spinal cord. Local effects may include inhibition of the release of nociceptive neurotransmitters such as substance P (presynaptic first-order neurons) and a decrease in the rate of depolarization (postsynaptic second-order neurons). Clonidine (alone or combined with baclofen) may relieve muscle spasms such as those in fibromyalgia, presumably by α_2-adrenergic-mediated presynaptic inhibition of spinal motor neurons.

Onset of Action: *Compounded ointment:* 30–60 minutes. *Transdermal systems:* Therapeutic plasma levels are achieved after 2 to 3 days. Therapeutic levels persist for about 8 hours following removal of the systems, then decline over several days.

Comments

May produce sedation, orthostatic symptoms. Monitor the blood pressure. May be compounded in combination with nonsteroidal anti-inflammatory drugs (NSAIDs), dimethyl sulfoxide (DMSO), dextromethorphan, capsaicin, or gabapentin.

CYCLOBENZAPRINE OINTMENT

Indication(s): Relief of acute and chronic pain associated with musculoskeletal conditions, especially back pain.

Concentration: 1.0–1.5% in a PLO ointment.

Dosing: Apply three to four times daily in the affected area. Titrate dose to patient response.

Gently rub ointment into the skin until absorbed.

Pharmacology

Cyclobenzaprine is structurally related to tricyclic antidepressants. The drug acts primarily at the brain stem to reduce tonic somatic motor activity, influencing both γ and α motor neurons. It does not have direct activity on skeletal muscle and does not act at the neuromuscular junction or the spinal cord (unlike baclofen or tizanidine).

Onset of Action: 30–60 minutes.

Comments

May be compounded in combination with nonsteroidal anti-inflammatory drugs (NSAIDs), dimethyl sulfoxide (DMSO), dextromethorphan, capsaicin, or gabapentin.

2-DEOXY-D-GLUCOSE OINTMENT

Indication(s): Decrease in duration of lesions and relief of pain for herpes zoster and postherpetic neuralgia, treatment of genital warts (in combination with salicylic acid 40% paste).

Concentration: 0.19% in a PLO gel.

Dosing: Apply three to four times daily. Gently rub ointment into the skin until absorbed.

Pharmacology

A glucose analogue, 2-deoxy-D-glucose interferes with viral cellular carbohydrate metabolism and inhibits the multiplication of herpes virus.

Onset of Action: 12 hours to 3 days.

Adverse Reactions: Dermatitis.

Comments

May be combined with oral antiviral medication or topical lidocaine, ketoprofen, or gabapentin.

DEXAMETHASONE OINTMENT

Indication(s): Relief of acute and chronic pain associated with inflammation, such as injury or arthritis, heel spurs, and bursitis.

Concentration: 0.1% in a PLO ointment.

Dosing: Apply two to four times daily in the affected area. Titrate dose to patient response. Gently rub ointment into the skin until absorbed.

Pharmacology

Dexamethasone ointment diffuses across cell membrane to interact with cytoplasmic receptors located in both dermal and intradermal cells. This glucocorticoid induces phospholipase A_2 inhibitory proteins in cells, thereby depressing the formation, release, and activity of endogenous mediators of inflammation such as prostaglandins, kinins, histamine, liposomal enzymes, and the complement system.

Onset of Action: 30–60 minutes.

Comments

Dexamethasone may be compounded with topical non-steroidal anti-inflammatory drugs (NSAIDs).

DEXTROMETHORPHAN OINTMENT

Indication(s): Relief of pain, enhancement of opioid analgesia.

Concentration: 1–10 mg/g.

Dosing: Apply every 3 to 4 hours. Titrate dose to patient response. Gently rub ointment into the skin until absorbed.

Pharmacology

An analogue of levorphanol, dextromethorphan is a noncompetitive *N*-methyl D-aspartate (NMDA) receptor antagonist. Opioid tolerance requires a functional NMDA receptor, and blockade of this receptor attenuates or reverses the development of opioid tolerance. Some patients who are poor metabolizers of dextromethorphan (or in whom the *O*-demethylation is competitively inhibited by other medication) may not experience any effect from the drug.

Onset of Action: 30–60 minutes.

Comments

Dextromethorphan has opioid-sparing activity. It enables a decrease (up to 50%) in the dose of opioid required to maintain pain control, with minimal side effects. It may be compounded with opioids such as morphine and codeine for oral administration.

DICLOFENAC OINTMENT

Indication(s): Relief of acute and chronic pain associated with musculoskeletal conditions and inflammation.

Concentration: 2–15% (20–150 mg/mL) in PLO gel or Vanishing Lecithin Organogel (VLO gel).

Dosing: Apply to the affected area two to four times daily. Titrate dose to patient response. Gently rub gel into the skin until absorbed.

Pharmacology

A nonsteroidal anti-inflammatory drug, topical diclofenac inhibits cyclooxygenase activity, thereby decreasing formation of prostaglandins and thromboxanes from arachidonic acid. Antibradykinin activity, combined with inhibition of synthesis of prostaglandins and other inflammatory neuropeptides, prevents the sensitization of peripheral pain receptors to mechanical or chemical stimulation. Peripheral interruption in afferent transmission may reduce centrally mediated hyperexcitability states. The topical route minimizes the dose-limiting side effects seen with systemic administration (e.g., gastrointestinal irritation).

Onset of Action: 30–60 minutes.

Adverse Reactions: Dermatitis, gastritis.

Comments

May be compounded in combination with baclofen, dimethyl sulfoxide (DMSO), dextromethorphan, capsaicin, clonidine, or gabapentin.

DIMETHYL SULFOXIDE (DMSO) GEL

Indication(s): Relief of sympathetic mediated pain, relief of a wide variety of musculoskeletal disorders and related collagen diseases, enhancement of the percutaneous absorption of drugs, symptomatic relief of interstitial cystitis.

Concentration: *Topical:* 2–25% in solution or vaseline-cetomacrogol cream. *Intravesical:* 50% solution.

Dosing: *Topical:* Apply gel three to five times daily. Titrate dose to patient response. Gently rub gel into the skin until absorbed.

Intravesical: Instill 50 mL of a 50% solution intravesically directly into the bladder by catheter or aspeto syringe and allow it to remain in the bladder for 15 minutes. Medication is expelled by spontaneous voiding. Dose may be repeated every 2 weeks until symptomatic relief is obtained.

Pharmacology

A scavenger of oxygen radicals, topical DMSO inhibits afferent conduction and decreases inflammatory swelling. DMSO's local anti-inflammatory effects provide symptomatic relief when the solution is applied intravesically in patients with interstitial cystitis.

Onset of Action: Within 10 minutes.

Adverse Reactions: *Intravesical:* Dysgeusia (garlic-like taste), transient chemical cystitis, bladder spasm, discomfort, anaphylactoid reaction. *Topical:* Dysgeusia, local dermatitis, sedation, nausea/vomiting, headache, burning eyes, ocular pain.

Comments

DMSO is available commercially in liquid form as Rimso-50 and in a variety of other forms, but purity is not controlled. Contaminants in nonpharmaceutical DMSO products can be transported into the body with topical application.

Do not administer IM or IV or in patients with urinary tract malignancies. Concomitant administration with sulindac may result in peripheral neuropathy.

DOXEPIN CREAM

Indication(s): Relief of neuropathic pain, including sympathetic mediated pain and postherpetic neuralgia; relief of pruritus.

Concentration: 5%.

Dosing: Apply cream four times daily and at bedtime. Safety and efficacy data are not available for use longer than 8 days. Chronic use beyond 8 days may result in higher systemic levels. Titrate dose to patient response. Gently rub cream into the skin until absorbed.

Pharmacology

Doxepin is a tertiary amine tricyclic antidepressant. Its antidepressant activity is partly due to inhibition of the amine-pump uptake of neurotransmitters (e.g., norepinephrine and serotonin) at the presynaptic neuron. The analgesic effects of doxepin may occur through the increase in serotonin and norepinephrine activity in descending pain-inhibitory pathways. Activation of these pathways decreases the transmission of nociceptive impulses from primary afferent neurons to first-order cells in laminae I and V of the spinal cord dorsal horn. The topical preparation has antipruritic effects, possibly due to the sedating and potent H_1 and H_2 receptor blocking activity. The cream may also be effective in relieving various neuropathic pain syndromes, for example, postherpetic neuralgia and sympathetic mediated pain.

Onset of Action: Several minutes.

Adverse Reactions: Drowsiness may occur when applied to greater than 10% body surface area.

Comments

Available commercially as Zonalon cream.

GABAPENTIN OINTMENT

Indication(s): Relief of neuropathic pain syndromes, including reflex sympathetic dystrophy, diabetic neuropathy; relief of arthritic and/or joint pain, including temporomandibular joint pain.

Concentration: 1.5–12.0% (15–120 mg/mL) in PLO gel.

Dosing: Apply to the affected area every 3 to 4 hours. Titrate dose to patient response. Gently rub gel into the skin until absorbed.

Pharmacology

A structural analogue of the neurotransmitter γ-aminobutyric acid (GABA), gabapentin has an unknown mechanism for its anticonvulsant activity. The beneficial effects of gabapentin in alleviating neuropathic and sympathetic mediated pain syndromes may be due to inhibitory action at its receptor sites and an increase in the bioavailability of serotonin, with consequent anti-depressant effects and decrease in catecholamine outflow.

Onset of Action: 30–60 minutes.

Adverse Reactions: Drowsiness, sedation.

Comments

May be compounded in combination with nonsteroidal anti-inflammatory drugs (NSAIDs), 2-deoxy-D-glucose, dimethyl sulfoxide (DMSO), dextromethorphan, capsaicin, or clonidine.

KETAMINE OINTMENT

Indication(s): Relief of neuropathic and sympathetic mediated pain, including complex regional pain syndrome types I and II involving the upper and lower extremities.

Concentration: 10–150 mg/mL (1–15%) in PLO gel placed in calibrated applicators.

Dosing: 10–700 mg (0.1–9.0 mg/kg) per single application. Apply one to three times daily until pain relief is obtained, then apply as needed. Other compounded combinations (e.g., gabapentin/clonidine/ketoprofen) may be applied regularly (e.g., three times daily), with ketamine ointment then applied for breakthrough pain. Gently rub gel into the skin until absorbed.

Pharmacology

An *N*-methyl D-aspartate (NMDA) receptor antagonist and a dissociative anesthetic, topical ketamine may interact with opioid receptors and sodium-potassium channels peripherally. This peripheral interruption in afferent transmission may reduce centrally mediated hyperexcitability states. Ketamine can relieve the burning dyesthesia and hyperesthesia associated with neuropathic and sympathetic mediated pain syndromes. Pain relief in some patients is superior to that obtained from sympathetic blocks (e.g., stellate ganglion blocks). The topical route minimizes the dose-limiting side effects seen with systemic administration (e.g., hallucinations, dysphoria, dissociative reactions, nausea). Opioid tolerance requires a functional NMDA receptor, and blockade of this receptor attenuates or reverses the development of opioid tolerance.

Adverse Reactions: High systemic levels may lead to hallucinations, dysphoria, dissociative reactions, and nausea.

Onset of Action: Within 5 minutes.

Comments

May be compounded in combination with dextromethorphan, gabapentin, or dimethyl sulfoxide (DMSO).

KETOPROFEN OINTMENT

Indication(s): Relief of arthritis, myofascial pain syndromes, fibromyalgia, postherpetic neuralgia, musculoligamentous sprains and strains, and sports injuries.

Concentration: 2–50% (20–500 mg/mL) in PLO gel or Vanishing Lecithin Organogel (VLO gel) placed in calibrated applicators.

Dosing: Apply 1 cc to the affected area every 6 hours. Titrate dose to patient response. Gently rub gel into the skin until absorbed.

Pharmacology

A nonsteroidal anti-inflammatory drug, topical ketoprofen inhibits cyclooxygenase activity, thereby decreasing formation of prostaglandins and thromboxanes from arachidonic acid. Antibradykinin activity, combined with inhibition of synthesis of prostaglandins and other inflammatory neuropeptides, prevents the sensitization of peripheral pain receptors to mechanical or chemical stimulation. Peripheral interruption in afferent transmission may reduce centrally mediated hyperexcitability states. The topical route minimizes the dose-limiting side effects seen with systemic administration (e.g., gastrointestinal irritation).

Onset of Action: 30–60 minutes.

Adverse Reactions: Dermatitis, gastritis.

Comments

May be compounded in combination with dimethyl sulfoxide (DMSO), dextromethorphan, capsaicin, clonidine, or gabapentin.

Neurolytic Agent

PHENOL

Class: Neurolytic Agent

Use(s): Neurolytic somatic and sympathetic nerve block.

Dosing: *Subarachnoid*

L1-L2: 1 mL 5% phenol in glycerin.

L4, L5, S1: 0.6 mL phenol in glycerin.

Thoracic: Maximum 1.2 mL phenol in glycerin.

Cervical: Maximum 1 mL phenol in glycerin.

Phenol is hyperbaric. The patient should be placed on the affected side with the spinal needle inserted in the lateral position. After cerebrospinal fluid is obtained, tilt the patient backward (about 40°) and slowly inject phenol. After injection, the patient should remain in the oblique position for 20 minutes and should remain supine (no sitting) for 24 hours.

Celiac plexus: 5 mL of 5–6% phenol in water.

Elimination: Hepatic, renal.

Preparations

Analytical-grade phenol is prepared by hospital pharmacists.

Pharmacology

Phenol is a nonselective neurolytic agent. It is poorly soluble in water at room temperature but very soluble in glycerin. The high solubility of phenol in glycerin enables it to be released slowly, which allows limited spread of the neurolytic and highly localized concentrations. Phenol produces nonselective degeneration of spinal cord roots. Concentrations greater than 5% cause protein coagulation and subsequent tissue necrosis. Initial selective effects on ummyelinated nerve fibers [A-γ (muscle tone), A-δ afferent (fast pain), C afferents (slow pain)] are caused by the local anesthetic properties. Subsequently, there is nonselective degeneration of all nerve fibers (including A-α and A-β). Neurolytic phenol procedures include subarachnoid and paravertebral somatic nerve blocks, and epidural, celiac plexus, and stellate ganglion blocks. Compared with the subarachnoid route, epidural phenol may produce patchy and unreliable analgesia. The neurolytic injections should be preceded by diagnostic local anesthetic nerve blocks and should be performed under fluoroscopic guidance to reduce the incidence of severe adverse effects. Peripheral phenol nerve injections may be associated with significant adverse effects resulting from the destruction of the motor, reflex, and sensory fibers.

Depending on the type of block, pain relief may last only a week or up to 3 to 6 months. Pain relief beyond 1 month is statistically unlikely. Recurrence of pain may be due to incomplete phenol-induced denervation, abolition of pain in one area unmasking pain in a previously unnoticed area, or the progressive spread of the tumor (in malignant pain). The neurolytic potency of 3% phenol is equivalent to that of 40% alcohol. Compared with alcohol, which diffuses rapidly and requires larger volumes, phenol enables more precise placement in lesion sites. However, alcohol is preferable in celiac plexus blocks because large volumes are required, and large volumes of phenol may result in toxicity and renal failure. Phenol injection is less painful than alcohol injection, which is a greater irritant on the musculature and other internal structures. Prior injection of long-acting local anesthetics (e.g., bupivacaine) enables assessment of the lesion site and a less painful neurolytic procedure.

Pharmacokinetics

Onset of Action: Epidural, 4–17 minutes; intrathecal, <1 minute.
Peak Effect: Infiltration/Epidural, 30–45 minutes; intrathecal, 15 minutes.
Duration of Action: 1 week to 6 months.

Interactions

Dilution in glycerin enables slow release and limited spread of phenol.

Toxicity

Toxic Range: Not routinely monitored.
Manifestations: Renal failure.
Antidote: No specific antidote.
Management: Discontinue or reduce medication. Support ventilation and circulation (patent airway, oxygen,

IV fluids, vasopressors). Benzodiazepines (diazepam IV 0.05–0.2 mg/kg, midazolam IV/IM 0.025–0.1 mg/kg) or barbiturates (thiopental sodium IV 0.5–2.0 mg/kg) to control seizures. Prolonged cardiopulmonary resuscitation with cardiac arrest: Sodium bicarbonate IV 1–2 mEq/kg to treat cardiac toxicity (sodium channel blockade); bretylium IV 5 mg/kg; DC cardioversion/defibrillation for ventricular arrhythmias.

Guidelines/Precautions

1. Fluoroscopic guidance is imperative for the safe administration of a neurolytic agent.
2. Before attempting a neurolytic block, diagnostic blocks should be performed with local anesthetics to predict the efficacy of the block and to assess potential serious side effects, such as pain, motor loss, and loss of bladder or bowel function.
3. In cancer patients, encasement of the nerve roots by tumor or inflammatory tissue may protect the nerves from the neurolytic agent and result in inadequate relief.
4. Due to the increased incidence of serious adverse effects, concentrations above 5% phenol in glycerin are not recommended for use.
5. Intravenous access is essential during major neurolytic block.
6. Use with caution in patients with hypovolemia, severe congestive heart failure, shock, or any form of heart block.
7. Phenol is contraindicated in patients with hypersensitivity to phenols.
8. Epidural or intrathecal injections should be avoided when the patient has hypovolemic shock, sep-

ticemia, infection at the injection site, or coagulopathy.

Principal Adverse Reactions

Cardiovascular: Hypotension, arrhythmias, cardiac arrest.

Pulmonary: Respiratory impairment, arrest.

CNS: Headache, numbness.

Musculoskeletal: Muscular weakness.

Genitourinary: Urinary incontinence, renal failure.

Allergic: Urticaria, angioneurotic edema, anaphylactoid symptoms.

Plexus/Epidural/Spinal: Paresthesia, hemiparesis, paraplegia, arachnoiditis, vascular thrombosis, spinal cord infarcts, nerve root damage, demyelination, lower extremity weakness and paralysis, loss of bowel and/or bladder sphincter control, backache, cranial nerve palsies.

Cancer Pain   *IV*

Pain is reported by about 50% of cancer patients at all stages of disease and by over 70% of those with advanced neoplasms (1). In the United States, cancer is diagnosed in more than 1 million patients annually, and more than 8 million have either cancer or a history of the disease.

The incidence of cancer pain is related to the type of cancer and the extent of disease. Bone cancer, pancreatic cancer, and primary neoplasms with bone metastasis are much more likely to be associated with pain than are the lymphomas or leukemias (2).

In cancer patients, pain may occur in several ways. In the majority (60% to 80%), pain is due to direct tumor involvement of bones, nerves, viscera, or soft tissue (3,4). There may be compression of nerve roots, trunks, or plexuses; infiltration of nerves and blood vessels by malignant cells; obstruction of hollow viscus; occlusion of blood vessels with venous engorgement or local ischemia; inflammation, swelling, or necrosis of invaded tissue; or raised intracranial pressure. In 20% to 25% of cancer patients, pain is associated with antineoplastic therapy as a result of surgery, chemotherapy, or radiation therapy. In 3% to 10% of cancer patients, pain is unrelated to cancer or its therapy and may include everyday maladies such as headaches or pain from arthritis or other concurrent disease.

The character of pain depends on the origin. Somatic pain (e.g., from bone metastasis) is due to activation of nociceptors in deep or cutaneous tissue. Such pain is well localized and perceived as a constant ache or gnawing sensation. Visceral pain (e.g., back and epigastric pain related to cancer of the pancreas and liver) is due to distention of thoracic and abdominal viscera. Such pain is poorly localized and perceived as a deep squeeze or pressure. Deafferentation or neuropathic pain (e.g., from brachial or lumbosacral plexopathy or postherpetic neuralgia) is due to neural infiltration or surgical intervention (phantom pain). This kind of pain is poorly localized and perceived as electric shock or burning.

Pain syndromes indirectly related or unrelated to cancer include myofascial pain due to excessive stress on muscles and involuntary splinting as a consequence of an adjacent nerve injury, pathologic fracture, or soft tissue infiltration. Herpes zoster may occur, especially in hematologic malignancies, and may be followed by postherpetic neuralgia.

Pain associated with cancer in adults and children is frequently undertreated and constitutes a serious health care problem. Studies have shown that 70% of patients treated in routine medical settings or at home have unrelieved pain (5,6). Patients with constant pain lose hope and have decreased confidence in the health care system, which may lead to treatment rejection and suicidal ideation. Diminished activity, decreased appetite, and loss of sleep weaken the already debilitated patient and lower the pain threshold. Even with a long life expectancy, productivity and quality of life decrease. Family and social relationships are stressed, eventually leading to demoralization and loss of hope.

The management of cancer pain begins with awareness, education, and changes in attitudes by health care providers and patients. The physician or nurse must believe that the patient's report of pain is real and that the severity of pain is whatever the patient reports. Pain is subjective; there are no objective parameters that may be relied on. Facial expressions, diaphoresis, pallor, or hemodynamic parameters (e.g., tachycardia) are unreliable. Pain relief may not be determined by the use of standard doses or measurement of drug levels (7). The cardinal rule is to give the patient the benefit of the doubt. Conversely, patients need to surmount fears of addiction and use prescribed medications for prevention and treatment of their pain. This requires education and reinforcement by health care providers. In short, effective analgesia is a joint effort of patients and their physicians.

The striking lack of emphasis on pain management in medical schools plays a significant role in physicans' lack of understanding and undertreatment of pain. There is no comparable therapeutic regimen that is so highly dependent on the individual bias of the physician. Inappropriate concerns about addiction by health care providers distort priorities and scientific judgment. Patients with poorly responding pain syndromes are quickly labeled as drug-seeking addicts. This is unfortunate, since multiple studies have shown that the incidence of addiction in patients receiving opioids for legitimate medical use is less than 1 in 3000 patients (8,9). Health care providers need better knowledge of pain pathophysiology, analgesic drug therapy, and techniques for pain management (10).

PRINCIPLES AND PROCEDURES OF PAIN MANAGEMENT

The perception of pain is complex and involves psychological and emotional processes in ascending neural pathways and descending pain-inhibiting pathways. Analgesic, antidepressant, local anesthetic, and adjuvant drugs may affect either or both of these pathways. Effective pain management involves assessment, treatment, reassessment of results, and sometimes referral. It entails continuity of professional care, including patient instruction and use of community resources (11).

Assessment

The goal of the initial assessment is to characterize the pain by location, intensity, and etiology. This involves a detailed history, physical examination, psychosocial assessment, and diagnostic evaluation. The history entails the patient's description of the quality and intensity of pain, utilizing pain intensity scales that include simple descriptive, numeric, and visual analogue scales (see Appendix 12). The location of the pain and aggravating or relieving factors should be documented. In patients who are cognitively impaired or who have communication problems relating to education, language, ethnicity, or culture, behavior suggestive of pain should be observed and more appropriate (i.e., simpler or translated) pain assessment tools should be used. Goals for pain control (as scores on a pain scale) should be documented in the patient's chart. The patient's preferred pain assessment tool should always be used.

Follow-up Assessment

Continual assessment of cancer pain is critical. Changes in pain pattern or the development of new pain may be due to development of tolerance or progression of the disease and should not be confused with addiction. Such changes indicate the need for a reevaluation of the diagnosis and modification of the treatment plan, for example, addition of adjuvant drugs or alternate therapies.

PHARMACOLOGIC TREATMENT

Recommendations for pharmacologic therapy begin with the World Health Organization (WHO) ladder—a three-step hierarchy for analgesic pain management (see Appendix 1). The cardinal rules for pharmacologic therapy include the following:

1. Use the simplest dosage schedules and least invasive pain management modalities first.
2. Prevention is better than cure. Schedule long-acting medications on an around-the-clock basis.
3. Provide for additional doses of short-acting medication for breakthrough pain.
4. Oral administration is convenient and cost effective. When indicated, alternative routes of administration include rectal, transdermal, intravenous, subcutaneous, transmucosal, epidural, and spinal routes.
5. Combined therapy of opioids, nonsteroidal anti-inflammatory drugs (NSAIDs), and adjuvant drugs

(e.g., antidepressant agents) provides for synergistic relief of moderate to severe pain with reduced risk of side effects.

Major Classes of Pain Medications
1. Acetaminophen and NSAIDs

Route: Oral, intravenous, intramuscular.

Use(s): Symptomatic treatment of mild to moderate pain, fever, inflammatory conditions (e.g., rheumatic fever, rheumatoid arthritis, osteoarthritis), chronic pain, and cancer pain (especially with bone metastasis).

Pharmacology: The analgesic activity of acetaminophen and the NSAIDs may be mediated by inhibition of the biosynthesis and release of prostaglandins that sensitize C fibers' nociceptors to mechanical stimuli and chemical mediators (e.g., bradykinin, histamine) and that may interfere with the endogenous descending pathways that inhibit pain transmission. Acetaminophen inhibits central prostaglandin synthesis, and the NSAIDs inhibit central and peripheral prostaglandin synthesis. The antipyretic activity of acetaminophen and NSAIDs may occur secondary to inhibition of pyrogen-induced release of prostaglandins in the central nervous system (including the hypothalamus) and possibly to centrally mediated peripheral vasodilatation. Unlike the NSAIDs, acetaminophen does not have anti-inflammatory activity, does not produce gastric irritation, does not interfere with platelet function, and has no uricosuric activity. The NSAIDs acetylate platelet cyclooxygenase and prevent the synthesis of thromboxane A_2, a potent vasoconstrictor and inducer of platelet aggregation. Thus, the drugs prolong bleeding time.

2. Opioids

Route: Oral, rectal, intravenous, intramuscular, epidural, intrathecal, subcutaneous, transdermal, transmucosal, intra-articular.

Use(s): Treatment of acute, chronic, and cancer pain.

Pharmacology: Opioids exert primary effects on the central nervous system and organs containing smooth muscle. Excitatory synaptic pain transmission is decreased by opioid receptor–mediated inhibition of neurotransmitter release (e.g., bradykinin at site of tissue injury, substance P in the dorsal horn, and dopamine in the basal ganglia). In addition, opioids may alter cognitive and emotional processing of painful input by acting on limbic and cortical opioid receptors. The pure agonists (e.g., morphine, meperidine) are potent analgesics and do not have ceiling effect for analgesia. The agonist-antagonists (e.g., pentazocine) are less potent and have ceiling effects for analgesia and respiratory depression. Spinal or epidural administration produces intensive analgesia by specific binding and activation of opioid receptors in the substantia gelatinosa. Once activated, the opioid receptors inhibit the release of substance P from nociceptive afferent C fibers. Analgesia is achieved without sensory, motor, or sympathetic blockade.

Drowsiness, euphoria, depression of the cough reflex, dose-dependent respiratory depression, and reduction in peripheral resistance (arteriolar and venous dilatation) may occur. Clinically important respiratory depression is rarely seen in patients with severe pain caused by malignant disease even with large doses, because pain and emotional stress are powerful antagonists to narcotic-induced respiratory depression. Development of new catheter materials and placement techniques has allowed long-term delivery of epidural and spinal opioids for months to years. The constipating effects of opioids result from induction of nonpropulsive contractions through the gastrointestinal tract. Emetic effects are due to opioid-induced stimulation of the chemoreceptor trigger zone in the floor of the fourth ventricle. Rostral spread and delivery of opioid molecules to the brain stem respiratory centers may lead to late-onset respiratory depression (occurring at 6 to 12 hours).

Adjuvant Drugs

3. Antidepressant Agents

Route: Oral, intramuscular, intravenous, topical.

Use(s): Treatment of neurotic and endogenous depression; adjunct treatment of neuropathic pain syndromes, including diabetic neuropathy, postherpetic neuralgia, tic douloureux, and cancer pain; anxiety disorders; migraine; phobias; panic disorders.

Pharmacology: The analgesic effects of antidepressant agents may occur partly through the alleviation of depression, which may be responsible for increased pain suffering, but also by mechanisms that are independent of mood effects. Serotonin and norepinephrine activity may be increased in descending pain-inhibitory pathways. Activation of these pathways decreases the transmission of nociceptive impulses from primary afferent neurons to first-order cells in laminae I and V of the spinal cord dorsal horn. Antidepressants may also potentiate the analgesic effect of opioids by increasing their binding efficacy to opioid receptors. The newer selective serotonin reuptake inhibitors (e.g., paroxetine) are preferable to the older tricyclic antidepressants (e.g., amitriptyline) because they have significantly fewer adverse effects (e.g., sedation, orthostatic hypotension, constipation, urinary retention). Topical application of antidepressants (e.g., doxepin cream) may be effective in treatment of postherpetic neuralgia and sympathetic mediated pain.

4. Bisphosphonate Agents

Route: Oral, intravenous.

Use(s): Treatment of hypercalcemia of malignancy; treatment of osteolytic bone metastasis of breast cancer and osteolytic bone lesions of multiple myeloma; slowing of bone disease progression and reduction of tumor-associated metastatic bone pain; treatment of osteoporosis and bone pain associated with reflex sympathetic dystrophy.

Pharmacology: Bisphosphonate drugs bind to bone hydroxyapatite and specifically inhibit the activity of osteoclasts, the bone-resorbing cells. Bone resorption is reduced with no direct effect on bone formation, although the latter process is ultimately reduced because bone resorption and formation are coupled during bone turnover. Bisphosphonate drugs thus reduce elevated rates of bone turnover. Osteoclastic activity resulting in excessive bone resorption is the underlying pathophysiologic derangement in metastatic bone disease and hypercalcemia of malignancy. In treatment of metastatic bone disease, pamidronate and other bisphosphonates (e.g., alendronate) treat hypercalcemia, reduce tumor-associated pain, reduce the incidence of pathologic fractures, and also slow bone disease progression.

Administration of bisphosphonates shortly after adjuvant chemotherapy can preserve bone density in female patients with chemotherapy-induced menopause. The bisphosphonate clodronate has been shown to reduce the incidence of bone metastasis in patients with early-stage breast cancer. There was no difference in the incidence of nonskeletal metastatic disease.

5. Local Anesthetic Agents

Route: Topical, infiltration, epidural, intrathecal, intravenous regional, intravenous.

Use(s): Regional anesthesia; systemic analgesia for treatment of painful conditions, such as neuropathic pain, reflex sympathetic dystrophy, burn or sickle cell pain, and pruritus.

Pharmacology: Local anesthetics stabilize the neuronal membrane and prevent the initiation and transmission of impulses. Sensory, motor, and autonomic blockade depend on the site of administration and the volume and concentration of the local anesthetic. The duration of action is prolonged by epinephrine, which reduces the rate of absorption and plasma concentration. Some local anesthetics (e.g., lidocaine) may be used for IV regional anesthesia. When administered as intravenous infusions, these local anesthetics may produce central analgesia. This may be due to the local anesthetic effects and central sympathetic blockade with decrease in pain-induced reflex vasoconstriction.

6. Phenothiazine Agents

Route: Oral, intramuscular, intravenous, rectal.

Use(s): Antipsychotic, antiemetic, relief of hiccups, treatment of phantom limb pain, adjunct treatment of neuropathic pain (e.g., diabetic neuropathy, postherpetic neuralgia).

Pharmacology: Phenothiazines have strong antiemetic, antiadrenergic, anticholinergic, and sedative effects. This class of drugs may be useful in chronic pain syndromes by altering the perception of pain and, where applicable, relieving psychosis and/or anxiety. Some phenothiazines (e.g., chlorpromazine) may be useful in postherpetic neuralgia and other neuropathies in which burning dyesthetic pain and lancinating sensations are prominent features. Due to the risk of serious adverse effects (e.g., permanent tardive dyskinesia), phenothiazines are not drugs of first choice for neuropathic pain. They should be used after initial therapy with antidepressants, narcotics, and/or nonsteroidal anti-inflammatory drugs. It is advisable to obtain informed consent before instituting phenothiazine therapy for chronic pain management.

7. Anticonvulsant Agents

Route: Oral, intravenous.

Use(s): Anticonvulsant; antidepressant; treatment of lancinating neuropathic pain, such as trigeminal neuralgia (tic douloureux) and other cranial neuralgias, postsympathectomy neuralgia, diabetic neuropathy, postherpetic neuralgia, phantom limb pain, the thalamic syndrome, or lightning tabetic pain; migraine.

Pharmacology: Anticonvulsants (e.g., gabapentin) may suppress the sharp lancinating and paroxysmal electrical shooting qualities common in neuropathic pain, such as in idiopathic trigeminal neuralgia, by decreasing synaptic transmission. The drugs are not as useful for the more chronic aching pains (e.g., in posttraumatic trigeminal pain). The antidepressant activity is comparable with that of the tricyclic antidepressants and may contribute to the analgesic effects.

8. Antiarrhythmic Agents
(e.g., Mexiletine)

Route: Oral.

Use(s): Treatment of lancinating neuropathic pain, such as trigeminal neuralgia (tic douloureux) and other cranial neuralgias, postsympathectomy neuralgia, postherpetic neuralgia, diabetic neuropathy, phantom limb pain, the thalamic syndrome, or lightning tabetic pain; symptomatic treatment of carpal tunnel syndrome.

Pharmacology: Mexiletine is a local anesthetic class 1B antiarrhythmic agent that is structurally similar to lidocaine but orally active. Mexiletine suppresses the sharp lancinating and paroxysmal electrical shooting qualities common in neuropathic pain such as in idiopathic trigeminal neuralgia.

9. Stool Softener Agents
(e.g., Docusate sodium)

Route: Oral, rectal.

Use(s): Prophylaxis and treatment of constipation (e.g., with chronic administration of opioids).

Pharmacology: Docusate softens fecal material and makes defecation easier secondary to a decrease in surface tension at the fecal oil-water interface, thus permitting water and lipids to penetrate. Increased fluid intake, a high-fiber diet, and use of fruits and fruit juices are also helpful in preventing an otherwise inevitable occurrence of severe constipation with chronic opioid therapy.

10. Antiemetic/Antihistamine Agents
(e.g., Hydroxyzine)

Route: Oral, intravenous, intramuscular.
Use(s): Antiemetic; sedative; adjunct treatment of acute, chronic, and cancer pain; treatment of pruritus due to allergic conditions (e.g., chronic urticaria and histamine-mediated pruritus).
Pharmacology: The sedative and tranquilizing effects of hydroxyzine may result principally from suppression of activity at subcortical levels of the CNS. The anti-emetic and anti-motion-sickness effects may result from central anticholinergic and CNS depressant properties. The sedative and analgesic effects of opioids may be potentiated, thus enabling a decrease in opioid dose and reduction of side effects such as nausea and vomiting.

11. Corticosteroid Agents

Route: Oral, intravenous, intramuscular, intratissue, epidural.
Use(s): Treatment of refractory bone pain; treatment of aching, burning, lancinating neuropathic pain, malignant spinal cord compression, and pain caused by malignant lesions of the brachial and lumbo-sacral plexus; treatment of inflammatory diseases, cerebral edema, aspiration pneumonitis, bronchial asthma, myofascial pain with trigger points, allergic reactions; prevention of rejection in organ transplantation; replacement therapy for adrenocortical insufficiency.
Pharmacology: Corticosteroids are useful in the management of acute and chronic cancer pain. In metastatic bone pain, corticosteroids may interfere with the

formation of prostaglandin E by inhibiting tumor-secreted phospholipase A_2, which catalyzes the release of arachidonic acid from plasma membranes. Corticosteroids may be oncolytic for certain tumors (e.g., lymphoma) and may ameliorate painful nerve or spinal cord compression by reducing edema in tumor and nerve tissue. Corticosteroids are effective in the treatment of malignant spinal cord compression. Short-term therapy (1 to 2 weeks) may be useful in the management of pain caused by malignant lesions of the brachial or lumbosacral plexus. Corticosteroids may suppress the hypothalamic-pituitary-adrenal axis.

NONPHARMACOLOGIC TREATMENT

Physical Modalities

Patients should be encouraged to remain active and participate in self-care when possible. Cutaneous stimulation, hot packs, ice packs, whirlpool, massage, and repositioning may relieve pain. Cold decreases pain by dulling the sensory nerves and decreasing blood flow, inflammation, and joint stiffness. Cold and ice work best for injuries and acute pain. The therapeutic effects of deep heat with diathermy or ultrasound occur when tissue temperature reaches 40° to 45°C (104°–112.7°F). Blood flow and cell membrane permeability increase, with enhanced transfer of metabolites. Other pain-relieving effects include decrease in muscle spasms and collagenous tissue tension, with an increase in range of motion. Heat therapy is helpful in chronic pain, joint stiffness, and muscle spasms. Exercises are useful in strengthening weak muscles, mobilizing stiff joints, and helping restore coordination and balance. Where possible, exercises should be coordinated with other interventions (e.g., nerve blocks).

Psychosocial Intervention

Psychological therapy includes behavioral modification, cognitive coping strategies, biofeedback, hypnosis, and psychotherapy. These therapies help give the patient a sense of control and develop coping skills to deal with the pain.

Psychosocial intervention may be required for problem solving or activation of the resources needed for patient care. Underlying motives (e.g., in worker's compensation cases) should be assessed and addressed. Information on local peer support groups and pastoral counseling should be offered to patients. The family should be mobilized to aid in the assessment, administration, and evaluation of pain control.

Radiation Therapy

Local or whole-body radiation may alleviate pain by reducing primary and metastatic tumor bulk. Radiation therapy is beneficial in controlling pain from radiosensitive tumors (e.g., undifferentiated carcinomas of the head and neck, and metastatic involvement of bone, soft tissues, and lymph nodes). The dosage of radiation should be carefully chosen to minimize damage to normal tissue, which may result in pain.

Surgery

Curative excision or tumor debulking may reduce pain directly, relieve symptoms of obstruction or compression, and improve prognosis. Open, percutaneous, and stereotactic ablative techniques may relieve pain by destruction of spinal, intercostal, or peripheral nerves and midbrain or pontine spinothalamic tracts. Serious adverse effects, including motor and sensory deficits, urinary incontinence, and death, may occur.

Electrical Therapy

Controlled low-voltage electrical stimulation may be applied proximal to the site of pain. The electrodes may be applied transcutaneously or implanted in the nerves, spinal cord, or deep brain. Pain transmission is inhibited by reversible neuronal blockade, activation of synaptic gating mechanisms, and/or the endogenous opiate pain suppression system.

Acupuncture

Pain is treated by inserting small solid needles at various points and depths in the skin. These needles may be manually manipulated or electrically stimulated. The pattern of needle placement is governed by various meridians that correspond to a series of anatomic points described in ancient Chinese texts. Each meridian represents the surface projection of an internal organ. The actual placement of the needles is based on the practitioner's interpretation of the distribution of the yin (cold or hypofunctionality) and yang (heat or hyperfunctionality) in a particular organ or organ system.

Local Anesthetic Blocks

Somatic or sympathetic nerve blocks may be performed with local anesthetic alone or in combination with corticosteroids or adrenergic blocking agents (e.g., guanethidine). These blocks may provide relief from nerve or root compression, causalgia, or reflex sympathetic dystrophy. Local anesthetic blocks are reversible and may provide prolonged pain relief by interrupting the afferent nociceptive barrage into the central nervous system and breaking the pain cycle.

Neurolytic Blocks

Neurolytic blocks with phenol or ethanol provide prolonged pain relief by nonselective destruction of neural tissue. These blocks should not be undertaken lightly. Proper technical application is required to avoid delivery to tissues outside the target area. Complications may include neuritis, hyperesthesias or dyesthesias (which may be worse than the original pain), distressing numbness (anesthesia dolorosa), prolonged motor paralysis, or perineal dysfunction.

REFERENCES

1. Bonica JJ. Treatment of cancer pain: current status and future needs. In: Fields HL, Dubner R, Cervero F, eds. Advances in pain research and therapy. vol. 9. Proceedings of the Fourth World Congress on Pain. New York: Raven Press, 1985.
2. Pannuti E, Rossi AP, Marraro D. Natural history of cancer pain. In: Twycross RG, Ventafridda V, eds. The continuing care of terminal cancer patients. New York: Pergamon, 1980.
3. Foley KM. Pain syndromes in patients with cancer. In: Bonica JJ, Ventafridda V, eds. Advances in pain research and therapy. vol. 2. New York: Raven Press, 1987.

4. Twycross RG, Fairfield S. Pain in far advanced cancer. Pain 1982;14:303–310.

5. Marks RM, Sacher EJ. Undertreatment of medical inpatients with narcotic analgesics. Ann Intern Med 1973;78:173–181.

6. Parkes CM. Home or hospital: terminal care as seen by the surviving spouse. J R Coll Gen Pract 1978;28:19–30.

7. Flexner JM. Management of cancer pain. Professional Education Newsletter 21(3). Nashville: American Cancer Society, 1993.

8. Porter J, Jick H. Addiction rare in patients treated with narcotics. N Engl J Med 1980;302:133.

9. Perry S, Heidrich G. Management of pain during debridement: a survey of U.S. burn units. Pain 1982;13:267–280.

10. Omoigui S. Sota Omoigui's anesthesia drugs handbook. 3rd ed. Malden, MA: Blackwell Science, 1999.

11. Jacox A, Carr DB, Payne R, et al. Management of cancer pain: adults quick reference guide 9. Rockville, MD: Department of Health and Human Services, Agency for Health Care Policy and Research, 1994. AHCPR Publication 94-0593.

Bibliography

Abram SE, Haddox DJ, Kettler RE, eds. The pain clinic manual. Philadelphia: JB Lippincott, 1990.

American Hospital Formulary Service. Drug information. Bethseda, MD: American Society of Hospital Pharmacists, 1999.

Bonica JJ, Loeser JD, Chapman CR, Fordyce WE, eds. The management of pain. Philadelphia: Lea and Febiger, 1990.

Carr DB, et al, eds. Clinical practice guideline for acute pain management: operative or medical procedures and trauma. Washington, DC: Agency for Health Care Policy and Research, 1992.

Cousins MJ, Bridenbaugh PO, eds. Neural blockade in clinical anesthesia and the management of pain. Philadelphia: JB Lippincott, 1998.

DiGregorio GJ, Barbieri EJ, Sterling GH, et al. Handbook of pain management. Westchester, PA: Medical Surveillance, 1991.

Drug facts and comparisons. Philadelphia: JB Lippincott, 1999.

Foley KM, Payne RM, et al, eds. Current therapy of pain. Philadelphia: BC Decker, 1989.

Omoigui S. Sota Omoigui's anesthesia drugs handbook. 3rd ed. Malden, MA: Blackwell Science, 1999.

Physician's desk reference. Oradell, NJ: Medical Economics, 1999.

Raj PP, et al, eds. Practical management of pain. St. Louis: Mosby–Year Book, 1992.

Scott DB, Hakansson L, eds. Techniques of regional anesthesia. Norwalk, CT: Appleton and Lange/Mediglobe, 1989.

Sinatra RS, et al, eds. Acute pain: mechanisms and management. St. Louis: Mosby–Year Book, 1993.

Tollison DC, Satterthwaite JR, Tollison JW, et al, eds. Handbook of pain management. Baltimore: Williams and Wilkins, 1994.

APPENDIX

Appendix

Appendix 1

WORLD HEALTH ORGANIZATION THREE-STEP ANALGESIC LADDER*

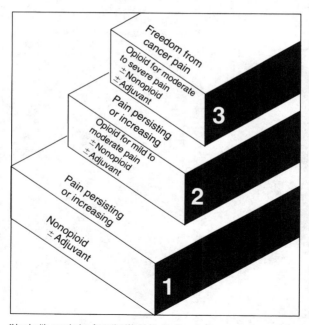

*Used with permission from the World Health Organization.

Appendix 2

DRUG TABLES

TABLE 2-1.
Opioids and Opioid Antagonists

Name	Potency (MS*)	Dose	Onset	Peak	Duration
Buprenorphine HCL (PA) **(Buprenex)**	30	IV/IM/SL 0.3–0.6 mg (6–12 µg/kg) q4–6 hr Epidural 50–60 µg (1 µg/kg)	IV < 1 min	IV 5–20 min IM 15 min	IV/IM/SL 6 hr IM 1 hr

Comments: Binds avidly to opioid receptors. Respiratory depression may not respond to naloxone; doxapram may be more suitable.

| Butorphanol Tartrate (Ag-An) **(Stadol)** | 3.5–7 | IV 0.5–2 mg (0.01–0.04 mg/kg) q3–4 hr IM 1–4 mg (0.02–0.08 mg/kg) q3–4 hr Nasal 1 mg Epidural 1–2 mg (20–40 µg/kg) | IV 1–5 min IM 10 min Nasal < 15 min | IV 5–10 min IM 30–60 min Nasal 1–2 hr | IV 2–4 hr IM 3–4 hr Nasal 4–5 hr Epidural 3–4 hr |

Comments: May be administered by epidural route for acute & chronic pain.

| Codeine Phosphate/ Sulfate (Ag) **(Codeine, in Tylenol with codeine, Phenaphen with codeine)** | 1/30–1/8 | PO/IM/IV 15–60 mg (0.5 mg/kg) q4 hr | PO 15–30 min | PO 30–60 min | PO 3–6 hr |

Comments: May be used with acetaminophen or aspirin for mild to moderate pain. Has analgesic & antitussive properties.

Key: *Potency, compared to oral morphine sulfate.
PA = Partial agonist; Ag-An = Agonist-Antagonist; Ag = Agonist; An = Antagonist; NA = Not applicable.

Continued.

671

TABLE 2-1 (cont.).

Name	Potency (MS*)	Dose	Onset	Peak	Duration
Fentanyl Citrate (Ag) **(Sublimaze)**	75–125	Oral (transmucosal) 200–400 μg (5–15 μg/kg) q4–6 hr	Oral 5–15 min	Oral 20–30 min	Oral 1–2 hr
		IV/IM 25–100 μg (0.7–2 μg/kg)	IV < 30 sec	IV 5–15 min	IV 30–60 min
			IM < 8 min	IM < 15 min	IM 1–2 hr
		Epidural 50–100 μg (1–2 μg/kg)	Epidural 4–10 min	Epidural < 30 min	Epidural 4–8 hr
		Spinal 5–20 μg (0.1–0.4 μg/kg)	Spinal 4–10 min	Spinal < 30 min	Spinal 4–8 hr
		Transdermal 25–100 μg/hr	Transdermal 12–18 hr		Transdermal 3 days

Comments: Potent opioid. Related to meperidine. Transdermal & oral transmucosal form useful in chronic pain.

Name	Potency (MS*)	Dose	Onset	Peak	Duration
Hydrocodone HCL (Ag) **(Lortab, Lorcet, Co-Gesic)**	1/30–1/8	PO 5–10 mg q4–6 hr	PO 15–30 min	PO 30–60 min	PO 4–8 hr

Comments: Mild analgesic. Potency similar to codeine. Used in combination with aspirin or acetaminophen.

Name	Potency (MS*)	Dose	Onset	Peak	Duration
Hydromorphone (Ag) HCL **(Dilaudid)**	7	PO 2–4 mg q4–6 hr	PO/IM/SC 15–30 min	PO/IM/SC 30–60 min	PO/IM/SC 4–6 hr
		IM/SC 2–4 mg (0.04–0.08 mg/kg)			
		Slow IV 0.5–2 mg (0.01–0.04 mg/kg)	IV < 30 sec	IV 5–20 min	IV 2–4 hr
		Epidural 1–2 mg (20–40 μg/kg)	Epidural 5 min	Epidural 30 min	Epidural 10–16 hr

Comments: Potent short-acting opioid. Used for breakthrough pain in conjunction with long-acting opioid, e.g., morphine. May be administered parenterally, rectally, or subcutaneously.

Drug	Potency*	Dose	Onset	Duration
Levorphanol Tartrate (Ag) (**Levo-Dromoran**)	5	PO/SC 2–4 mg q4–6 hr Slow IV 1 mg (0.02 mg/kg)	IV 10–15 min	SC 60–90 min IV < 20 min	SC 6–8 hr IV 6–8 hr

Comments: Highly concentrated. Useful for subcutaneous infusions which require small volumes.

Meperidine HCL (Ag) (**Demerol**)	0.1	PO/IM/IV/SC 50–150 mg (1–3 mg/kg) Slow IV 25–100 mg (0.5–2 mg/kg) Epidural 50–100 mg (1–2 mg/kg) Spinal 0.2–1 mg (4–20 µg/kg)	PO 10–45 min IM 1–5 min IV < 1 min Epidural 2–12 min Spinal 2–12 min	PO < 1 hr IM 30–50 min IV 5–20 min	IV/IM/PO 2–4 hr Epidural 1–8 hr Spinal 1–8 hr

Comments: Only opioid with local anesthetic properties and direct myocardial depressant effects.

Methadone HCL (Ag) (**Dolophine**)	1–3	PO/IM/SC 2.5–10 mg (0.05–0.1 mg/kg) q3–4 hr then 5–20 mg q6–8 hr Epidural 1–5 mg (20–100 µg/kg)	IV 30–60 min IV < 1 min IM 1–5 min Epidural 5–10 min	IV 5–20 min IM 30–60 min	IV/IM 4–6 hr PO 22–48 hr Epidural 6–10 hr

Comments: Long-acting opioid analgesic; accumulates with use, and dosing frequency may be decreased.

Key: *Potency, compared to oral morphine sulfate.
PA = Partial agonist; Ag-An = Agonist-Antagonist; Ag = Agonist; An = Antagonist; NA = Not applicable.

Continued.

673

TABLE 2-1 (cont.).

Name	Potency (MS*)	Dose	Onset	Peak	Duration
Morphine Sulfate (Ag) (**Morphine, MS Contin, Duramorph, Astramorph**)	1	PO 10–60 mg q4 hr PO (M.S. Contin) 15–100 mg q12 hr IM/SC 2.5–20 mg q4 hr Rectal 10–20 mg q4 hr IV 2.5–15 mg Epidural 2–5 mg (40–100 μg/kg) Spinal 0.2–1 mg (4–20 μg/kg)	PO < 60 min IM 1–5 min IV < 1 min Epidural 15–60 min Spinal 15–60 min	PO < 60 min IM 30–60 min SC 50–90 min Rectal 20–60 min IV 5–20 min Epidural 30 min Spinal 30 min	IV/IM/SC 2–7 hr Epidural 6–24 hr Spinal 6–24 hr

Comments: Principal alkaloid of opium. Prototype of the opiate agonists. Long-acting preparation used for chronic pain.

Name	Potency (MS*)	Dose	Onset	Peak	Duration
Nalbuphine HCL (Ag-An) (**Nubain**)	1	IV/IM/SC 5–10 mg (0.1–0.3 mg/kg) q3–6 hr	IV 2–3 min IM/SC < 15 min	IV 5–15 min	IV/IM/SC 3–6 hr

Comments: Effective in reversing ventilatory depression of agonist opioids (e.g., morphine) while maintaining reasonable analgesia.

Name	Potency (MS*)	Dose	Onset	Peak	Duration
Naloxone HCL (An) (**Narcan**)	NA	IV/IM/SC 0.1–2 mg (10–100 μg/kg)	IV 1–2 min IM/SC 2–5 min	IV/IM 5–15 min	IV/IM/SC 1–4 hr

Comments: Reverses the side effects (e.g., respiratory depression and pruritis) of opioid agonists, and the psychotomimetic and dysphoric effects of agonists-antagonists (e.g., pentazocine).

Drug	Potency*	Dose/Route	Onset	Peak	Duration
Naltrexone HCL (An) **(Trexan)**	NA	PO 12.5–50 mg daily	PO 15–30 min	PO 6–12 hr	PO 24–72 hr

Comments: May reverse the hypotension and cardiovascular instability secondary to endogenous endorphins (potent vasodilators) released in patients with septic or cardiogenic shock.

Drug	Potency*	Dose/Route	Onset	Peak	Duration
Oxycodone HCL (Ag) **(OxyContin, Roxicodone, in Percocet, Percodan, Roxicet, Tylox)**	2	PO 5–10 mg q4–6 hr	PO 10–15 min	PO 30–60 min	PO 3–6 hr

Comments: Potency similar to morphine. Used often in combination with aspirin and acetaminophen.

Drug	Potency*	Dose/Route	Onset	Peak	Duration
Oxymorphone HCL (Ag) **(Numorphan)**	10	IV 0.5 mg q4–6 hr IM/SC 0.5–1.5 mg q4–6 hr Rectal 5 mg q4–6 hr	IV 5–10 min IM/SC 10–15 min	IV/IM 30–60 min	IV/IM 3–6 hr

Comments: Derivative of hydromorphone, with similar effects.

Drug	Potency*	Dose/Route	Onset	Peak	Duration
Pentazocine HCL (Ag-An) **(Talwin)**	1/3	PO 50–100 mg (1–2 mg/kg) q3–4 hr IM/SC 30–60 mg (0.5–1 mg/kg) q3–4 hr IV 15–30 mg (0.3–0.5 mg/kg) q3–4 hr	PO 15–30 min IM/SC 15–20 min IV 2–3 min	PO 1–3 hr IM 1 hr IV 15 min	PO 3–6 hr IM 2 hr IV 1 hr

Comments: Oldest agonist-antagonist opioid. Like other agonist-antagonists, may be associated with psychotomimetic effects.

Key: *Potency, compared to oral morphine sulfate.
PA = Partial agonist; Ag-An = Agonist-Antagonist; Ag = Agonist; An = Antagonist; NA = Not applicable.

Continued.

TABLE 2-1 (cont.).

Name	Potency (MS*)	Dose	Onset	Peak	Duration
Propoxyphene HCL (Ag) **(Darvon, in Genagesic, Wygesic)**	1/50–1/25	PO 65 mg q4 hr	PO 15–60 min	PO 2–3 hr	PO 4–6 hr

Comments: Derivative of methadone. Weak analgesic. Used in combination with other analgesics (e.g., acetaminophen).

Name	Potency (MS*)	Dose	Onset	Peak	Duration
Sufentanil Citrate (Ag) **(Sufenta)**	500–700	IV/IM 10–30 μg (0.2–0.6 μg/kg)	IV 1–3 min	IV 3–5 min	IV 20–45 min IM 2–4 hr
		Epidural 10–30 μg (0.2–0.6 μg/kg)	Epidural 4–10 min	Epidural < 30 min	Epidural 2–4 hr
		Spinal 1–4 μg (0.02–0.08 μg/kg)	Spinal 4–10 min	Spinal < 30 min	Spinal 2–4 hr

Comments: Most potent opioid in clinical use, 700 times more potent than morphine. Use by epidural or spinal route for chronic pain. Parenteral route used for general anesthesia.

Name	Potency (MS*)	Dose	Onset	Peak	Duration
Tramadol (Ag) **(Ultram)**	1/8	PO 50–100 mg q4–6 hr Max 400 mg daily	PO < 1 hr	PO 2–3 hr	PO 3–6 hr

Comments: Unique dual mechanism of action. Acts on opioid receptors and acts like a mild anti-depressant by inhibiting the reuptake of serotonin and norepinephrine.

Key: *Potency, compared to oral morphine sulfate.
PA = Partial agonist;   Ag-An = Agonist-Antagonist;   Ag = Agonist;   An = Antagonist;   NA = Not applicable.

TABLE 2-2.
Nonsteroidal Anti-inflammatory Drugs (NSAIDs)

Name	Potency (ASA*)	Dose	Onset	Peak	Duration
Acetaminophen (**Tylenol, Panadol, Phenaphen, Tempra, in Anacin-3, Excedrin, Vicodin, Tylox, Percocet, Darvon-N, etc.**)	1	PO/rectal 325–650 mg (6–12 mg/kg) q4 hr	PO 5–30 min	PO 0.5–2 hr	PO 3–7 hr

Comments: Most commonly available analgesic. Does not produce gastric irritation, does not interfere with platelet function.

| Aspirin (**Aspirin, in Bufferin, Buffaprin, Alka-Seltzer, Anacin, Percodan, Taiwin, etc.**) | 1 | PO 325–650 mg (6–12 mg/kg) q4–8 hr | PO 5–30 min | PO 0.5–2 hr | PO 3–7 hr |

Comments: Irreversibly inhibits platelet aggregation for the life of the platelet (7–10 days) and prolongs bleeding time. Enhances urinary excretion of uric acid & useful for treatment of gout. May prevent arterial & possible venous thrombosis. Increased risk of developing Reye's syndrome, if used in children with Influenza or chickenpox.

| Celecoxib (**Celebrex**) | 3 | PO 100–200 mg once or twice daily | PO 15–30 min | PO 24–48 hr | PO half-life 11 hr |

Comments: A COX-2 inhibitor. At therapeutic concentrations, does not inhibit COX-1 isoenzyme. May be administered orally without regard to meals. Better tolerated than diclofenac, naproxen, or ibuprofen, and equipotent doses are associated with less gastric mucosal abnormalities.

Key: *Potency, as compared to aspirin.

Continued.

677

TABLE 2-2 (cont.).

Name	Potency (ASA*)	Dose	Onset	Peak	Duration
Choline Salicylate (Arthropan)	1	PO 435–870 mg or 2.5–5 mL (8–16 mg/kg) or 0.05–0.1 mL/kg) q4 hr	PO 5–30 min	PO 0.5–2 hr	PO 3–7 hr
Comments: Does not inhibit platelet aggregation. Useful in patients with GI intolerance to aspirin.					
Diclofenac Sodium (Voltaren)	15	PO 100–200 mg (2–4 mg/kg) daily in 2 to 4 divided doses	PO 15–30 min	PO 1–3 hr	PO 4–6 hr
Comments: Structurally related to mefenamic acid but more potent.					
Diflunisal (Dolobid)	3.5–13	PO 1 gram then 500 mg q8–12 hr	PO < 60 min	PO 2–3 hr	PO 3–7 hr
Comments: May be administered twice daily. In contrast to the prolonged effects of aspirin, platelet aggregation returns to normal within 24 hours.					
Etodolac (Lodine)	3	PO 200–400 mg (4–8 mg/kg) q6–12 hr	PO 15–30 min	PO 1–2 hr	PO 4–6 hr
Comments: Better tolerated than indomethacin, naproxen, or ibuprofen, and equipotent doses are associated with less gastric mucosal abnormalities.					
Fenoprofen Calcium (Nalfon)	3	PO 200 mg (4 mg/kg) q4–6 hr	PO 15–30 min	PO 1–2 hr	PO 4–6 hr
Comments: Better tolerated than aspirin, and equipotent doses are associated with less gastric mucosal abnormalities.					
Ibuprofen (Advil, Motrin)	1	PO 200–800 mg (8–16 mg/kg) q6 hr	PO < 30 min	PO 2–4 hr	PO 6–8 hr
Comments: Better tolerated than aspirin or naproxen, and equipotent doses are associated with less gastric mucosal abnormalities.					
Indomethacin (Indocin)	20	PO 25–50 mg (0.5–1 mg/kg) q6–12 hr	PO 15–30 min	PO 1–2 hr	PO 4–6 hr
Comments: Potent NSAID. More effective than aspirin in relieving the pain of primary dysmenorrhea. Indomethacin has antiinflammatory effects comparable with colchicine in the treatment of gouty arthritis.					

	Potency[*]		Onset	Peak	Duration
Ketoprofen (**Orudis**)	20	PO 25–50 mg (0.5–1 mg/kg) q6–8 hr	PO 15–30 min	PO 1–2 hr	PO 3–4 hr

Comments: Potent NSAID. Better GI tolerance than indomethacin or aspirin.

Ketorolac Tromethamine (**Toradol**)	60 (PO)	Loading: IM/IV 30–60 mg (0.5–1 mg/kg) Maintenance: IM/IV 15–30 mg (0.25–0.5 mg/kg) PO 10 mg q4–6 hr	IV < 1 min IM < 10 min PO < 1 hr	IV 1–3 hr IM 1–3 hr PO 1–3 hr	IV 3–7 hr IM 3–7 hr PO 3–7 hr

Comments: The only NSAID approved for parenteral administration for analgesia. To minimize serious adverse effects, duration of use should not exceed 5 days for parenteral and 14 days for oral administration.

Meclofenamate Sodium (**Meclomen**)	3	PO 200–300 mg (4–6 mg/kg) daily in 3 or 4 divided doses	PO 30–60 min	PO 1–2 hr	PO 3–7 hr

Comments: Structurally related to mefenamic acid, but fewer incidences of hematologic abnormalities.

Mefenamic Acid (**Ponstel**)	3	PO 500 mg (10 mg/kg), then 250 mg (5 mg/kg) daily q6 hr	PO 30–60 min	PO 1–2 hr	PO 3–7 hr

Comments: May be associated with hematologic abnormalities (e.g., decreased hematocrit, leukopenia, agranulocytosis, & pancytopenia).

Nabumetone (**Relafen**)	3	PO 1000–2000 mg per day (20–40 mg/kg/day) once daily or in two divided doses	PO 15–30 min	PO 1–2 hr	PO 4–6 hr

Comments: May be administered orally without regard to meals. Better tolerated than indomethacin, naproxen, or ibuprofen, and equipotent doses are associated with less gastric mucosal abnormalities.

Key: *Potency, as compared to aspirin.

Continued.

TABLE 2-2 (cont.).

Name	Potency (ASA*)	Dose	Onset	Peak	Duration
Naproxen (**Naprosyn, Aleve**)	3	PO 500 mg (10 mg/kg), then 250 mg (5 mg/kg) q6–12 hr	PO 30–60 min	PO 1–2 hr	PO 3–7 hr
Comments: Medium-potency NSAID; better GI tolerance than aspirin. Available over the counter in the U.S.					
Piroxicam (**Feldene**)	3	PO 20–40 mg (0.4–0.8 mg/kg) daily, in 1 or 2 divided doses	PO 30–60 min	PO 1–2 hr	PO 48–72 hr
Comments: May be administered once daily. Structurally unrelated to other NSAIDs. Medium potency and long duration of action.					
Salsalate (**Disalcid, Argesic**)	1	PO 2–4 grams (40–80 mg/kg) daily in 2 or 3 divided doses	PO 5–30 min	PO 0.5–2 hr	PO 3–7 hr
Comments: Useful in patients with GI intolerance to aspirin. Does not inhibit platelet aggregation. Increased risk of developing Reye's syndrome if used in children with influenza or chickenpox.					
Sulindac (**Clinoril**)	20	PO 150–200 mg (3–4 mg/kg) b.i.d.	PO 15–30 min	PO 1–2 hr	PO 3–4 hr
Comments: Equipotent to indomethacin but associated with less gastric mucosal abnormalities.					
Tolmetin Sodium (**Tolectin**)	20	PO 400–600 mg (8–12 mg/kg) q8 hr	PO 15–30 min	PO 1–2 hr	PO 3–4 hr
Comments: Equipotent to indomethacin but associated with less gastric mucosal abnormalities.					

Key: *Potency, as compared to aspirin.

TABLE 2-3.
Antidepressant Agents

Name	Dosing: Pain Syndromes & Depression	Onset	Peak	Duration
Amitriptyline HCL (**Elavil**)	**Pain:** Initial PO 10–25 mg (0.2–0.5 mg/kg) daily @ bedtime. Titrate up q3–4 wks by 10–25 mg as necessary. Maintenance: PO 10–150 mg (0.2–3 mg/kg) daily @ bedtime	Analgesic: PO < 5 days		
	Depression: Initial PO 75–100 mg (1.5–2 mg/kg) daily in 1–4 doses	Antidepress: PO 1–2 wks	PO 2–4 wks	PO variable
	Maintenance: PO 25–150 mg (0.5–3.0 mg/kg) daily in 1–4 doses			
	IM 20–30 mg QID, then replace w/oral. Do not use intravenously			

Comments: Classic tricyclic antidepressant. Like other tricyclics produces anticholinergic, antihistaminic, & sedating effects. Potentiates analgesic effects of opioids. May enhance ulcer healing (antihistaminic effect).

| Amoxapine HCL (**Asendin**) | **Pain:** Initial PO 50–150 mg (1–3 mg/kg) daily @ bedtime. Titrate dose up q3–4 wks by 25–50 mg as necessary. Maintenance: PO 50–300 mg (1–6 mg/kg) daily @ bedtime | Analgesic: PO < 5 days | | |

Continued.

TABLE 2-3 (cont.).

Name	Dosing: Pain Syndromes & Depression	Onset	Peak	Duration
	Depression: Initial PO 100–150 mg (2–3 mg/kg) daily in 1–3 doses. Maintenance: PO 100–400 mg (2–8 mg/kg) daily in 1–3 doses. Doses that exceed 300 mg should be administered in 2–3 doses.	Antidepress: PO 4–7 days	PO 2–4 wks	PO variable

Comments: Tricyclic antidepressant. Moderately sedating and has little anticholinergic effect. Rapid onset of activity. May be associated with the development of extrapyramidal symptoms. Toxic levels produce CNS manifestations rather than cardiovascular effects (as compared to other tricyclics).

Name	Dosing: Pain Syndromes & Depression	Onset	Peak	Duration
Desipramine HCL **(Pertofrane)**	**Pain:** Initial PO 50–100 mg (1–2 mg/kg) daily @ bedtime. Titrate dose up q3–4 wks by 25–50 mg as necessary. Maintenance: PO 50–200 mg (1–4 mg/kg) daily @ bedtime	Analgesic: PO < 5 days		
	Depression: Initial PO 75–100 mg daily in 1–4 doses. Maintenance: PO 50–300 mg in 1–4 doses. Doses >200 mg not recommended for outpatients. IM 100 mg daily in divided doses, then replace with oral.	Antidepress: PO 2–5 days	PO 2–3 wks	PO variable

Comments: Tricyclic antidepressant. Low incidence of anticholinergic or antihistaminic effects. It is not sedating for most patients and may even stimulate some. Thus it may be given in the morning.

| Doxepin HCL (Sinequan) | **Pain:** Initial PO 25–50 mg (0.5–1 mg/kg) daily @ bedtime
Titrate dose up q3–4 wks by 25–50 mg as necessary.
Maintenance: PO 25–150 mg (0.5–3 mg/kg) daily @ bedtime | Analgesic:
PO < 5 days | |
| | **Depression:** Initial 30–150 mg daily in 1–3 doses.
Maintenance PO 25–300 mg daily in 1–4 doses.
Doses >150 mg daily are not recommended for outpatients | Antidepress:
PO 1–2 wks | PO 2–4 wks PO variable |

Comments: Tricyclic antidepressant. Compared with amitriptyline, doxepin may have less anticholinergic effects.

| Fluoxetine HCL (Prozac) | **Pain:** Initial 5–20 mg (0.1–0.4 mg/kg) daily in the morning
Titrate dose up q3–4 wks by 5–10 mg as necessary
Maintenance: PO 5–60 mg (0.1–1 mg/kg) daily in the morning | Analgesic:
PO < 5 days | |
| | **Depression:** Initial 5–20 mg daily in 1–2 doses.
Maintenance: PO 5–80 mg daily in 1–2 doses
(morning & noon)
Second dose may be given @ bedtime if sedation occurs.
Doses >20 mg daily may be associated with adverse effects | Antidepress:
PO 1–3 wks | PO 4 wks PO variable |

Comments: Selective serotonin reuptake inhibitor. Antidepressant activity is comparable or superior to tricyclics with fewer adverse effects. May be associated with some anxiety and activation of mania/hypomania. Unlike the tricyclics, sedating, anticholinergic, and cardiovascular effects are minimal.

Continued.

TABLE 2-3 (cont.).

Name	Dosing: Pain Syndromes & Depression	Onset	Peak	Duration
Imipramine HCL (Tofranil)	**Pain:** Initial PO 25–100 mg (0.5–2 mg/kg) daily @ bedtime Titrate dose q3–4 wks by 25–50 mg as necessary. Maintenance: PO 25–200 mg (0.5–4 mg/kg) daily @ bedtime	Analgesic: PO < 5 days		PO variable
	Depression: Initial PO 75–100 mg daily in 1–4 doses. Maintenance: PO 50–300 mg daily in 1–4 doses Doses >200 mg are not recommended for outpatients. IM 100 mg daily in divided doses, then replace with oral.	Antidepress: PO 1–2 wks	PO 2–4 wks	

Comments: Structurally related to the phenothiazine antipsychotic agents. Compared with doxepin or amitriptyline, imipramine produces less sedation or hypotension.

Name	Dosing: Pain Syndromes & Depression	Onset	Peak	Duration
Nortriptyline HCL (Pamelor)	**Pain:** Initial PO 10–50 mg (0.5–1 mg/kg) daily @ bedtime Titrate dose up q3–4 wks by 10–25 mg as necessary. Maintenance: PO 10–150 mg (0.2–3 mg/kg) daily @ bedtime	Analgesic: PO < 5 days		PO variable
	Depression: Initial PO 50–100 mg (1.5–2 mg/kg) daily in 1–4 doses. Maintenance: PO 50–150 mg (1–3 mg/kg) daily in 1–4 doses Monitor serum levels with doses that exceed 100 mg daily	Antidepress: PO 1–2 wks	PO 2–4 wks	

Comments: Compared with the parent drug (amitriptyline), nortriptyline has fewer side effects. The only tricyclic antidepressant with a therapeutic window for serum levels (50–150 ng/mL).

Paroxetine HCL (**Paxil**)	**Pain:** Initial PO 10–20 mg daily preferably in the morning Titrate dose up q weekly by 10 mg as necessary Maintenance: PO 10–50 mg daily in the morning	Analgesic: PO < 5 days
	Depression: Initial PO 20 mg daily preferably 1 dose in AM Titrate dose up by 10 mg/day by weekly intervals as necessary Maintenance: PO 20–50 mg daily in 1 dose in AM	Antidepress: PO 1–2 wks PO 3–4 wks PO variable

Comments: Selective serotonin reuptake inhibitor. Antidepressant activity is comparable to fluoxetine and superior to doxepin or trazadone with fewer adverse effects. Unlike the tricyclics, sedating, anticholinergic, and cardiovascular effects are minimal.

Protriptyline HCL (**Vivactil**)	**Pain:** Initial PO 5 mg (0.1 mg/kg) three times daily Maintenance: PO 5–10 mg (0.1–0.2 mg/kg) t.i.d.	Analgesic: PO < 5 days
	Depression: Initial PO 5 mg (0.1 mg/kg) t.i.d. Maintenance: PO 5–20 mg (0.1–0.4 mg/kg) t.i.d.	Antidepress: PO < 7 days PO 2–4 wks PO variable

Comments: Tricyclic antidepressant. Protriptyline may have a more rapid onset of action than imipramine or amitriptyline. Like other secondary amines (e.g., amoxapine, nortriptyline, and desipramine), it is more effective in patients with low norepinephrine levels compared with serotonin-deficient patients.

Continued.

TABLE 2–3 (cont.).

Name	Dosing: Pain Syndromes & Depression	Onset	Peak	Duration
Sertraline HCL (**Zoloft**)	**Pain:** Initial PO 25–50 mg daily, preferably in the morning or evening Titrate dose q weekly by 50 mg/day as necessary Maintenance: PO 50–200 mg daily in the morning or evening	Analgesic: PO < 5 days		
	Depression: Initial PO 25–50 mg daily, preferably in the morning or evening Titrate dose q weekly by 50 mg/day as necessary Maintenance: PO 50–200 mg daily in the morning or evening	Antidepress: PO 1–2 wks	PO 3–4 wks	PO variable

Comments: Selective serotonin reuptake inhibitor. Differs structurally from other SSRIs or tricyclic antidepressant drugs. Antidepressant activity is comparable to fluoxetine or paroxetine and superior to doxepin or trazodone with fewer adverse effects. Unlike the tricyclics, sedating, anticholinergic, and cardiovascular effects are minimal.

Name	Dosing: Pain Syndromes & Depression	Onset	Peak	Duration
Trimipramine Maleate (**Surmontil**)	**Pain:** Initial PO 25–100 mg (0.5–2 mg/kg) daily @ bedtime Titrate dose up q3–4 wks by 25–50 mg as necessary Maintenance: PO 25–200 mg (0.5–4 mg/kg) daily @ bedtime	Analgesic: PO < 5 days		
	Depression: Initial PO 75–100 mg daily in 1–4 doses. Maintenance: PO 50–300 mg daily in 1–4 doses. Doses >200 mg daily are not recommended for outpatients Do not administer intravenously.	Antidepress: PO 1–2 wks	PO 2–4 wks	PO variable

Comments: Tricyclic antidepressant. Structurally related to imipramine.

Appendix 3

INFUSION TABLES

TABLE 3-1.
Epidural Hydromorphone, 5 mg in
100 mL Local Anesthetic
(50 µg/mL)

mg/hr	mL/hr
0.15	3.0
0.2	4.0
0.25	5.0
0.3	6.0

Data from *The Anesthesia Drugs
Software*. Redondo Beach, CA: State-
of-the-Art Technologies, 1990.

TABLE 3-2.
Epidural Meperidine, 100 mg in
50 mL Local Anesthetic (2 mg/mL)

mg/hr	mL/hr
10	5
12	6
14	7
16	8
18	9
20	10

Data from *The Anesthesia Drugs
Software*. Redondo Beach, CA: State-
of-the-Art Technologies, 1990.

TABLE 3-3.
Epidural Morphine, 10 mg in
100 mL Local Anesthetic
(0.1 mg/mL)

mg/hr	mL/hr
0.1	1.0
0.2	2.0
0.3	3.0
0.4	4.0
0.5	5.0
0.6	6.0
0.7	7.0
0.8	8.0
0.9	9.0
1.0	10.0

Data from *The Anesthesia Drugs Software*. Redondo Beach, CA: State-of-the-Art Technologies, 1990.

TABLE 3-4.
Epidural Sufentanil, 100 μg in
100 mL (1 μg/mL)

μg/hr	mL/hr
5	5
10	10
15	15
20	20
25	25
30	30

Data from *The Anesthesia Drugs Software*. Redondo Beach, CA: State-of-the-Art Technologies, 1990.

TABLE 3–5.
Epidural Fentanyl, 500 µg in
100 mL Local Anesthetic (5 µg/mL)

µg/hr	mL/hr
20	4
25	5
30	6
35	7
40	8
45	9
50	10
55	11
60	12

Data from *The Anesthesia Drugs
Software*. Redondo Beach, CA: State-
of-the-Art Technologies, 1990.

Appendix 4

RELATIVE POTENCIES OF OPIOIDS

TABLE 4–1.
Equianalgesic Dose (in mg)

	IM	PO	Rectal
Codeine phosphate	130	200	
Diacetylmorphine HCL (heroin)	5	60	
Fentanyl citrate	0.1	—	
Hydromorphone HCL	1.5	7.5	
Levopharnol tartrate	2	4	
Meperidine HCL	75	300	
Methadone HCL	10	20	
Morphine sulfate	10	60	
Oxycodone HCL	15	30	
Oxymorphone HCL	1	6	10
Propoxyphene HCL	—	130	
Sufentanil HCL	0.02	—	
Tramadol HCL	—	150	

TABLE 4–2.
Equianalgesic Dose (Morphine/Transdermal Fentanyl)

PO Morphine sulfate (mg/day)	IM Morphine sulfate (mg/day)	Transdermal Fentanyl (μg/hr)
45–134	8–22	25
135–224	23–37	50
225–314	38–52	75
315–404	53–67	100
405–494	68–82	125
495–584	83–97	150
585–674	98–112	175
675–764	113–127	200
765–854	128–142	225
855–944	143–157	250
945–1034	158–172	275
1035–1124	173–187	300

The Federal Clinical Practice Guideline on the Management of Cancer Pain advocates regularly scheduled administration of opioid analgesics. Such administration results in a 3 : 1 oral to parenteral dose ratio. Thus the equianalgesic doses of fentanyl may be two times that stated above (obtained from the Duragesic™ package labeling).

Appendix 5

PREVENTION AND MANAGEMENT OF OPIOID SIDE EFFECTS

Unmanageable side effects are the major reason why patients stop taking opioids, often without their physician's knowledge. Patient compliance is thus dependent on the physician's ability to prevent these side effects and to treat them when they occur.

Constipation

Long-term opioid administration will inevitably lead to constipation.

Prevention: Increase regular exercise and oral fluids and administer stool softeners daily, for example, Colace (docusate sodium) 100 mg twice daily or a bowel stimulant/stool softener such as Senokot-S (senna concentrate plus docusate sodium) at bedtime (two tablets). Do not administer bulk-forming agents that contain methylcellulose, polycarbophil, or psyllium (e.g., Metamucil). Temporary arrest in the passage through the gastrointestinal tract may lead to fecal impaction or bowel obstruction.

Use adjuvant drugs (e.g., antidepressants, dextromethorphan) to increase the effectiveness of lower opioid doses.

Treatment

> No bowel movement in any 24-hour period: Senokot-S, two to four tablets once, twice, or three times daily.
>
> No bowel movement in any 48-hour period: Add Dulcolax (bisacodyl), two to three tablets at bedtime or two to three times daily.
>
> No bowel movement in any 72-hour period: Increase the daily dose of Senokot-S and Dulcolax.
>
> If nonimpacted, add one of the following:
>> Haley's MO (milk of magnesia and mineral oil) PO 45–60 mL.
>>
>> Duphalac (lactulose) PO 45–60 mL.
>>
>> Fleet Phospho-Soda (sodium phosphates) PO 20–45 mL.
>>
>> Fleet Bisacodyl Laxative Tablets, two or three tablets once daily.
>>
>> Dulcolax suppository, one per rectum.
>>
>> Fleet Bisacodyl Enema, one per rectum.
>
> If impacted, disimpact and continue enemas until clear.

Nausea

Prevention: Relieve constipation.
Treatment

> Metoclopramide (Reglan) PO 10 mg every 8 hours and at bedtime as needed.
>
> Cisapride (Propulsid) PO 10 mg every 8 hours and at bedtime as needed.
>
> Prochlorperazine (Compazine) PO 5 mg every 4 hours as needed.

Sedation

Sedation and/or confusion may occur during the first 24 to 48 hours after the initiation of opioid therapy or after a significant dose increase. Patients will usually develop a tolerance within 2 to 3 days after a stable dose has been established.

Prevention: Use adjuvant drugs (e.g., antidepressants, dextromethorphan) to increase the effectiveness of lower opioid doses. Utilize regional opioids and/or anesthetics (e.g., epidural analgesia).

Treatment

> For persistent sedation, CNS stimulants may be administered to increase alertness:
>
> Caffeine 100–200 mg every 4 hours.
>
> Methylphenidate (Ritalin) PO 5–10 mg with breakfast (may repeat the dosage with lunch).
>
> Dextroamphetamine (Dexedrine) PO 2.5–7.5 mg twice daily.
>
> Pemoline (Cylert) PO 18.75–37.5 mg twice daily.
>
> Opioid antagonists may be administered to reverse the sedative (and analgesic) effects, as follows:
>
> Naltrexone (ReVia) PO 12.5–50.0 mg daily as necessary.
>
> Naloxone SC/IM/IV 0.1–0.8 mg or IV infusion 1–5 µg/kg/hr. (Dilute 0.4–0.8 mg naloxone in 1000 mL IV fluid.)
>
> For persistent confusion: Haloperidol (Haldol) PO 0.5–1.0 mg twice or three times daily.

Respiratory Depression

Pain is a powerful stimulant, and respiratory depression rarely occurs in chronic pain patients when there has been careful titration of the opioid dose. With repeated doses, tolerance develops to this effect. Respiratory depression is more likely to occur in elderly, debilitated patients and in those with decreased pulmonary reserve (e.g., patients with chronic obstructive pulmonary disease or cor pulmonale).

Prevention: Use adjuvant drugs (e.g., antidepressants, dextromethorphan) to increase the effectiveness of lower opioid doses.

Treatment

> Naltrexone (ReVia) PO 12.5–50.0 mg daily as necessary.
>
> Naloxone SC/IM/IV 0.1–2.0 mg. IV infusion, 5–15 µg/kg/hr. (Dilute 1 mg naloxone in 100 mL IV fluid.)

Pruritus

This is often transient in nature and may be managed with antihistamine medications as needed.

Prevention/Treatment

> Diphenhydramine (Benadryl) PO/IM/IV 12.5–25.0 mg every 6 hours as needed.
>
> Promethazine PO/IM/IV 12.5–25.0 mg every 6 hours as needed.
>
> Naltrexone (ReVia) PO 12.5–50.0 mg daily as necessary.
>
> Naloxone SC/IM/IV 0.1–0.8 mg. IV infusion, 1–5 µg/kg/hr. (Dilute 0.4–0.8 mg naloxone in 1000 mL IV fluid.)

Urinary Retention

This may occur with high parenteral opioid doses and in men with prostatism or in patients with pelvic tumors and bladder outlet obstruction.

Treatment

>Discontinue adjuvant drugs with anticholinergic effects (which may potentiate urinary retention), for example, tricyclic antidepressants.
>
>Change to another opioid or route of administration.
>
>Bethanechol (Urecholine) PO 15–30 mg or SC 5 mg.
>
>Naltrexone (ReVia) PO 12.5–50.0 mg daily as necessary.
>
>Naloxone SC/IM/IV 0.1–0.8 mg. IV infusion: 1–5 μg/kg/hr. (Dilute 0.4–0.8 mg naloxone in 1000 mL IV fluid.)
>
>Straight bladder catheterization as needed.

Appendix 6

RELATIVE POTENCIES OF STEROIDS

TABLE 6–1.
Glucocorticold Equivalencies and Potencies

Glucocorticoid	Equivalent Dose (mg)	Anti-inflammatory (Glucocorticold) Potency	Mineralocorticoid Potency
Short Acting			
Cortisone	25	0.8	2
Hydrocortisone	20	1	2
Intermediate Acting			
Methylprednisolone	4	5	0
Prednisolone	5	4	1
Prednisone	5	4	1
Triamcinolone	4	5	0
Long Acting			
Betamethasone	0.6-0.75	20-30	0
Dexamethasone	0.75	20-30	0

Appendix 7

INTRAVENOUS PCA STANDARD ORDERS — MODE (CHOOSE ONE): ☐ PCA ONLY ☐ PCA + CONTINUOUS INFUSION ☐ CONTINUOUS INFUSION ONLY

	☐ MORPHINE 1 mg/ml (Pediatric Dose By Weight)	☐ MEPERIDINE 10 mg/ml (Peds Dose By Weight) PCA MODE ONLY for Peds Pts	☐ OTHER ___ mg or mcg/ml (Pediatric Dose By Weight)
DRUG Select Only One			
	PCA MODE		
LOADING DOSE	___ mg (N.R. 1-3 mg or 0.02 - 0.06 mg/kg)	___ mg (N.R. 10 - 30 mg or 0.2 - 0.6 mg/kg)	___ mg or mcg
PCA DOSE	___ mg (N.R. 0.5 - 3 mg or 0.01 - 0.06 mg/kg)	___ mg (N.R. 5 - 30 mg or 0.1 - 0.6 mg/kg)	___ mg or mcg
LOCKOUT TIME	___ min. (N.R. 5 - 15 minutes)	___ min. (N.R. 5 - 15 minutes)	___ minutes
4 HOUR LIMIT (OPTIONAL)	___ mg (N.R. 20 - 30 mg or 0.4 - 0.6 mg/kg)	___ mg (N.R. 200 - 300 mg or 4 - 6 mg/kg)	
	INFUSION MODE (OPTIONAL)		
INFUSION RATE	___ mg/hr (N.R. 0.5 - 2 mg/hr or 0.01 - 0.04 mg/kg/hr)	___ mg/hr (N.R. 5 - 10 mg/hr or 0.1 - 0.2 mg/kg/hr)	___ mg or mcg/hr
INFUSION INSTRUCTIONS (SELECT ONLY ONE)	☐ Continuous Infusion ☐ Infuse from 2200 - 0600 hours	☐ Continuous Infusion ☐ Infuse from 2200 - 0600 hours	☐ Continuous Infusion ☐ Infuse from 2200 - 0600 hours
	INADEQUATE PAIN RELIEF		
FIRST OCCURRENCE (SELECT ONLY ONE)	☐ Call Acute Pain Service ☐ Repeat loading dose — May increase by 0.5 - 1 mg or 0.01 - 0.02 mg/kg	☐ Call Acute Pain Service ☐ Repeat loading dose — May increase by 5 - 10 mg or 0.1 - 0.2 mg/kg	☐ Call Acute Pain Service ☐ Repeat loading dose — May increase within the normal range
1 HOUR AFTER THE FIRST OCCURRENCE (SELECT ONLY ONE)	☐ Call Acute Pain Service ☐ Repeat previous loading dose and increase PCA dose By 0.5 - 1 mg or 0.01 - 0.02 mg/kg	☐ Call Acute Pain Service ☐ Repeat previous loading dose and increase PCA dose By 5 - 10 mg or 0.1 - 0.2 mg/kg	☐ Call Acute Pain Service ☐ Repeat previous loading dose and increase PCA dose By ___ mg or mcg
2 HOURS AFTER THE FIRST OCCURRENCE (SELECT ONLY ONE)	☐ Call Acute Pain Service ☐ Decrease lockout time by 1–5 min. Minimum lockout time is 5 minutes	☐ Call Acute Pain Service ☐ Decrease lockout time by 1–5 min. Minimum lockout time is 5 minutes	☐ Call Acute Pain Service ☐ Decrease lockout time by ___ min. Minimum lockout time is 5 minutes
STILL INADEQUATE PAIN RELIEF	Call Acute Pain Service	Call Acute Pain Service	Call Acute Pain Service

STANDARD ORDERS

1. Discontinue all systemic narcotics and other CNS depressants except as ordered by the Acute Pain Service.

2. Vital Signs (blood pressure, pulse and respiration) should be obtained prior to PCA therapy.

3. Monitoring - Respiratory rate, analgesia level, sedation scale and BP should be assessed every 2 hrs for 8 hrs, then every 4 hrs and whenever the loading dose is repeated.

4. NOTE: The oncoming RN is to perform the first evaluation within the first hour of the beginning of the shift.

5. For ALL complications with pediatric patients, notify pediatric physician and Acute Pain Service immediately.

6A. Sedation Scale = 2, RR <8 per min (<14 per min pediatric) or PCO2 >50 mm Hg

Call Acute Pain Service and primary physician

6B. Sedation scale = 3, RR <8 per min (<14 per min pediatric)

Naloxone 0.1 - 0.4 mg IV stat (0.02 - 0.08 mg/kg) and call Acute Pain Service and primary physician

6C. Nausea or Vomiting

Metoclopramide 10 mg IV q 6 hrs pm (not recommended for children) or Promethazine 12.5-25 mg IV/M/Rectal q 6 hrs pm (0.25 - 0.5 mg/kg)

6D. Severe Itching

Diphenhydramine 12.5 - 25 mg IV/M q 6 hrs pm (0.25 - 0.5 mg/kg) or Naloxone 0.1 - 0.4 mg IV stat (0.02 - 0.08 mg/kg)

NOTE: N.R. = Normal Range

TIME	DATE	PHYSICIAN'S SIGNATURE
		X

MARTIN LUTHER KING, JR./DREW MEDICAL CENTER
County of Los Angeles • Department of Health Services
Department of Anesthesiology Acute Pain Service

DISTRIBUTION
GREEN ..... Patient Chart
CANARY ... Acute Pain Serv
WHITE ...... Pharmacy

IMPRINT PATIENT'S I.D.

NAME

MLK NO

D O B

INTRAVENOUS P.C.A. STANDARD ORDERS   MLK-1913   76449S

Appendix 8

MARTIN LUTHER KING, JR/DREW MEDICAL CENTER
DEPARTMENT OF ANESTHESIOLOGY
ACUTE PAIN SERVICE

DEPARTMENT OF HEALTH SERVICES

DATE	TIME	INITIALS	RESP. RATE	SEDATION	ANALGESIA	B.P.	LOCKOUT TIME	4 HR. LIMIT	LOADING DOSE	PCA DOSE	PCA INJECTED	PCA PARTIAL	PCA DEMANDS

Comments

TOTAL DOSAGE GIVEN DURING SHIFT

DATE	TIME	INITIALS	RESP. RATE	SEDATION	ANALGESIA	B.P.	LOCKOUT TIME	4 HR. LIMIT	LOADING DOSE	PCA DOSE	PCA INJECTED	PCA PARTIAL	PCA DEMANDS

Comments

TOTAL DOSAGE GIVEN DURING SHIFT

DATE	TIME	INITIALS	RESP. RATE	SEDATION	ANALGESIA	B.P.	LOCKOUT TIME	4 HR. LIMIT	LOADING DOSE	PCA DOSE	PCA INJECTED	PCA PARTIAL	PCA DEMANDS

Comments

TOTAL DOSAGE GIVEN DURING SHIFT

SIGNATURES - SHIFT 1	SIGNATURES - SHIFT 2	SIGNATURES - SHIFT 3	SIGNATURES - SHIFT 4
✗	✗	✗	✗
✗	✗	✗	✗

ANALGESIA SCALE
Adults (0-10)
0 = No pain
10 = Worst pain

CHILDREN
(Checkers are little pieces of hurt)
0 = No hurt
5 = The most hurt you can have

SEDATION SCALE
0. **None** Awake, alert & oriented
1. **Mild** Drowsy, arousable with verbal stimuli
2. **Moderate** Lethargic, arousable with physical stimuli, disoriented
3. **Severe** Somnolent, difficult to arouse
S. **Sleep** Normal sleep, easy to arouse

IMPRINT PATIENT S I D

NAME

MLK NO

D O B

DISTRIBUTION
WHITE ... Pt. Chart
CANARY ... A.P.S.

PATIENT CONTROLLED ANALGESIA FLOWSHEET
MLK-1914   76A499T

Appendix 9

PROLOTHERAPY

Prolotherapy is defined as the treatment of injured ligaments and tendons by injection of an irritant solution, resulting in fibroblastic stimulation, hyperplasia of the connective tissue, and healing.

Dextrose Proliferant Solution

Use a 15% dextrose and 0.2% lidicaine solution constituted as follows:

Lidocaine 1%	2 mL
Sterile water for injection	5 mL
Dextrose 50%	3 mL
	10 mL

or

Lidocaine 2%	1 mL
Sterile water for injection	6 mL
Dextrose 50%	3 mL
	10 mL

For intra-articular injections, use 25% dextrose (obtained by diluting 50% dextrose equally with local anesthetic solution and sterile water for injection).

References

1. Hackett GS, Hemwall GA, Montgomery GA. Ligament and tendon relaxation treated by prolotherapy. Oakbrook: Thomas & Hemwall, 1991.
2. Dorman AT, et al. Prolotherapy in the lumbar spine and pelvis. Spine: state of the art reviews. vol. 9. Philadelphia: Hanley and Belfus, 1995.

Appendix 10

Martin Luther King, Jr/Drew Medical Center
Department of Anesthesiology
Acute Pain Service

Epidural Analgesia Monitoring Orders

Epidural Bolus

Drug _____ Mg/Mcg in _____ mls _____
Time Given _____

(check applicable two boxes or fill in blank spaces above)

☐ Fentanyl 50-100 mcg in 15-20 mls   ☐ Presv. Free NS or   ☐ 0.1% Bupivacaine
☐ Hydromorphone 1-2 mg in 10 mls   ☐ Presv. Free NS or   ☐ 0.1% Bupivacaine
☐ Meperidine 50-100 mg in 15-20 mls   ☐ Presv. Free NS or   ☐ 0.1% Bupivacaine
☐ Morphine 3-5 mg in 10 mls   ☐ Presv. Free NS or   ☐ 0.1% Bupivacaine
☐ Sufentanil 10-30 mcg in 15-20 mls   ☐ Presv. Free NS or   ☐ 0.1% Bupivacaine

Epidural Infusion

Drug _____ Mg/Mcg in _____ mls _____
Run at _____ Mg/Mcg/Hour _____ Mls/Hour
Start Time _____

(check applicable two boxes or fill in blank spaces above)

☐ Fentanyl 200 mcg   ☐ Presv. Free NS or   ☐ 0.1% Bupivacaine (2 mcg/ml). Run
  in 100 mls   at 25-60 mcg/hr or 10-30 mls/hr
☐ Hydromorphone 5 mg   ☐ Presv. Free NS or   ☐ 0.1% Bupivacaine 50 (mcg/ml). Run
  in 100 mls   at 0.15-0.3 mg/hr or 3-6 mls/hr
☐ Meperidine 200 mg   ☐ Presv. Free NS or   ☐ 0.1% Bupivacaine (2 mg/ml). Run at
  in 100 mls   10-20 mg/hr or 3-6 mls/hr
☐ Morphine 10 mg   ☐ Presv. Free NS or   ☐ 0.1% Bupivacaine (0.1 mg/ml). Run
  in 100 mls   at 0.1-1 mg/hr or 1-10 mls/hr
☐ Sufentanil 100 mcg   ☐ Presv. Free NS or   ☐ 0.1% Bupivacaine (1 mcg/ml). Run
  in 100 mls   at 5-30 mg/hr or 5-20 mls/hr

Standard Orders

---

1. No Systemic narcotics or other CNS depressants to be given except as ordered by the Acute Pain Service
2. Maintain IV access for 24 hours after last dose of the epidural drug
3. Monitoring. Vital signs (BP, P, R) should be obtained on admission. Respiratory rate and sedation scale should be assessed hourly for 12 hours then q 4 hrs until discharge from the Acute Pain Service. Analgesia level and BP should be assessed q 2 hrs for 8 hrs then q 4 hrs until discharge from the Acute Pain Service.

   NOTE: the oncoming RN is to perform the first evaluation within the first hour of the beginning of the shift.

4. Record all parameters on the first seven columns of the PCA Flow Sheet.
5. Naloxone (Narcan) 0.4 mg with syringe taped to the head of the bed.
6. A. For sedation scale = 2, RR<8 per minute, or pCO2>50 mmHg, call APS
   B. For sedation scale = 3 or 4 plus RR<8/minute, administer Naloxone 0.1-0.4 mg IV stat (0.02-0.08 mg/kg), and call APS and the primary physician. While waiting, administer supplemental oxygen (Nasal cannula or Face Mask at 2-4 litres/min)
   C. For nausea or vomiting, administer
      Metoclopramide 10 mg IV q 6 hrs prn (not recommended for children) or Promethazine IV/IM 12.5-25 mg IV (0.25-0.5 mg/kg) q 6 hrs prn or Naloxone 0.1-0.4 mg IV stat (0.02-0.08 mg/kg) or Naloxone infusion 5-15 mcg/kg/hr
   D. For severe itching, administer
      Diphenhydramine 12.5-25 mg IV/IM q 6 hrs prn (0.25-0.5 mg/kg) or Naloxone 0.1-0.4 mg IV stat (0.02-0.08 mg/kg) or Naloxone infusion 5-15 mcg/kg/hr
   E. For urinary retention, administer
      Naloxone 0.4-0.8 mg IV titrated (0.08-0.16 mg/kg) or Naloxone infusion 5-15 mcg/kg/hr or Bethanechol (urecholine) 15-30 mg PO or 5 mg SC or 'In and out' bladder catheterization p.r.n.
7. **For inadequate analgesia, or other complications related to the Epidural Narcotic, call the Acute Pain Service.**
8. **For Respiratory/CNS depression, notify primary physician and Acute Pain Service immediately.**

OPTIONAL ORDERS (PHYSICIAN MUST CHECK OFF BOXES)

---

1. Opioid Side Effects

Prophylaxis
☐ Naloxone IV infusion
   (Add 0.4 mg in 1000 mls of the patient's maintenance IV if the IV
   maintenance rate is less than 100 mls/minute)

Treatment
☐ Naloxone IV 0.2-0.8 mg and/or
☐ Naloxone IV infusion at 5 mcg/kg/hr
   (Add 4 mg naloxone in 50 mls D5W or NS and run at 5-10 mls/hr
   in adult patients.)

2. Supplemental Oxygen:
   ☐ Nasal Cannula   _____ litres/min
   ☐ Face Mask   _____ litres/min
   ☐ Other   _____ litres/min

        Signature _____

        Date _____

Appendix 11

CONTROLLED DRUG SCHEDULES

Schedule I

Schedule II
Codeine
Fentanyl
Hydrocodone
Hydromorphone
Levorphanol
Meperidine
Methadone
Morphine
Oxycodone
Oxymorphone
Remifentanil
Sufentanil

Schedule III
Hydrocodone
Morphine (when available as a fixed-combination preparation in a concentration
of 0.5 mg or less per milliliter or per gram with a therapeutic amount of one or
more nonopiate drugs)

Schedule IV
Propoxyphene
Nasal butorphanol

Schedule V
Buprenorphine

No Schedule
Nalbuphine
Butorphanol

Appendix 12

PAIN RATING SCALES

TABLE 12–1 Pain intensity scales

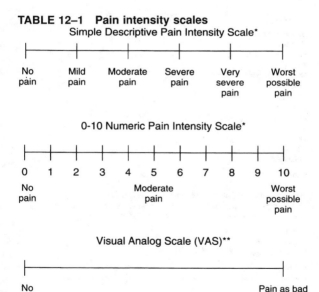

Simple Descriptive Pain Intensity Scale*

No pain	Mild pain	Moderate pain	Severe pain	Very severe pain	Worst possible pain

0-10 Numeric Pain Intensity Scale*

0	1	2	3	4	5	6	7	8	9	10
No pain					Moderate pain					Worst possible pain

Visual Analog Scale (VAS)**

No pain — Pain as bad as it could possibly be

* If used as a graphic rating scale, a 10-cm baseline is recommended.
** A 10-cm baseline is recommended for VAS scales.

TABLE 12–2 Pain distress scales

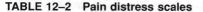

Simple Descriptive Pain Distress Scale*

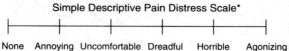

None Annoying Uncomfortable Dreadful Horrible Agonizing

0-10 Numeric Pain Distress Scale*

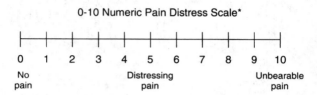

0   1   2   3   4   5   6   7   8   9   10

No
pain

Distressing
pain

Unbearable
pain

Visual Analog Scale (VAS)**

No
distress

Unbearable
distress

* If used as a graphic rating scale, a 10-cm baseline is recommended.
** A 10-cm baseline is recommended for VAS scales.

TABLE 12–3   Initial pain assessment tool

Date _____

Patient's Name _____ Age ____ Room ____
Diagnosis _____ Physician _____
Nurse _____

I. Location: Patient or nurse mark drawing.

II. Intensity: Patient rates the pain. Scale used _____
　　　Present: _____
　　　Worst pain gets: _____
　　　Best pain gets: _____
　　Acceptable level of pain: _____
III. Quality: (Use patient's own words, e.g. prick, ache, burn, throb, pull, sharp)_____

IV. Onset, duration variations, rhythms: _____

V. Manner of expressing pain: _____

VI. What relieves the pain? _____

VII. What causes or increases the pain? _____

VIII. Effects of pain: (Note decreased function, decreased quality of life.)
　　　Accompanying symptoms (e.g. nausea) _____
　　　Sleep _____
　　　Appetite _____
　　　Physical activity _____
　　　Relationship with others (e.g. irritability) _____
　　　Emotions (e.g. anger, suicidal, crying) _____
　　　Concentration _____
　　　Other _____
IX. Other comments: _____

X. Plan: _____

May be duplicated for use in clinical practice. Used with permission from McCaffery, M. and Beeebe A. *Pain: Clinical Manual for Nursing Practice.* (1989), St. Louis: C.V. Mosby.

TABLE 12–4 Flow sheet—pain

Patient _____ Date _____

* Pain rating scale used _____

Purpose: to evaluate the safety and effectiveness of the analgesic(s).

Analgesic(s) prescribed: _____

Time	Pain rating	Analgesic	R	P	BP	Level of arousal	Other†	Plan & comments

* *Pain rating:* A number of different scales may be used. Indicate which scale is used and use the same one each time. For example, 0-10 (0 = no pain, 10 = worst pain).

† *Possibilities for other columns:* bowel function, activities, nausea and vomiting, other pain relief measures. Identify the side effects of greatest concern to patient, family, physician, and nurses.

May be duplicated for use in clinical practice. Used with permission from McCaffery, M. and Beeebe, A. *Pain: Clinical Manual for Nursing Practice.* (1989), St. Louis: C.V. Mosby.

Appendix 13

CPR ALGORITHMS

13-1 Universal Algorithm for Adult*
Emergency Cardiac Care

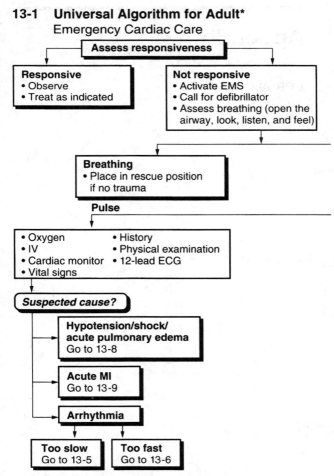

*From Guidelines for Cardiopulmonary Resuscitation and Emergency Cardiac Care, Committee of the American Heart Association, *JAMA* 1992: 268: 2171-2302.

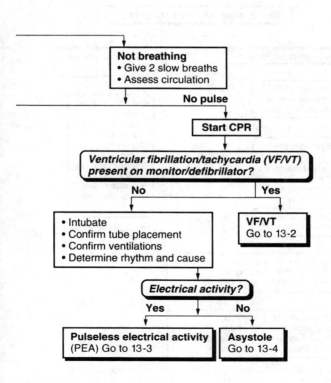

Not breathing
- Give 2 slow breaths
- Assess circulation

No pulse

Start CPR

Ventricular fibrillation/tachycardia (VF/VT) present on monitor/defibrillator?

No **Yes**

- Intubate
- Confirm tube placement
- Confirm ventilations
- Determine rhythm and cause

VF/VT
Go to 13-2

Electrical activity?

Yes **No**

Pulseless electrical activity
(PEA) Go to 13-3

Asystole
Go to 13-4

13-2 Ventricular Fibrillation/Pulseless Ventricular Tachycardia Algorithm (VF/VT)*

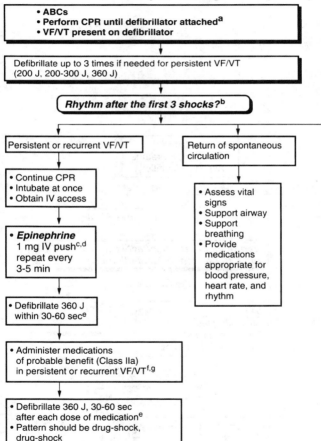

*From Guidelines for Cardiopulmonary Resuscitation and Emergency Cardiac Care, Committee of the American Heart Association. *JAMA* 1992: 268: 2171-2302.

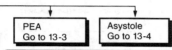

PEA
Go to 13-3

Asystole
Go to 13-4

Class I: definitely helpful
Class IIa: acceptable, probably helpful
Class IIb: acceptable, possibly helpful
Class III: not indicated, may be harmful

(a) Precordial thump is a Class IIb action in witnessed arrest, no pulse, and no defibrillator immediately available.
(b) Hypothermic cardiac arrest is treated differently after this point. *See section on hypothermia.*
(c) The recommended dose of *epinephrine* is 1 mg IV push every 3-5 min.
If this approach fails, several Class IIb dosing regimens can be considered:
 • Intermediate: *epinephrine* 2-5 mg IV push, every 3-5 min
 • Escalating: *epinephrine* 1 mg-3 mg-5 mg IV push, 3 min apart
 • High: *epinephrine* 0.1 mg/kg IV push, every 3-5 min
(d) *Sodium bicarbonate* (1 mEq/kg) is Class I if patient has known preexisting hyperkalemia.
(e) Multiple sequenced shocks (200, 200-300 J, 360 J) are acceptable here (Class I), especially when medications are delayed.
(f) Medications:
 • *Lidocaine* 1.5 mg/kg IV push. Repeat in 3-5 min to total loading dose of 3 mg/kg; then use
 • *Bretylium* 5 mg/kg IV push. Repeat in 5 min at 10 mg/kg
 • *Magnesium sulfate* 1-2 g IV in torsades de pointes or suspected hypomagnesemic state or severe refractory VF
 • *Procainamide* 30 mg/min in refractory VF (maximum total 17 mg/kg)
(g) *Sodium bicarbonate* (1 mEq/kg IV):
 Class IIa
 • If known preexisting bicarbonate-responsive acidosis
 • If overdose with tricyclic antidepressants
 • To alkalinize the urine in drug overdoses
 Class IIb
 • If intubated and continued long arrest interval
 • Upon return of spontaneous circulation after long arrest interval
 Class III
 • Hypoxic lactic acidosis

13-3   Pulseless Electrical Activity (PEA) Algorithm*
(Electromechanical Dissociation [EMD])

Includes:
- Electromechanical dissociation (EMD)
- Pseudo-EMD
- Idioventricular rhythms
- Ventricular escape rhythms
- Bradyasystolic rhythms
- Postdefibrillation idioventricular rhythms

- Continue CPR
- Intubate at once
- Obtain IV access
- Assess blood flow using Doppler ultrasound

↓

Consider possible causes
(parentheses = possible therapies and treatments)

- Hypovolemia (volume infusion)
- Hypoxia (ventilation)
- Cardiac tamponade (pericardiocentesis)
- Tension pneumothorax (needle decompression)
- Hypothermia (see hypothermia algorithm)

- Massive pulmonary embolism (surgery, ***thrombolytics***)
- Drug overdoses such as tricyclics, digitalis, beta-blockers, calcium channel blockers
- Hyperkalemia[a]
- Acidosis[b]
- Massive acute myocardial infarction (go to 13-9)

↓

- ***Epinephrine*** 1 mg IV push[a,c] repeat every 3-5 min

↓

- If absolute bradycardia (<60 beats/min) or relative bradycardia, give ***atropine*** 1 mg IV
- Repeat every 3-5 min to a total of 0.04 mg/kg[d]

---

*From Guidelines for Cardiopulmonary Resuscitation and Emergency Cardiac Care, Committee of the American Heart Association. *JAMA* 1992: 268: 2171-2302.

Class I: definitely helpful
Class IIa: acceptable, probably helpful
Class IIb: acceptable, possibly helpful
Class III: not indicated, may be harmful

(a) *Sodium bicarbonate* 1 mEq/kg is
    Class I if patient has known
    preexisting hyperkalemia.
(b) *Sodium bicarbonate* (1 mEq/kg):
    Class IIa
    • If known preexisting
      bicarbonate-responsive acidosis
    • If overdose with tricyclic
      antidepressants
    • To alkalinize the urine in drug
      overdoses
    Class IIb
    • If intubated and long arrest interval
    • Upon return of spontaneous
      circulation after long arrest interval
    Class III
    • Hypoxic lactic acidosis
(c) The recommended dose of
    epinephrine is 1 mg IV push every
    3-5 min. If this approach fails,
    several Class IIb dosing regimens
    can be considered:
    • Intermediate: *epinephrine* 2-5 mg
      IV push, every 3-5 min
    • Escalating: *epinephrine* 1 mg-
      3 mg-5 mg IV push, 3 min apart
    • High: *epinephrine* 0.1 mg/kg
      IV push, every 3-5 min
(d) Shorter *atropine* dosing intervals
    are possibly helpful in cardiac
    arrest (Class IIb).

13-4 Asystole Treatment Algorithm*

- **Continue CPR**
- **Intubate at once**
- **Obtain IV access**
- **Confirm asystole in more than one lead**

↓

Consider possible causes
- Hypoxia
- Hyperkalemia
- Hypokalemia
- Preexisting acidosis
- Drug overdose
- Hypothermia

↓

Consider immediate transcutaneous pacing (TCP)[a]

↓

- ***Epinephrine*** 1 mg IV push[b,c]
  repeat every 3-5 min.

↓

- ***Atropine*** 1 mg IV
  repeat every 3-5 min up to a total of 0.04 mg/kg[d,e]

↓

Consider termination of efforts[f]

Class I: definitely helpful
Class IIa: acceptable, probably helpful
Class IIb: acceptable, possibly helpful
Class III: not indicated, may be hamful

(a) TCP is a Class IIb intervention. Lack of success may be due to delays in pacing. To be effective TCP must be performed early, simultaneously with drugs. Evidence does not support routine use of TCP for asystole.
(b) The recommended dose of ***epinephrine*** is 1 mg IV push every 3-5 min. If this approach fails, several Class IIb dosing regimens can be considered:
- Intermediate: ***epinephrine*** 2-5 mg IV push, every 3-5min
- Escalating: ***epinephrine*** 1 mg-3 mg -5 mg IV push, 3 min apart
- High: ***epinephrine*** 0.1 mg/kg IV push every 3-5 min
(c) ***Sodium bicarbonate*** 1 mEq/kg is Class I if patient has known preexisting hyperkalemia.
(d) Shorter ***atropine*** dosing intervals are Class IIb in asystolic arrest.
(e) ***Sodium bicarbonate*** 1 mEq/kg:
Class IIa
- if known preexisting bicarbonate-responsive acidosis
- if overdose with tricyclic anti-depressants
- to alkalinize the urine in drug overdoses
Class IIb
- if intubated and continued long arrest interval
- upon return of spontaneous circulation after long arrest interval
Class III
- hypoxic lactic acidosis
(f) If patient remains in asystole or other agonal rhythms after successful intubation and initial medications and no reversible causes are identified, consider termination of resuscitative efforts by a physician. Consider interval since arrest.

---

*From Guidelines for Cardiopulmonary Resuscitation and Emergency Cardiac Care, Committee of the American Heart Association. *JAMA* 1992: 268: 2171-2302.

13-5 Bradycardia Algorithm*
(Patient is not in cardiac arrest)

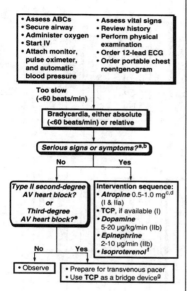

- Assess ABCs
- Secure airway
- Administer oxygen
- Start IV
- Attach monitor, pulse oximeter, and automatic blood pressure
- Assess vital signs
- Review history
- Perform physical examination
- Order 12-lead ECG
- Order portable chest roentgenogram

Too slow
(<60 beats/min)

Bradycardia, either absolute (<60 beats/min) or relative

Serious signs or symptoms?[a,b]

No / Yes

Type II second-degree AV heart block?
or
Third-degree AV heart block?[e]

Intervention sequence:
- *Atropine* 0.5-1.0 mg[c,d] (I & IIa)
- TCP, if available (I)
- *Dopamine* 5-20 µg/kg/min (IIb)
- *Epinephrine* 2-10 µg/min (IIb)
- *Isoproterenol*[f]

No / Yes

- Observe

- Prepare for transvenous pacer
- Use **TCP** as a bridge device[g]

(a) Serious signs or symptoms must be related to the slow rate. Clinical manifestations include:
  - symptoms (chest pain, shortness of breath, decreased level of consciousness)
  - signs (low BP, shock, pulmonary congestion, CHF, acute MI).
(b) Do not delay TCP while awaiting IV access or for *atropine* to take effect if patient is symptomatic.
(c) Denervated transplanted hearts will not respond to *atropine*. Go at once to pacing, *cactecholamine* infusion, or both.
(d) *Atropine* should be given in repeat doses in 3-5 min up to total of 0.04 mg/kg. Consider shorter dosing intervals in severe clinical conditions. It has been suggested that *atropine* should be used with caution in atrioventricular (AV) block at the His-Purkinje level (type II AV block and new third-degree block with wide QRS complexes) (Class IIb).
(e) Never treat third-degree heart block plus ventricular escape beats with *lidocaine*.
(f) *Isoproterenol* should be used, if at all, with extreme caution. At low doses it is Class IIb (possibly helpful); at higher doses it is Class III (harmful).
(g) Verify patient tolerance and mechanical capture. Use analgesia and sedation as needed.

*From Guidelines for Cardiopulmonary Resuscitation and Emergency Cardiac Care, Committee of the American Heart Association. *JAMA* 1992: 268: 2171-2302.

13-6 Tachycardia Algorithm*

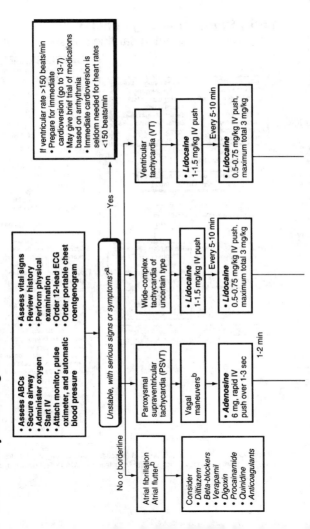

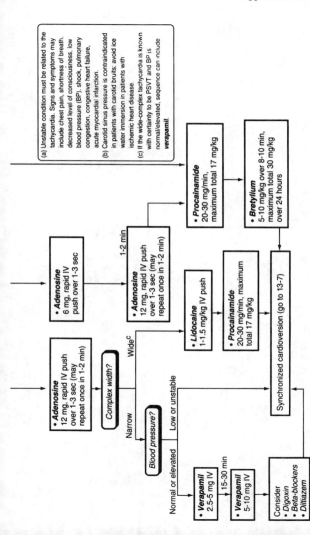

(a) Unstable condition must be related to the tachycardia. Signs and symptoms may include chest pain, shortness of breath, decreased level of consciousness, low blood pressure (BP), shock, pulmonary congestion, congestive heart failure, acute myocardial infarction.

(b) Carotid sinus pressure is contraindicated in patients with carotid bruits; avoid ice water immersion in patients with ischemic heart disease.

(c) If the **wide-complex tachycardia** is known with certainty to be PSVT and BP is normal/elevated, sequence can include **verapamil**.

• **Procainamide**
20-30 mg/min, maximum total 17 mg/kg

• **Bretylium**
5-10 mg/kg over 8-10 min, maximum total 30 mg/kg over 24 hours

• **Adenosine**
6 mg, rapid IV push over 1-3 sec

• **Adenosine**
12 mg, rapid IV push over 1-3 sec (may repeat once in 1-2 min)

1-2 min

• **Adenosine**
12 mg, rapid IV push over 1-3 sec (may repeat once in 1-2 min)

Complex width?

Wide[c]

• **Lidocaine**
1-1.5 mg/kg IV push

• **Procainamide**
20-30 mg/min, maximum total 17 mg/kg

Narrow

Blood pressure?

Low or unstable

Synchronized cardioversion (go to 13-7)

Normal or elevated

• **Verapamil**
2.5-5 mg IV

15-30 min

• **Verapamil**
5-10 mg IV

Consider
• **Digoxin**
• **Beta-blockers**
• **Diltiazem**

*From Guidelines for Cardiopulmonary Resuscitation and Emergency Cardiac Care, Committee of the American Heart Association. JAMA 1992: 268: 2171-2302.

13-7   Electric Cardioversion Algorithm*
(Patient is not in cardiac arrest)

Tachycardia
With serious signs and symptoms
related to the tachycardia

If ventricular rate is >150 beats/min, prepare
for IMMEDIATE CARDIOVERSION. May give
brief trial of medications based on specific
arrhythmias. Immediate cardioversion is
generally not needed for rates <150 beats/min.

Check
- Oxygen saturation
- Suction device
- IV line
- Intubation equipment

Premedicate whenever possible[a]

Synchronized cardioversion[b,c]
VT[d]
PSVT[e]   100 J, 200 J
Atrial fibrillation   300 J, 360 J
Atrial flutter[e]

(a) Effective regimens have included a sedative (e.g. *diazepam, midazolam, barbiturates, etomidate, ketamine, methohexital*) with or without an analgesic agent (e.g. *fentanyl, morphine, meperidine*). Many experts recommend anesthesia if service is readily available.
(b) Note possible need to resynchronize after each cardioversion.
(c) If delays in synchronization occur and clinical conditions are critical, go to immediate unsynchronized shocks.
(d) Treat polymorphic VT (irregular form and rate) like VF: 200 J, 200-300 J, 360 J.
(e) PSVT and atrial flutter often respond to lower energy levels (start with 50 J).

*From Guidelines for Cardiopulmonary Resuscitation and Emergency Cardiac Care, Committee of the American Heart Association. *JAMA* 1992: 268: 2171-2302.

13-8   Hypotension/Shock/Acute Pulmonary Edema Algorithm*

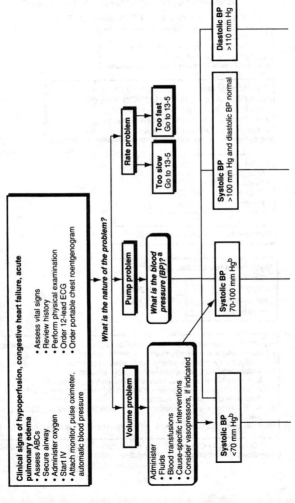

Clinical signs of hypoperfusion, congestive heart failure, acute pulmonary edema
- Assess ABCs
- Secure airway
- Administer oxygen
- Start IV
- Attach monitor, pulse oximeter, automatic blood pressure
- Assess vital signs
- Review history
- Perform physical examination
- Order 12-lead ECG
- Order portable chest roentgenogram

What is the nature of the problem?

Volume problem   **Pump problem**   **Rate problem**

What is the blood pressure (BP)? [a]

Too fast Go to 13-5
Too slow Go to 13-5

Administer
- Fluids
- Blood transfusions
- Cause-specific interventions
- Consider vasopressors, if indicated

Systolic BP <70 mm Hg[b]

Systolic BP 70-100 mm Hg[b]

Systolic BP >100 mm Hg and diastolic BP normal

Diastolic BP >110 mm Hg

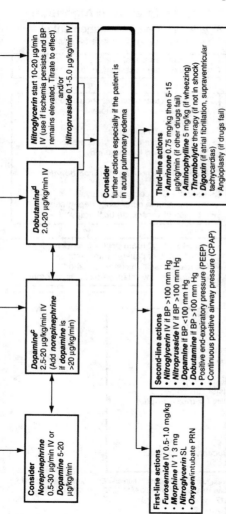

Consider
Norepinephrine IV
0.5-30 µg/min IV or
Dopamine 5-20
µg/kg/min

Dopamine[c] 2.5-20 µg/kg/min IV
(Add *norepinephrine* if *dopamine* is >20 µg/kg/min)

Dobutamine[d] 2.0-20 µg/kg/min IV

Nitroglycerin start 10-20 µg/min IV (use if ischemia persists and BP remains elevated. Titrate to effect)
and/or
Nitroprusside 0.1-5.0 µg/kg/min IV

Consider
further actions especially if the patient is
in acute pulmonary edema

First-line actions
• *Furosemide* IV 0.5-1.0 mg/kg
• *Morphine* IV 1.3 mg
• *Nitroglycerin* SL
• *Oxygen*/intubate PRN

Second-line actions
• *Nitroglycerin* IV if BP >100 mm Hg
• *Nitroprusside* IV if BP >100 mm Hg
• *Dopamine* if BP <100 mm Hg
• *Dobutamine* if BP >100 mm Hg
• Positive end-expiratory pressure (PEEP)
• Continuous positive airway pressure (CPAP)

Third-line actions
• *Amrinone* 0.75 mg/kg then 5-15 µg/kg/min (if other drugs fail)
• *Aminophylline* 5 mg/kg (if wheezing)
• *Thrombolytic* therapy (if not in shock)
• *Digoxin* (if atrial fibrillation, supraventricular tachycardias)
• Angioplasty (if drugs fail)
• Intra-aortic balloon pump (bridge to surgery)
• Surgical interventions (valves, coronary artery bypass grafts, heart transplant)

(a) Base management after this point on invasive hemodynamic monitoring if possible.
(b) Fluid bolus of 250-500 mL normal saline should be tried. If no response, consider sympathomimetics.
(c) Move to *dopamine* and stop *norepinephrine* when BP improves.
(d) Add *dopamine* when BP improves. Avoid *dobutamine* when systolic BP <100 mm Hg.

*From Guidelines for Cardiopulmonary Resuscitation and Emergency Cardiac Care, Committee of the American Heart Association. JAMA 1992: 268: 2171-2302.

13-9 **Acute Myocardial Infarction Algorithm***

Recommendations for early management of patients with chest pain and possible AMI

COMMUNITY	**Community emphasis on "Call First, Call Fast, Call 911"**

EMS SYSTEM	EMS system approach that should address • Oxygen-IV-cardiac monitor-vital signs • *Nitroglycerin* • Pain relief with narcotics • Notification of emergency department • Rapid transport to emergency department • Prehospital screening for *thrombolytic* therapy* • 12-lead ECG, computer analysis, transmission to emergency department* • Initiation of *thrombolytic* therapy*

EMERGENCY DEPARTMENT	**"Door-to-drug" team protocol approach** • Rapid triage of patients with chest pain • Clinical decision maker established (emergency physician, cardiologist, or other)

Assessment

Immediate:
• Vital signs with automatic BP
• Oxygen saturation
• Start IV
• 12-lead ECG (MD review)
• Brief, targeted history and physical
• Decide on eligibility for *thrombolytic* therapy

Soon:
• Chest x-ray
• Blood studies (electrolytes, enzymes, coagulation studies)

*From Guidelines for Cardiopulmonary Resuscitation and Emergency Cardiac Care, Committee of the American Heart Association. *JAMA* 1992: 268: 2171-2302.
† See *JAMA* 1992:268:2171–2302.
‡ See *JAMA* 1992:268:2171–2302.

†For information on the National Heart Attack Alert Program, contact the National Institutes of Health Information Center, P.O. Box 30105, Bethesda, MD 20824-0105

†Optional guidelines

Time interval in emergency department

Treatments to consider if there is evidence of coronary thrombosis plus no reasons for exclusion:
(some but not all may be appropriate)
- *Oxygen* at 4 L/min
- *Nitroglycerin* SL, paste or spray (if systolic blood pressure >90 mm Hg)
- *Morphine* IV
- *Aspirin* PO
- *Thrombolytic* agents
- *Nitroglycerin* IV (limit systolic BP drop to 10% if normotensive; 30% drop if hypertensive; never drop below 90 mm Hg systolic)
- *Beta-blockers* IV
- *Heparin* IV
- Routine *lidocaine* administration is **NOT** recommended for all patients with AMI
- *Magnesium sulfate* IV
- Percutaneous transluminal coronary angioplasty

30-60 min to *thrombolytic* therapy

Appendix 14

TABLE 14–1 Pediatric CPR Drugs Table

Drug	Concentration	Dose	Frequency	Route/Comments
Atropine	1 mg/ml	0.02 mls/kg IV or ET (0.02 mg/kg)	Every 5 min	Min. dose 0.1 mg. May dilute 1 : 1 with NS if given ET
Bretylium	50 mg/ml	5-10 mg/kg IV	Every 15-30 min	Max dose 30 mg/kg
Calcium Chloride	100 mg/ml (10%)	0.1 ml/kg IV (10 mg/kg)	Every 10 min	Indicated for treatment of hypocalcemia, hyper-magnesemia or hy-pokalemia with cardiac toxicity
Calcium Gluconate	100 mg/ml (10%)	0.3 ml/kg IV (30 mg/kg)	Every 10 min	Indicated for treatment of hypocalcemia, hyper-magnesemia or hy-pokalemia with cardiac toxicity
Cardiover-sion (synchro-nized)	0.5-1 watt/sec/kg	Double dose if necessary. For optimal effect, check oxygeni-zation, acid/base status and correct.		Indicated for ventricular rate >150 beat/min with serious signs and symptoms (not sinus tachycardia). The synchronizer circuit must be activated. On some older models, the QRS complex must be upright for proper acti-vation.
Defibrillation		2 watt/sec/kg	Double dose if necessary. For optimal effect, check acid/base status and correct	Max 4 watt/sec/kg (ven-tricular fibrillation only)
Epinephrine	1 : 10,000	0.1 ml/kg IV or ET (0.01 mg/kg)	Every 5 min	Dilute 1 : 1 with NS if given ET
Glucose	50%	1-2 ml/kg IV		Monitor blood glucose
Lidocaine	10 mg/ml	Loading 1 mg/kg IV or ET (0.01 mls/kg)	Maint. 0.5 mg/kg every 5 min or infusion 20-50 μg/kg/min	May dilute 1 : 1 with NS if given with ET

TABLE 14–1—cont'd

Drug	Concentration	Dose	Frequency	Route/Comments
Naloxone	0.4 mg/ml	0.025-0.25 mls/ kg IV, ET, IM, SQ (0.01-0.1 mg/kg)	Every 2-3 min	Max dosage 10 mg
Sodium Bicarbonate	1 mEq/ml	1-2 mEq/kg IV	Every 10-15 min of arrest	By ABG values
Volume expanders	Whole blood 5% albumin Normal Saline Lactated Ringer's, Hespan	10 mls/kg IV	Give over 5-10 min	Give by syringe or infusion

INFUSIONS*

Dobutamine	50 mg/ml	0.5-30 µg/kg/ min		
Dopamine	40 mg/ml	1-50 µg/kg/min		
Isoproterenol	0.2 mg/ml	0.02-0.15 µg/ kg/min		
Norepinephrine	1 mg/ml	0.04-0.4 µ/kg/min		

*To achieve the desired dose (µg/kg/min) the following amount of drug is added to 100 mls D5W of NS:

$$\text{mg in 100 mls} = \frac{6 \times \text{wt (kg)} \times \text{dose (µg/kg/min)}}{\text{desired infusion rate (ml/hr)}}$$

or

To determine the infusion rate at a desired dose (µg/kg/min) and concentration (mg/ml):

$$\text{infusion rate (mls/hr)} = \frac{\text{wt (kg)} \times 60 \times \text{dose (µg/kg/min)}}{\text{conc (mg/ml)} \times 1000}$$

or

Utilize the infusion table.

Note: ET = Endotracheal Tube
IV = Intravenous
IM = Intramuscular
SQ = Subcutaneous
NS = Normal Saline
ABG = Arterial Blood Gas

Appendix 15

TRADE NAME TABLE

Trade Name	Generic Name
Acephen	Acetaminophen
Aceta	Acetaminophen
Acetaminophen Elixir	Acetaminophen
Acetaminophen Uniserts	Acetaminophen
Adalat	Nifedipine
Adrenaline	Epinephrine HCL
Adreno-Mist	Epinephrine HCL
Advil	Ibuprofen
Alfenta	Alfentanil HCL
Alka-Seltzer	Aspirin with buffers
Aleve	Naproxen sodium
Amoxapine	Amoxapine
Anacin	Aspirin with caffeine
Anacin-3	Acetaminophen
Anaguard Epinephrine	Epinephrine HCL
Anaprox	Naproxen sodium
Anergan	Promethazine HCL
Anexsia	Hydrocodone bitartrate and acetaminophen
Anodynos-DHC	Hydrocodone bitartrate and acetaminophen
Ansaid	Flurbiprofen
Antrocol	Atropine sulfate and phenobarbital
Anxanil	Hydroxyzine HCL
Arava	Leflunomide
Aredia	Pamidronate
Argesic	Salsalate
Arthra-G	Salsalate
Arthropan	Choline salicylate
Ascriptin	Aspirin with buffers
Ascriptin A/D	Aspirin with buffers
Asendin	Amoxapine
Aspergum	Aspirin

Trade Name	Generic Name
Aspirin Uniserts	Aspirin
AsthmaHaler	Epinephrine bitartrate
Asthma-nefrin	Racepinephrine HCL
Astramorph	Morphine sulfate (preservative free)
Atarax	Hydroxyzine HCL
Ativan	Lorazepam
Atropine Sulfate	Atropine sulfate
Atropine and Demerol Carpuject	Atropine sulfate and meperidine
Atropine and Neostigmine Min-I-Mix	Atropine sulfate and neostigmine methylsulfate
Aventyl	Nortriptyline HCL
Azdone	Hydrocodone bitartrate and aspirin
Azotal	Aspirin with butalbital
Bayer Aspirin	Aspirin (film coated)
Bayer Children's Aspirin	Aspirin
Bayer Timed Release	Aspirin (extended release)
Bellergal-S	Ergotamine tartrate, levorotatory belladonna alkaloids, and phenobarbital
Bel-Phen-Ergot S	Ergotamine tartrate, levorotatory belladonna alkaloids, and phenobarbital
Betachron	Propranolol HCL
Bilax	Docusate sodium and dehydrocholic acid
Breatheasy	Racepinephrine HCL
Bretylol	Bretylium tosylate
Bronitin Mist	Epinephrine bitartrate
Bronkaid Mist	Epinephrine
Buffaprin	Aspirin with buffers
Buffered Aspirin	Aspirin with buffers
Bufferin	Aspirin with buffers
Buffex	Aspirin with buffers
Buffinol	Aspirin with buffers
Buprenex	Buprenorphine HCL
Cafergot	Ergotamine tartrate and caffeine
Calan	Verapamil HCL
Calan SR	Verapamil HCL (slow release)
Capital and Codeine	Codeine phosphate and acetaminophen
Carafate	Sucralfate
Carbocaine	Mepivacaine HCL
Catapres	Clonidine HCL
Catapres TTS	Clonidine HCL (transdermal therapeutic system)

Trade Name	Generic Name
Children's Aspirin	Aspirin
Chloroprocaine HCL	Chloroprocaine HCL
Citanest	Prilocaine HCL
Clinoril	Sulindac
Clonopin	Clonazepam
Co-Advil	Ibuprofen and pseudoephedrine HCL
Cocaine	Cocaine HCL
Codeine Phosphate	Codeine phosphate
Codeine Sulfate	Codeine sulfate
Codoxy	Oxycodone HCL and aspirin
Co-Gesic	Hydrocodone bitartrate and acetaminophen
Colace	Docusate sodium
Colace Liquid	Docusate sodium
Combipres	Clonidine HCL
Compazine	Prochlorperazine
Correctol	Docusate sodium and phenolphthalein
Cortan	Prednisone
Cytotec	Misoprostol
Dalalone Decaject	Dexamethasone sodium phosphate
Dalalone D.P.	Dexamethasone acetate
Dalalone L.A.	Dexamethasone acetate
Damason-P	Hydrocodone bitartrate and aspirin
Dapa	Acetaminophen
Darvocet-N	Acetaminophen with propoxyphene napsylate
Darvon	Propoxyphene HCL
Darvon Compound	Propoxyphene HCL, aspirin, and caffeine
Darvon-N	Propoxyphene napsylate
Daypro	Oxaprozin
DC 240	Docusate calcium
Decadrol	Dexamethasone sodium phosphate
Decadron	Dexamethasone
Decadron-L.A.	Dexamethasone acetate
Decadron Phosphate	Dexamethasone sodium phosphate
Decadron Phosphate with Xylocaine	Dexamethasone sodium phosphate and lidocaine HCL
Decadron Respihaler	Dexamethasone sodium phosphate
Dekasol	Dexamethasone sodium phosphate
Dekasol-L.A.	Dexamethasone acetate
Deltasone	Prednisone
Demerol	Meperidine HCL
Depa	Valproic acid

Trade Name	Generic Name
Depakene	Valproic acid
Depakote	Valproic acid
Depakote Sprinkle	Valproic acid
Desyrel	Trazodone HCL
Dexacene-4	Dexamethasone sodium phosphate
Dexamethasone	Dexamethasone
Dexamethasone Intensol	Dexamethasone
Dexamethasone Sodium Phosphate	Dexamethasone sodium phosphate
Dexasone	Dexamethasone sodium phosphate
Dexone	Dexamethasone
Dexone L.A.	Dexamethasone acetate
D.H.E. 45 (R)	Dihydroergotamine mesylate
Dialose	Docusate potassium
Dialose Plus	Docusate potassium and casanthranol
Diazepam Solution	Diazepam
Dilantin	Phenytoin sodium
Dilantin Kapseals	Phenytoin sodium (extended release)
Dilaudid	Hydromorphone HCL
Dilaudid HP	Hydromorphone HCL (high potency)
Dilocaine	Lidocaine HCL
Dioctocal	Docusate calcium
Diocto-K	Docusate potassium
Diocto-K Plus	Docusate potassium and casanthranol
Diocto Liquid	Docusate sodium
Dioctolose Plus	Docusate potassium and casanthranol
Dioeze	Docusate sodium
Dionex	Docusate sodium
Diosuccin	Docusate sodium
Diphenylan Sodium	Phenytoin sodium (prompt release)
Disalcid	Salsalate
Disanthrol	Docusate sodium and casanthranol
Disolan	Docusate sodium and phenolphthalein
Disolan Forte	Docusate sodium, carboxymethylcellulose sodium, and casanthranol
Disonate	Docusate sodium
Disonate Liquid	Docusate sodium
Disoplex	Docusate sodium and carboxymethylcellulose
Di-Sosul	Docusate sodium
Dolacet	Hydrocodone bitartrate and acetaminophen
Dolobid	Diflunisal

Trade Name	Generic Name
Dolophine	Methadone HCL
DOS	Docusate sodium
Doxidan Liquigel	Docusate calcium and phenolphthalein
Doxinate	Docusate sodium
Doxinate Solution	Docusate sodium
D-S-Duosol	Docusate sodium
DSMC	Docusate potassium
DSMC Plus	Docusate potassium and casanthranol
D-S-S Plus	Docusate sodium and casanthranol
Duentric	Aspirin (delayed release, enteric coated)
DuoCet	Hydrocodone bitartrate and acetaminophen
Duract	Bromfenac sodium
Duradyne DHC	Hydrocodone bitartrate and acetaminophen
Duragesic	Fentanyl citrate (topical transdermal system)
Duramorph	Morphine sulfate (preservative free)
Duranest	Etidocaine
Easprin	Aspirin (delayed release, enteric coated)
Ecotrin	Aspirin (delayed release, enteric coated)
Elavil	Amitriptyline HCL
E-Lor	Propoxyphene HCL and acetaminophen
Elmiron	Pentosan polysulfate sodium
EMLA	Lidocaine and prilocaine
Empirin with Codeine	Codeine phosphate and aspirin
Enbrel	Etanercept
Endep	Amitriptyline HCL
Enovil	Amitriptyline HCL
Ephedrine Sulfate	Ephedrine sulfate
Epinephrine	Epinephrine HCL
Epinephrine Mist	Epinephrine
Epi-Pen	Epinephrine HCL
Epitol	Carbamazepine
Equagesic	Aspirin with meprobamate
Equazine-M	Aspirin with meprobamate
Ercaf	Ergotamine tartrate and caffeine
Esimil	Guanethidine monosulfate and hydrochlorothiazide
Excedrin P.M.	Acetaminophen and diphenhydramine citrate
Ex-Lax Extra Gentle	Docusate sodium and phenolphthalein
Feen-A-Mint	Docusate sodium and phenolphthalein
Feldene	Piroxicam

Trade Name	Generic Name
Fentanyl Oralet	Fentanyl citrate (oral transmucosal system)
Fioricet	Acetaminophen, butalbital, and caffeine
Fioricet with Codeine	Acetaminophen, butalbital, caffeine, and codeine
Fiorinal	Aspirin, butalbital, and caffeine
Fiorinal with Codeine	Aspirin, butalbital, caffeine, and codeine
Fluphenazine Decanoate	Fluphenazine decanoate
Fosamax	Alendronate sodium
Gemnisyn	Acetaminophen with aspirin
Genacote	Aspirin (delayed release, enteric coated)
Genagesic	Acetaminophen and propoxyphene HCL
Genapap	Acetaminophen
Genapap Children's	Acetaminophen
Genebs	Acetaminophen
Genpril	Ibuprofen
Genprin	Aspirin (film coated)
Gentlax S	Docusate sodium and senna concentrate
Haldol	Haloperidol lactate
Haldol Decanoate	Haloperidol decanoate
Halenol	Acetaminophen
Haloperidol	Haloperidol lactate
Hexadrol	Dexamethasone
Hexadrol Phosphate	Dexamethasone sodium phosphate
Hydrocet	Hydrocodone bitartrate and acetaminophen
Hy-Pam	Hydroxyzine pamoate
Hy-Phen	Hydrocodone bitartrate and acetaminophen
Hyzine	Hydroxyzine HCL
Ibuprin	Ibuprofen
Imitrex	Sumatriptan succinate
Inderal	Propranolol HCL
Inderide	Propranolol HCL and hydrochlorothiazide
Inderide LA	Propranolol HCL and hydrochlorothiazide
Indocin	Indomethacin
Indocin SR	Indomethacin (slow release)
Infumorph	Morphine sulfate (preservative free)
Ismelin	Guanethidine monosulfate
Isoptin	Verapamil HCL
Isoptin SR	Verapamil HCL (slow release)
Janimine	Imipramine HCL
Kasof	Docusate potassium
Lanatrate	Ergotamine tartrate and caffeine

Trade Name	Generic Name
Levo-Dromoran	Levorphanol
Libritabs	Chlordiazepoxide
Librium	Chlordiazepoxide HCL
Lidoject	Lidocaine HCL
Limbitrol	Amitriptyline HCL and chlordiazepoxide
Lioresal	Baclofen
Lodine	Etodolac
Lopressor	Metoprolol tartrate
Lopressor HCT	Metoprolol tartrate and hydrochlorothiazide
Lorazepam Intensol	Lorazepam
Lorcet	Hydrocodone bitartrate and acetaminophen
Lortab	Hydrocodone bitartrate and acetaminophen
Lortab ASA	Hydrocodone bitartrate and aspirin
Magnaprin	Aspirin with buffers
Marcaine	Bupivacaine HCL
Maxiprin	Aspirin (delayed release, enteric coated)
Meclomen	Meclofenamate sodium
Medipren	Ibuprofen
Megaprin	Aspirin (delayed release, enteric coated)
Menadol	Ibuprofen
Mepergan	Promethazine HCL and meperidine HCL
Mepro-Analgesic	Aspirin with meprobamate
Meticorten	Prednisone
Mexitil	Mexiletine HCL
microNefrin	Racepinephrine HCL
Migranal Nasal Spray	Dihydroergotamine mesylate
Modane Plus	Docusate sodium and phenolphthalein
Modane Soft	Docusate sodium
Motrin	Ibuprofen
MS Contin	Morphine sulfate (slow release)
MSIR	Morphine sulfate
Nalfon	Fenoprofen
Naprelan	Naproxen sodium (controlled release)
Naprosyn	Naproxen
Naropin	Ropivacaine HCL
Neopap Supprettes	Acetaminophen
Nephron	Racepinephrine HCL
Nervocaine	Lidocaine HCL
Nesacaine	Chloroprocaine HCL
Nesacaine-MPF	Chloroprocaine HCL
Neucalm	Hydroxyzine HCL
Norcet	Hydrocodone bitartrate and acetaminophen

Trade Name	Generic Name
Norwich	Aspirin
Novocain	Procaine HCL
Nubain	Nalbuphine HCL
Numorphan	Oxymorphone HCL
Nuprin	Ibuprofen
Oramorph SR	Morphine sulfate (slow release)
Orasone	Prednisone
Orudis	Ketoprofen
Oxycet	Oxycodone HCL and acetaminophen
OxyContin	Oxycodone HCL
Pamelor	Nortriptyline HCL
Panadol	Acetaminophen
Panadol Children's	Acetaminophen
Panasol	Prednisone
Paxil	Paroxetine HCL
Pepcid	Famotidine
Percocet	Oxycodone HCL and acetaminophen
Percodan	Oxycodone HCL and aspirin
Percodan-Demi	Oxycodone HCL and aspirin
Perestan	Docusate potassium and casanthranol
Peri-Colace	Docusate sodium and casanthranol
Peri-DOS	Docusate sodium and casanthranol
Permitil	Fluphenazine HCL
Pertofrane	Desipramine HCL
Phenaphen	Acetaminophen
Phenaphen with Codeine	Codeine phosphate and acetaminophen
Phenazine 25	Promethazine HCL
Phencen	Promethazine HCL
Phenerbel-S	Ergotamine tartrate, levorotatory belladonna alkaloids, and phenobarbital
Phenergan	Promethazine HCL
Phenergan VC	Promethazine HCL and phenylephrine HCL
Phenoject	Promethazine HCL
Phenytoin Sodium	Phenytoin sodium
Pherazine	Promethazine HCL
Phillips LaxCaps	Docusate sodium and phenolphthalein sodium
Polocaine	Mepivacaine HCL
Ponstel	Mefenamic Acid
Pontocaine	Tetracaine HCL
Prednicen-M	Prednisone
Primatene Mist	Epinephrine

Trade Name	Generic Name
Pro-Cal-Sof	Docusate calcium
Procardia	Nifedipine
Procardia XL	Nifedipine
Prolixin	Fluphenazine HCL
Prolixin Decanoate	Fluphenazine decanoate
Prolixin Enanthate	Fluphenazine enanthate
Promethegan	Promethazine HCL
Propranolol HCL Intensol	Propranolol HCL
Prorex	Promethazine HCL
Prozac	Fluoxetine HCL
Quiess	Hydroxyzine HCL
Reglan	Metoclopramide HCL
Regutol	Docusate sodium
Relafen	Nabumetone
ReVia	Naltrexone
RMS	Morphine sulfate
Robaxin	Methocarbamol
Robaxisal	Methocarbamol and aspirin
Roxanol	Morphine sulfate
Roxanol SR	Morphine sulfate (slow release)
Roxicet	Oxycodone HCL and acetaminophen
Roxicodone	Oxycodone HCL
Roxilox	Oxycodone HCL and acetaminophen
Roxiprin	Oxycodone HCL and aspirin
S-2 Inhalant	Racepinephrine HCL
Senokot S	Docusate sodium and senna concentrate
Sensorcaine	Bupivacaine HCL
Sereen	Chlordiazepoxide HCL
Sinequan	Doxepin HCL
Sloprin	Aspirin (extended release)
Solurex L.A.	Dexamethasone acetate
Stadol	Butorphanol
Sublimaze	Fentanyl citrate
Sufenta	Sufentanil citrate
Suppap	Acetaminophen
Surfak	Docusate calcium
Surmontil	Trimipramine HCL
Sus-Phrine	Epinephrine
Tagamet	Cimetidine HCL
Talacen Caplets	Pentazocine HCL with acetaminophen
Talwin	Pentazocine lactate
Talwin Compound Caplets	Pentazocine HCL with aspirin

Trade Name	Generic Name
Talwin Nx Caplets	Pentazocine HCL and naloxone HCL
Tegretol	Carbamazepine
Therevac Plus Enema	Docusate sodium and benzocaine
Therevac S.B. Enema	Docusate sodium
Tofranil	Imipramine HCL
Tofranil-PM	Imipramine pamoate
Tolectin	Tolmetin sodium
Toradol	Ketorolac tromethamine
Trexan	Naltrexone HCL
Triavil	Perphenazine and amitriptyline HCL
Tri-buffered Bufferin	Aspirin with buffers
Trilafon	Perphenazine
Trilax	Docusate sodium, dehydrocholic acid, and phenolphthalein
Trisilate	Choline salicylate with magnesium salicylate
Tylenol	Acetaminophen
Tylenol with Codeine	Acetaminophen and codeine phosphate
Tylenol Children's	Acetaminophen
Tylox	Acetaminophen and oxycodone HCL
Uni Ace	Acetaminophen
Valium	Diazepam
Valproic Acid	Valproate sodium
Valrelease	Diazepam
Vaponefrin	Racepinephrine HCL
Verelan	Verapamil HCL
Versed	Midazolam HCL
V-Gan	Promethazine HCL
Vicodin	Hydrocodone bitartrate and acetaminophen
Vicodin ES	Hydrocodone bitartrate and acetaminophen
Vistacon	Hydroxyzine HCL
Vistaject	Hydroxyzine HCL
Vistaril	Hydroxyzine HCL
Vistaril	Hydroxyzine pamoate
Vistazine	Hydroxyzine HCL
Vivactil	Protriptyline HCL
Voltaren	Diclofenac sodium
Wigraine	Ergotamine tartrate and caffeine
Wygesic	Propoxyphene HCL and acetaminophen
Xanax	Alprazolam
Xylocaine	Lidocaine HCL
Zantac	Ranitidine
Zetran	Diazepam

Trade Name	Generic Name
Zofran	Ondansetron HCL
Zoloft	Sertraline HCL
Zomig	Zolmitriptan
Zonalon	Doxepin HCL cream
ZORprin	Aspirin (extended release)
Zostrix	Capsaicin
Zostrix HP	Capsaicin
Zovirax	Acyclovir
Zydon	Hydrocodone bitartrate and acetaminophen

Appendix 16

OXYCONTIN TITRATION GUIDE

Continue titrating, if necessary, using the principles outlined on page 744.

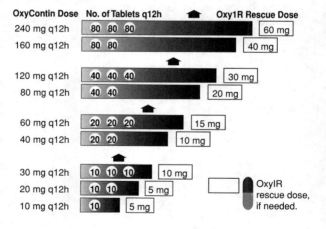

Figure modified from *24 hours of pain control the hard way*. Norwalk, CT: Purdue Pharma L.P., 1997.

Titrate patients every 1–2 days if necessary.

Increase the OxyContin (Oxycodone HCL Sustained Release) dose by 25–50% if necessary.

There is no maximum daily dose or "ceiling" to analgesic efficacy.

Some patients may tolerate an increase in dosing frequency (e.g., q 8 hours) better than an increase in dose.

Manage breakthrough pain with a short-acting opioid preparation such as OxyIR (Oxycodone HCL Immediate Release) at one-half to one-third of the 12-hour OxyContin dose.

Increase the OxyContin dose if more than two OxyIR rescue doses per day are required.

Use adjuvant agents.

Appendix 17

CONVERTING OTHER OPIOIDS TO OXYCONTIN

Fixed-Combination Opioid/ ──────────► OxyContin
Nonopioid Products

Dose of regular-strength products (e.g., Percocet, Percodan, Tylox, Vicodin, Lortab, Lorcet, and Tylenol with Codeine)	Recommended OxyContin conversion dose range	OxyIR rescue dose for breakthrough pain, if necessary
1–5 tablets/capsules/ caplets per day	10 or 20 mg q12 h	5 mg
6–9 tablets/capsules/ caplets per day	20 or 30 mg q12 h	5 or 10 mg
10–12 tablets/capsules/ caplets per day	30 or 40 mg q12 h	10 mg

The nonopioid ingredient (NSAID or APAP) may be continued as a separate drug. Discontinue all other around-the-clock opioids when initiating OxyContin therapy.

Modified from *24 hours of pain control the hard way*. Norwalk, CT: Purdue Pharma L.P., 1997.

Index

Note: Bold page numbers indicate a major discussion of a drug.

Opioid analgesia, enhancement of
  dextromethorphan for, 161
  dextromethorphan ointment for, 633
Opioid antagonists, 671–676
Opioids, 671–676
  for cancer pain, 652–653
  conversion to OxyContin of, 745
  relative potencies of, 690–691
  side effects of
    naltrexone for, 426
    prevention and management of, 692–696
  tolerance to, dextromethorphan for, 161, 163
  withdrawal from, clonidine for, 130, 132
Organic headache, tizanidine for, 581
Organ transplantation
  corticosteroid agents for, 658
  dexamethasone for, 156
  methylprednisolone for, 372
  prednisone for, 497
Osteoarthritis
  acetaminophen for, 651
  aspirin for, 42
  capsaicin for, 89
  choline salicylate for, 117
  diflunisal for, 174
  NSAIDs for, 651
  salsalate for, 545
  sodium hyaluronate for, 557
Osteolytic bone lesions, of multiple myeloma
  bisphosphonate agents for, 654
  pamidronate for, 462
Osteolytic bone metastasis, of breast cancer, bisphosphonate agents for, 654
Osteoporosis
  alendronate sodium for, 13, 14
  bisphosphonate agents for, 654
  pamidronate for, 462, 465
Oxycodone HCL, **450–457**, 675
  adverse reactions to, 456–457
  class of, 450
  dosing for, 451
  elimination of, 451
  equianalgesic dose of, 690
  guidelines/precautions with, 455–456
  interactions with, 454
  pharmacokinetics of, 454
  pharmacology of, 452–453
  preparations of, 451–452
  toxicity of, 454–455
  uses of, 450
OxyContin
  conversion of other opioids to, 745
  titration guide for, 743–744
Oxymorphone HCL, **457–461**, 675

OTHER PUBLICATIONS BY
SOTA OMOIGUI

Title: *Sota Omoigui's Anesthesia Drugs Handbook*, Third Edition
Publisher: Blackwell Science, Malden, MA
Description: Dosing information and guidelines for drugs used in anesthesia.
Order Info: 1-800-9-MEDIC-9 or at the website www.medicinehouse.com

Title: *The Universal Drug Infusion Ruler*
Publisher: S.O.T.A. Technologies, Redondo Beach, CA
Description: This unique slide ruler incorporates an infusion data guide and enables infusion calculations for any drug at any dose and at any concentration.
Order Info: 1-800-9-MEDIC-9 or at the website www.medicinehouse.com

Title: *Pain Relief - The L.A. Pain Clinic Guide*
Publisher: S.O.T.A. Technologies, Redondo Beach, CA
Description: Presents in an easy-to-read, concise format the latest treatment and medications for common pain syndromes including arthritis, back pain, cancer pain, diabetes and HIV pain, interstitial cystitis, migraine and tension headache, menstrual and labor pain, herpes zoster and postherpetic neuralgia, reflex sympathetic dystrophy (chronic regional pain syndrome), sickle cell pain, and vulvodynia.
Order Info: 1-800-9-MEDIC-9 or at the website www.medicinehouse.com

Title: *Pain Medicine Letter*
Publisher: S.O.T.A. Technologies, Redondo Beach, CA
Description: A monthly newsletter containing the latest information on medication and treatment in pain medicine.
Order Info: 1-800-9-MEDIC-9 or at the website www.medicinehouse.com

Title: *A Medical Guide to Herbs and Supplements*
Publisher: S.O.T.A. Technologies, Redondo Beach, CA
Description: An easy-to-read guide on herbs and supplements describing their use, pharmacology, side-effects, drug interactions, etc. Scientific studies that validate traditional uses of the herbs and supplements are included.
Order Info: 1-800-9-MEDIC-9 or at the website www.medicinehouse.com